MAP K

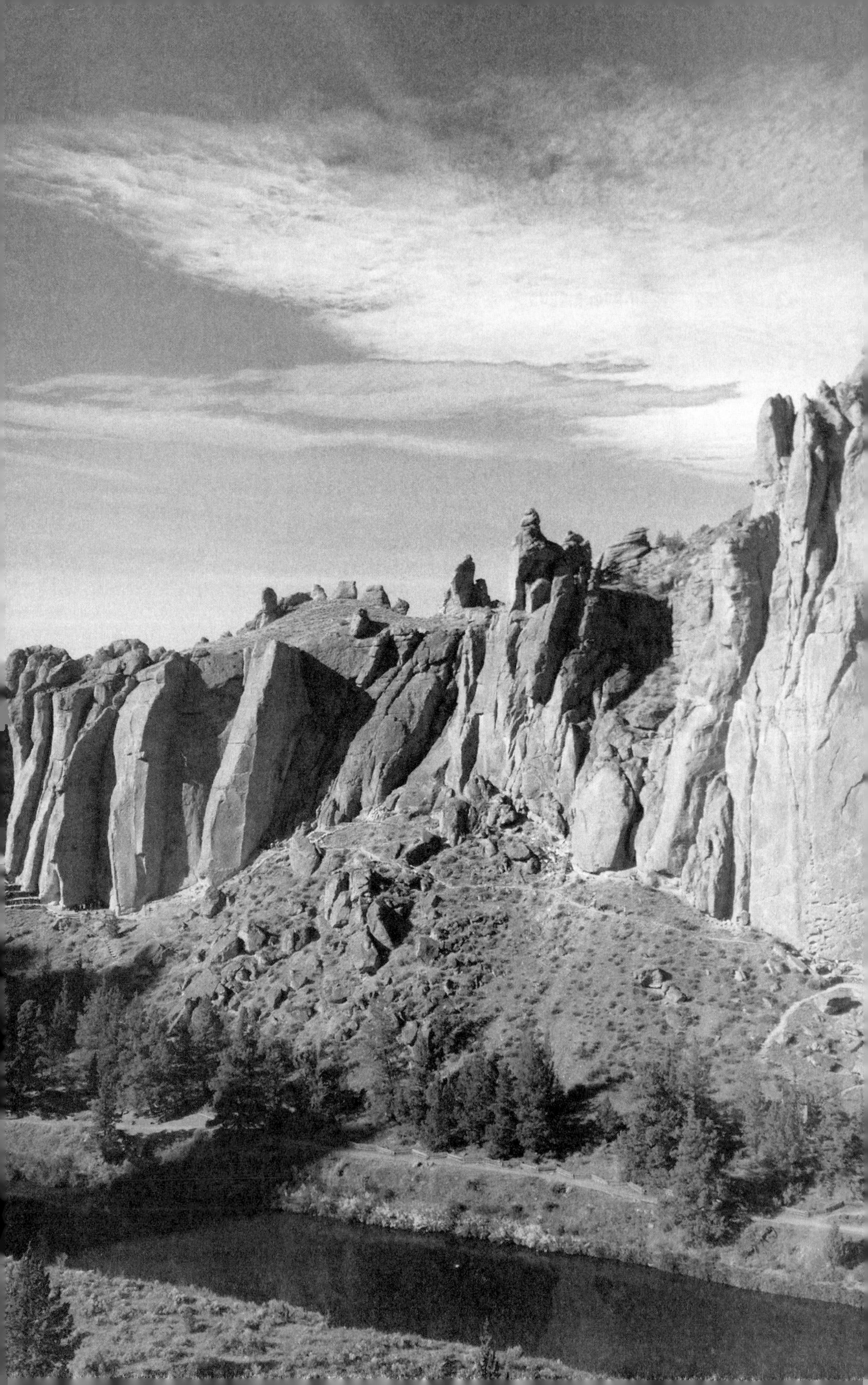

TRAIL RUNNING BEND AND CENTRAL OREGON

GREAT LOOP TRAILS FOR EVERY SEASON

LUCAS ALBERG

WILDERNESS PRESS . . . *on the trail since 1967*

Trail Running Bend and Central Oregon

First edition, first printing

Project editor: Ritchey Halphen
Cover photos: © 2016 by Nate Wyeth (front), © Aurora Photos /Alamy Stock Photo (back)
Interior photos: © 2016 by Lucas Alberg, except where noted
Cartography and cover design: Scott McGrew
Text design: Annie Long
Copyeditor: Kerry Smith
Proofreader: Rebecca Henderson
Indexer: Sylvia Coates

Cataloging-in-Publication Data is on file with the Library of Congress.
ISBN: 978-0-89997-823-9; eISBN: 978-0-89997-824-6

Manufactured in the United States of America

Distributed by Publishers Group West

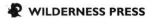

WILDERNESS PRESS
An imprint of AdventureKEEN
2204 1st Ave. S., Suite 102
Birmingham, AL 35233

Visit **wildernesspress.com** for a complete listing of our books and for ordering information. Contact us at **info@wildernesspress.com, facebook.com/wildernesspress 1967,** or **twitter.com/wilderness1967** with questions or comments.

Frontispiece: A view of the River Trail alongside the Crooked River from the Smith Rock State Park Day-Use Area *(see Smith Rock State Park, page 96)*

SAFETY NOTICE Although Wilderness Press and the author have made every attempt to ensure that the information in this book is accurate at press time, they are not responsible for any loss, damage, injury, or inconvenience that may occur to anyone while using this book. You are responsible for your own safety and health while in the wilderness. The fact that a trail is described in this book does not mean that it will be safe for you. Be aware that trail conditions can change from day to day. Always check local conditions and know your own limitations.

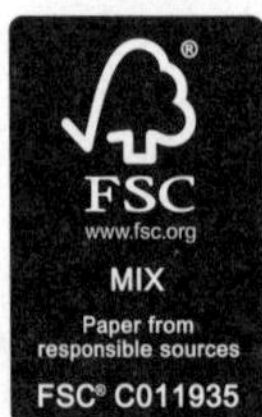

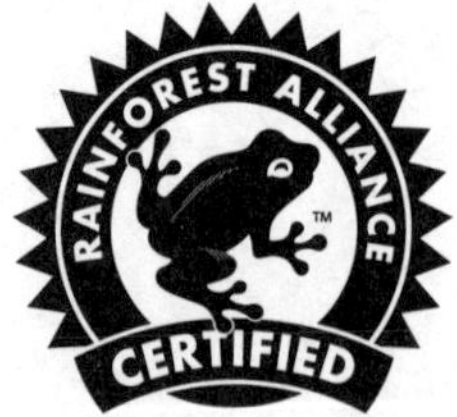

TABLE OF CONTENTS

CHAPTER 5 FALL RUNS 185

ACKNOWLEDGMENTS

THIS BOOK HAS BEEN A LONG TIME in the making, and it wouldn't have been possible without the help of a lot of people. First and foremost, I would like to thank my wife, Rae, who has supported this endeavor throughout, for her patience, edits, input, advice, and rides to and from trailheads. A big thanks also goes out to John Zilly, who helped me navigate the guidebook world and provided helpful advice on everything from formatting proposals to providing introductions. My initial proposals wouldn't have had an impact were it not for the help from friends and fellow runners Nate Pedersen, who helped with edits, and Dustin Gouker, who shared his talents for layout and design. A big thanks also goes out to Nate Wyeth, who provided his photography talents for the cover and additional runs, and his wife, Danielle, who happily jumped onboard the cover-photo shoot.

I would also like to thank the many local Central Oregon runners who (either knowingly or unknowingly) answered my many questions about trail running in the area. Special thanks go out to local runner extraordinaire Max King, who was kind enough to write the foreword for this book. And finally, I would like to extend my thanks to the folks at Wilderness Press/AdventureKEEN for publishing this book—in particular, Tanya Sylvan for kicking off the process and Tim Jackson for accepting the proposal and shaping the manuscript.

—**LUCAS ALBERG**

A NOTE FROM THE AUTHOR

IT'S NOT ATYPICAL FOR ME to start a weekend morning poring over maps at the dining room table. I've spent countless hours over the years tracing the contours of ridgelines and peaks, rivers and lakes, piecing together trails to make a mountain running loop to explore later that day.

To the surprise and bewilderment of my lovely wife, this is something I actually enjoy. In fact, reading maps is right up there with trail running as one of my favorite hobbies. There's something about envisioning the journey of a run, first through a map and then later playing it out on the trails, that strikes a resonant chord with me.

I've realized over time that not everyone shares this passion, however, and this is one of the sparks that led me to write this guidebook. I hope that through my work and love of maps, loops, and trails, this guidebook can be a spark to others for pursuing their interest and love of trail running in the wilderness.

FOREWORD

BY MAX KING

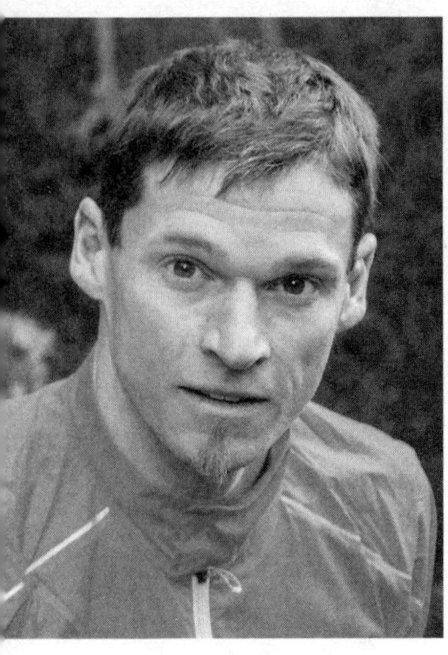

PHOTO: PAUL NELSON PHOTOGRAPHY

I'VE HAD THE PLEASURE OF CALLING CENTRAL OREGON HOME SINCE 2002. I graduated from college, packed up a U-Haul, and drove straight here. The reason was for the outdoor recreation opportunities, the lifestyle, and the trail running. I've put in more than 50,000 miles over the years on Central Oregon trails and explored most, but not all, of the corners of the region. During that time, I've had the opportunity to explore trails around the world, and I can say without a doubt that we have one of the best trail systems for running anywhere. From our miles of buff singletrack to wild mountain escapes to loops through towering ponderosa pine forests, we have such a variety of trails that you'll never get bored and you'd be lucky to be able to explore it all in a lifetime.

It's also the proximity to our homes that makes Central Oregon trails so unique. Many places around the country require you to put in a good amount of windshield time to get to the trailhead, but we're lucky enough here to be able to reach our destinations quickly by comparison. For someone like me who runs for a living, this means more time doing the things that matter, such as training and spending time with my family.

Finding some of these trails, especially for visitors, has often required some degree of unknown adventure or not being able to find them at all. Trying to explain to a visitor where to go for the best trail runs can require two maps, talking them through where to go on the trail once they get there, and worrying that you just sent them on a wild goose chase. A guidebook like this one helps to alleviate this challenge.

The Central Oregon running community is one of the strongest I've seen, and this close-knit community loves to share the best of what it has to offer. Until now, there has never been a comprehensive guide for our trail-running Mecca. Lucas has combined his love of trail running with his love of the Central Oregon region to bring this long-overdue book to life.

Lucas presents all the routes that we, as locals, love running throughout the year in a way that clearly explains the route, with maps, elevation profiles, distances, and beautiful photos. The beauty of our region is that the trails we run in the winter are completely different from the ones that we run in the summer. Lucas gives the runner the best trails for the season, the ones that we like to hit for a winter long run, a quick jaunt before an evening at the pub, or where we go for a summer run through the wildflowers and mountain views.

This will be an indispensable guide for runners visiting the area and a great resource for everyone looking for a new trail to explore. Whether you're from the area or just passing through, I hope you'll take advantage of this book to get out, explore, and push your boundaries.

Max King *won the individual 2011 World Mountain Running Championship in Albania and the 2014 IAU 100K World Championship in Qatar. He also participated in the 2012 Olympic track-and-field trials, finishing sixth in the 3,000-meter steeplechase, and is a three-time Xterra World Trail Run champion. In addition, he was named both the 2014 Men's Ultra Trail Runner of the Year and 2014 Men's Road Ultra Runner of the Year by USA Track & Field.*

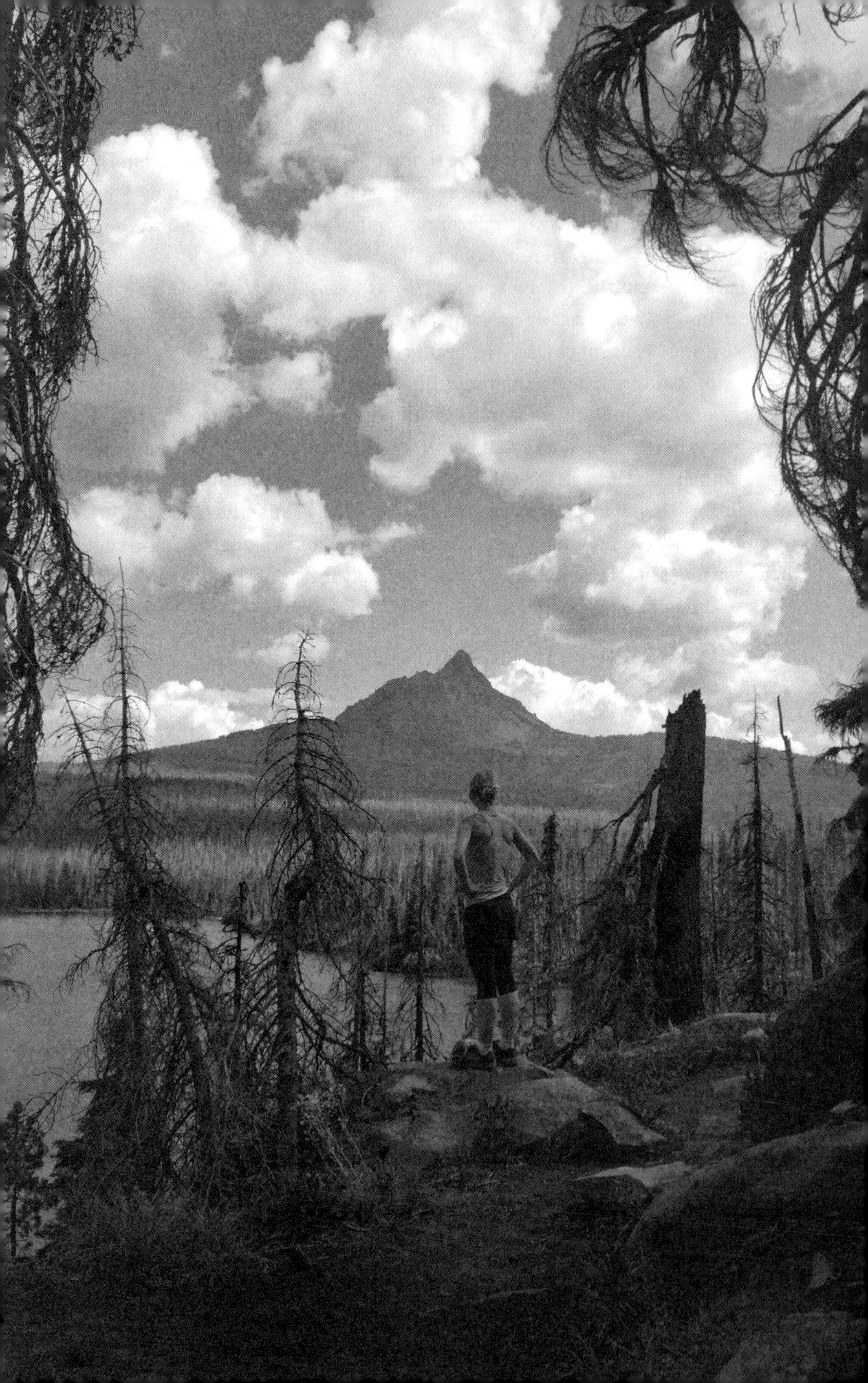

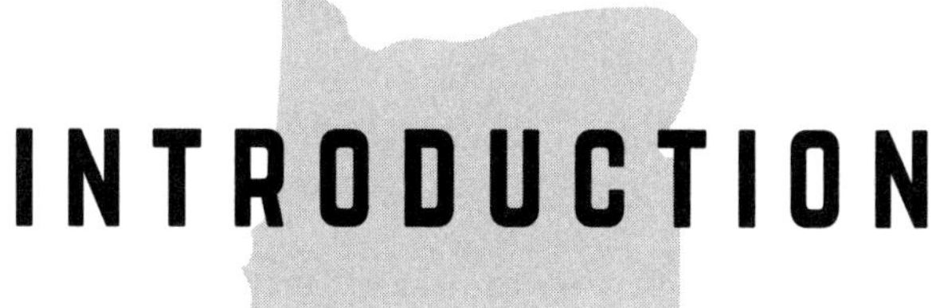

INTRODUCTION

THE STATE OF OREGON is typically known for its lush green forests, singular volcanic peaks jutting up from the evergreens, and the constant drizzle of rain nine months out of the year. While this is true for the western one-third of the state, it's a different story altogether on the east side of the Cascade Mountains.

Lying in a rain shadow opposite the verdant Willamette Valley on the other side of the Cascades, dry and sunny Central Oregon sees approximately 300 days of sunshine per year. For those keeping count, that's more than double the sun of Portland, the state's largest city. The typical bright and arid climate of Central Oregon, combined with the region's close proximity to nature, help to make it a veritable Shangri-La for outdoor recreationalists.

Outdoor adventure beckons year-round in Central Oregon. From skiing on the dry, fluffy powder that is typical of Mount Bachelor to kayaking and fly-fishing on the Deschutes River, there's something for everyone. And for trail runners, it simply doesn't get any better: The varied landscape in Central Oregon provides excellent options for all seasons, and the sheer number of trail miles equates to innumerable choices for those who like to continually explore.

During the summer, access to the high-country trails gives runners up-close-and-personal views of pristine alpine lakes and mountain peaks. The shoulder seasons provide ideal running temperatures, along with abundant wildflowers in the spring and autumnal colors in the fall. For those willing to brave the colder temperatures in wintertime, the conditions prove the perfect setting to explore the hard-packed sand trails of the Oregon Badlands Wilderness and the arid deserts east of Bend. No matter your preference or style, you'll find a trail to your liking in Central Oregon.

So grab those trail runners, pack your maps and your essentials, and get ready to experience some of the nation's best trail running in Central Oregon!

OPPOSITE: *Looking out over Big Lake to Mount Washington*

Why This Book?

Trail Running Bend and Central Oregon was written with several goals in mind. First and foremost, my intention was to write a guidebook that would make runners feel safe, comfortable, and confident in pursuing their interest in the sport. Running in the wilderness can be intimidating and scary for those just starting out, and for those unprepared, it can also be dangerous.

The runs in this book include very specific turn-by-turn directions and callouts to landmarks down to the tenth of a mile. Routes with an abundance of confusing or unmarked intersections were not included in the book; instead, I've focused on routes that are easily navigated and generally well marked. All of the trailheads can be reached in passenger cars without having to endure miles and miles of rough forest roads, and all are located within 65 miles of Bend, Oregon.

Likewise, the book was written with usability in mind, from quickly retrieving information from the pages to an understanding of the intended route on the trail. Information for elevation and distances is included for each run, along with ratings for scenery, crowds, and difficulty (according to the author). Permits and fees, maps, contact information, special rules and trail closures, dog accessibility, and open seasons are included with each running route. *Please note that since the date of publication, some trails may have changed. You're encouraged to check with the appropriate contact beforehand regarding any trail closures or special circumstances.*

Being a regional guidebook, the book was also written with the local running community in mind. With the growing popularity in trail running and the already existing strong community of runners in the area, my hopes were that this book would provide both inexperienced and experienced local- and regional-trail runners alike with a one-stop guide for where to go, when to go, and how to get to the trails. Some of the routes are already well known to locals, while others are infrequently used and some are new routes altogether.

Finally, the book was written to fill a void for one of the premier destinations in the country for trail running. This is the first trail-running book dedicated solely to Central Oregon, and it extensively highlights the region's outstanding geography and terrain. Runners from all over the country come to explore Central Oregon trails. With this book, my hope is to make these explorations that much easier.

Trail Running in Central Oregon

Trail running is a small but growing sport in the United States and around the world. Fueled by the success of the 2009 book *Born to Run* and the subsequent rise of ultra running, the number of trail runners in the United States rose more than 33% between 2006 and 2012 and is expected to rise even more in the coming years, according to a study by the Outdoor Industry Association. In Central Oregon, the area has a higher-than-average percentage of athletes and trail runners, and it's no surprise why.

Bend, Central Oregon's largest city, is consistently named one of America's top outdoor towns by publications such as *Outside* magazine, and it was named the nation's best trail-running town by the publication in 2006. *Trail Runner* magazine included Bend among its "Top Trail Towns" in 2013, and the popular ultra-running blog iRunFar.com called out Bend as one of its "Best Trail Running Cities" in 2011.

Bend has also won awards and recognition for its other outdoor sports, including best mountain biking town (*Mountain Biking* magazine), best stand-up-paddleboarding destination (*Outside* magazine), best town for sportsmen (*Outdoor Life*), best place to raise outdoor children (*Backpacker*), and numerous others.

The region's competition, topography, and abundance of incredible trails attract hordes of professional runners and trail runners. In fact, it's not unusual to run a 5K or 10K race in Central Oregon and run alongside—and soon behind—Olympic and professional athletes. Top runners like Lauren Fleishman, Stephanie Howe, Jeff Browning, Ryan Bak, Mario Mendoza, Ian Sharman, and Max King (whose running resume reads like the credits of a 3-hour movie) call the area home.

The beauty of trail running—and the running community in general—is that the spirit of competition is tempered with a strong sense of community and friendship. Most races are concluded with celebratory microbrews, and the fastest finishers tend to stick around to encourage others across the finish line. Likewise, many of the well-known athletes in the area take time to coach, mentor, and train local runners. All in all, the trail-running community seems to fall right in line with the slogan on a popular bumper sticker around the state: BE NICE, YOU'RE IN OREGON.

Trail Etiquette

When out enjoying the trails, runners should always respect the surrounding environment and leave it as good—or better—than when they first encountered

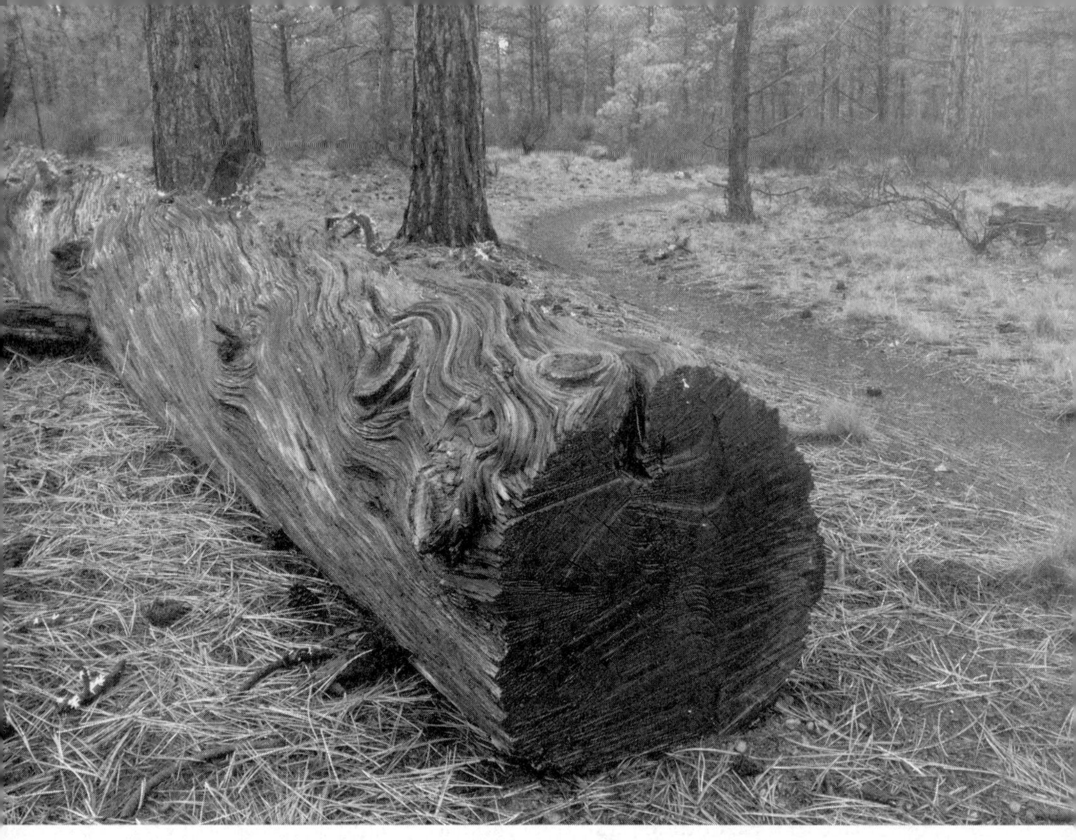

An aged log lies beside flowing singletrack on the Lower Peterson Ridge Trail (see page 43).

it. Most trails are created and maintained by volunteers and other trail lovers (and users). Nobody is paid to clean up after you as in many cities and neighborhoods, making it all the more important to pick up after yourself. Never litter, pack out what you bring in, and be especially mindful of small items like gel packets that are easy to lose track of while on the go. Leave what you find out on the trail, including wildflowers, rocks, and other tempting objects (plus, these will slow you down!), and never remove or alter trail markers (this can lead to steep fines). Keep yourself up to date on Leave No Trace principles (see **lnt.org**) or the American Trail Running Association's "Rules on the Run" (see **tinyurl.com/rulesontherun**).

Abide by the golden rule and respect other trail users by being aware of how your actions are affecting the quality of their experience. If running with a partner, be mindful of the volume of your voices—many people go into the wilderness seeking quiet and tranquility. Stay on the trails when in groups, and avoid cutting corners and running outside the singletrack lanes, which widen the paths over time and destroy vegetation. Likewise, run through mud if possible and over roots, rocks, and limbs to avoid widening of the trail. If the trail is excessively muddy, consider another route to avoid damaging it with "potholes"—the footstep equivalent of a mountain bike tire's rut.

If you're running with a dog, please leash it—it's the law. Though you love your pet, not everyone may, and likewise, your pet may not love others the way it loves you. Be respectful of others on the trail by obeying leash laws and cleaning up after your companion.

In general, faster trail users should yield to slower users—that is, bikes yield to runners, both yield to hikers, passing on the left. In most cases, you should yield to uphill traffic, though occasionally it's easier (and safer) to step aside for mountain bikers and fast runners who are careening down a mountainside. The notable exception is to always yield to horses. When you encounter horseback riders, slow down as you approach, step to the downhill side of the trail, and stop running, allowing them to pass.

Don't startle people! As a runner, chances are you will be traveling much faster than hikers (in some cases, even mountain bikers when traveling uphill). Let them know you are coming well ahead of time by announcing yourself (in an audible and courteous fashion) and your intention to pass. A simple statement such as "Runner on your left" works quite well.

Run only on open or public trails, unless specific permission is given. Leave gates as you found them, or adhere to any posted signs with specific instructions or requests (Gray Butte, page 100, is an example).

Last but not least: *Be nice!* You're in Oregon, after all, and you're out in the wilderness and enjoying nature—that should put a smile on your face. If you are a frequent trail-user, consider giving back through volunteering for trail cleanups, maintenance, or building. You'll replenish your own trail karma and feel good in the process.

Safety Concerns

Any wilderness adventure carries with it some degree of risk. The best way to mitigate it is to always plan ahead and be prepared. Be aware of your surroundings, of others, of wildlife, weather, regulations, and special concerns with the area. Carry proper gear, nutrition, and maps, and most of all, know yourself and your limits. If you're unfamiliar with the area, don't push yourself beyond your capabilities. Trail running is supposed to be fun, after all.

When running in the backcountry, always let a friend or spouse know where you are going and when you expect to get back. If possible, run with a partner or in small groups. Run prepared, and carry an up-to-date map and a compass on longer runs, along with the knowledge of how to use them. Cell phones and GPS units are useful, though battery-operated devices eventually run out of juice and coverage is spotty at best when you're up in the mountains.

The "10 Essentials" are often associated with hiking and backpacking, but distance runners should consider them as well. When you're out in the wilderness for hours, it's paramount to take along the right gear. Proper clothing for adverse and changing weather conditions, enough food to get you through your run, water (and a means of purification such as iodine tablets, a filter, or a LifeStraw as a backup), a lightweight first-aid kit, a map and compass, matches or a lighter, a small flashlight or headlamp, sunscreen, insect repellent, and toilet paper for when nature calls.

Know your route, and be aware of any possible obstacles such as treacherous river crossings or snowy passes. If you're running alone, don't try to be a hero: Turn around and retrace your steps to the trailhead if you don't feel comfortable or confident in your abilities to navigate the route safely.

Weather

Never underestimate the power of Mother Nature—weather can change very quickly in the mountains, and hypothermia is a legitimate concern even in the middle of summer. In fact, it's not unheard of for Central Oregon to get snow in the upper elevations during August. Always know the weather forecast, be prepared, and bring along additional layers of clothing.

In the fall and winter, running in snow can be peaceful and picturesque. Nothing makes a scene more magical than a lovely white blanket of snow covering rocks, limbs, and trees. Hidden wildlife suddenly seems all around you, with visible tracks of all sizes through the forest. Unfortunately, once all the surroundings are covered, it can also be completely disorienting and difficult to find your way back. The trail suddenly disappears, and you're left to your own navigational abilities. For this reason, if there's any chance you may encounter snow on your run, be sure that your orientation skills can get you back to the trailhead.

The summer months in the High Desert of Oregon can bring intense heat and piercingly strong sunrays in the higher elevations. Avoid heat exhaustion by staying hydrated, wearing proper skin protection in the form of clothing and sunscreen, and, most importantly, knowing your limits. Electrolyte-replacement drinks or tablets can help to replenish the salt you lose through sweating. Everybody is different, though, so test through your trainings until you find the right balance of nutrition that suits your needs.

During the summer and shoulder seasons, thunderstorms can also be a possibility in Central Oregon. These storms tend to move in quickly, so it's important to be aware of the forecast ahead of time and plan accordingly. If you find yourself in a lightning storm in higher elevations, get below the treeline as soon as you can. Reduce your risk of being struck by avoiding tall objects, lakes, rivers, and other bodies of water, as well as natural lightning rods such as metal fences and power lines. Ideally, you should aim to get inside a car or building as soon as possible, but in the wilderness your next best bet often tends to be getting lower and seeking shelter in a group of trees (rather than a singular tree). For protection against hail, keep a hat handy.

Animal Precautions and Wildlife Safety

The Central Oregon region is chock-full of wildlife throughout its mountains, deserts, and valleys. Remember that when running in the wilderness, you're a visitor to the home of these creatures and not the other way around. Always be respectful of wildlife and observe from a distance. Do not approach, follow, or intentionally interact with animals. Doing so can alter their natural behaviors and endanger them.

Please don't feed animals—not even the cute ones like ground squirrels and chipmunks. Feeding wildlife can damage the animals' health, alter their natural feeding routines, and possibly render them dependent on human interaction; plus, it can spoil the environment for future trail-users. Remember that not-so-peaceful family picnic at a campground where your table was set upon by squirrels? That was most likely because previous picnic-goers had fed them. Protect wildlife, and your own food and experience in the process, by storing your food and packing your trash securely and out of the reach of animals.

Be aware that during certain times of the year, some natural areas are closed to trail users due to sensitive times of breeding, mating, nesting, and raising young.

Pay attention to postings and respect the warnings by seeking out other, open trails. A few of the trails in this book, such as Otter Bench (page 212) and the Castle Trail in the Badlands (part of the Badlands Rock run, page 57), are among those with seasonal closures. Though such closures are pointed out where they apply, it's best to double-check with the managing agency online or by phone before you go.

Part of the excitement of being in the wilderness is the chance that you may see wildlife in its natural habitat. Though Central Oregon is home to a few larger predatory animals, your chances of encountering them are low. That said, if you're a regular backcountry-trail runner, sooner or later you're going to have an unexpected meet and greet, so it's best to be prepared.

A small number of **black bears** roam the east side of the Cascade Mountains. Most bears will run away upon seeing you and are likely more scared of you than you of them. If you encounter a bear, give it plenty of room and be calm. If the bear is on the trail, back away slowly and take an alternate route if you can. The worst thing to do is to corner a bear—make sure it has an escape route. Be extra-cautious of cubs and young bears, as mothers will most likely be nearby. The chances of a bear attacking you are extremely slim, but if it does happen, stand tall, be loud, and *fight back*.

Cougars also roam the mountains, deserts, and lower elevations of Central Oregon. Cougar sightings are very rare, encounters even rarer. If you see a cougar in the wild, count yourself lucky—you must be extremely light on your feet and quick with the eye. In all my days of running all over the state, I've never seen or come across a cougar. On the slim chance that you *do* encounter a cougar, raise your arms above your head to make yourself appear large and threatening. Maintain eye contact with the cougar, be calm, and slowly back away (do not run!). If attacked, do whatever you can to fight back—punch, kick, and claw.

In the deserts of Central and Eastern Oregon, **rattlesnakes** are common. Though not large in numbers, chances are if you spend enough time running the trails in those environments, you'll come across one eventually. As is the case with most animals, snakes want to be left alone and very rarely attack unprovoked. With this in mind, watch your footing (most snake bites come from when they are stepped on), and if you see a rattlesnake, give it a wide berth and a clear path for retreat.

In Central Oregon, we're very fortunate not to have a lot of **biting insects.** Sure, there are plenty of mosquitoes in the early summer months, along with a few biting flies, but compared with trail runners in other parts of the country, we can count ourselves lucky. Fortunately for us, the best way to avoid biting insects is simply to do what you came out to do: run. Most insects simply won't be able to keep pace with you. Likewise, if you happen to come across a beehive, simply keep running to put distance between you and the bees.

Waste Management

As the saying goes, "When you gotta go, you gotta go." Though it's smart to take care of business before you leave home, sometimes the urge comes during the middle of your run, miles from the nearest restroom. If this happens to you, please be considerate and dispose of solid waste properly: Pick a spot at least 200 feet from the nearest water source and trail; dig a hole of 6 inches or more with your heel, a rock, or a stick; and cover the waste well when done—nobody likes to look at poop. Bury your (biodegradable) toilet paper as well, or pack it out. Urinate on bare ground or rocks so that the liquid absorbs quickly and vegetation (such as wildflowers) is unaffected. Finish with hand sanitizer.

A Word About Technology

Technology has its place in the outdoors, and it can certainly help runners achieve their goals. With the evolution of apps, most smartphones can help runners track mileage, calories, heart rate, and so on. Runners can also utilize their phones' map software on closer-in trails. And let's be honest, it's nice to have a smartphone handy simply for taking pictures—most phones these days take great photos, and they're more convenient than lugging a separate camera around. In fact, many of the photos in this book, and nearly all of the field notes for it, were taken or entered from my phone.

All of that said, technology has its limitations in the wilderness. A phone or GPS is great to have on hand, but it shouldn't be your primary means of navigation. Up in the mountains and out in the backcountry, cellular reception can be spotty, even nonexistent. And although a dedicated GPS unit is more reliable than a smartphone, it too can have coverage limitations in canyons, ravines, and deep forest. What's more, battery-operated devices eventually run out of power. Guess what doesn't? You guessed it—a map and compass! When in the backcountry, always carry both in addition to your electronic device(s), and know how to use them. Each trail run includes a recommendation for a supplementary map in addition to the maps in this book.

Different people run for different reasons. Likewise, different runners have different preferences and idiosyncrasies—for example, wearing headphones to listen to music. Though enjoyable, this practice is generally discouraged while running in the wilderness. The American Trail Running Association advises against using headphones and music players, mainly because they make it hard to hear the approach of other trail users or wildlife. Plus, if the volume is too high, the sound can bleed from your headphones and disrupt the peacefulness of the wilderness for others. Perhaps worst of all, headphones make for awkward passing: I can't count the number of times I've passed other runners and hikers who were wearing headphones and scared the living daylights out of them, even after I announced myself two or three times prior. If you just can't do without music while you run, at least make sure that the volume is low enough that you can still hear what's going on around you.

Running Shoes and Clothing

These days, if you ask a dozen people for advice on what shoes to buy for trail running, you're likely to get a dozen answers. From "minimalist" shoes like Vibram's Trek Ascent to heavily cushioned "maximalists" like the HOKA ONE ONE and the Brooks Cascadia series in between, runners have a wide spectrum to choose from. Truth is, there is no cut-and-dried correct choice. Finding the right shoe for you depends on a lot of factors, and it helps to ask a few questions beforehand.

Do you have wide feet or skinny feet? High arch or no arch? Do you pronate? Are you a heel, midfoot, or forefoot striker? Also, ask yourself what type of terrain you'll be running in most frequently: Will it be rocky, technical terrain or mostly smooth river paths? If rocky, what types of rock? Will you be running on some of the high Cascade trails that contain the notoriously sharp lava rock? These types of questions will help guide you. Most importantly, though, when looking for a trail-running shoe, go with what feels best and works best for you. Everyone's anatomy, physiology, interests, and tastes are different, and the right shoe for you may not be the right shoe for your running partner.

Trail-running shoes stand apart from road-running and cross-training shoes for a number of reasons. Most notably, trail-specific shoes have a more rugged outer sole to provide better traction on the myriad rocks, roots, and terrain types you're likely to encounter. These features provide protection and stability to help your feet handle changing impact points. Trail shoes have a more durable toe and tougher (or sometimes all-weather) construction to offset changing surface conditions and adverse weather. When buying your shoes, keep in mind that it's good to give yourself a little extra toe-box room for the downhills as well as to compensate for swelling during a longer run.

Though the minimalist movement is starting to fade somewhat, it's important to understand your running form and what type of foot strike you have if you choose to go this route. Wearing minimalist shoes and running with poor form can lead to serious injuries and hamper your zest for running. Utilize the various clinics, workshops, and classes at local running shops to help you learn proper form and mechanics. If you do buy a pair of minimalist shoes, start with very short distances and work your way up from there. The biggest cause of injury while wearing minimalist shoes is pushing yourself too hard and too far without allowing your body enough time to adjust.

In direct response to the minimalist movement, so-called maximalist shoes have become a permanent fixture on running-store shelves. These shoes provide abundant cushioning and are good for running over technical terrain and for long distances. One argument against wearing maximalists is that the cushioning hampers your ability to feel the terrain under your feet and thus your ability to be responsive on the trails. Conversely, proponents argue that these shoes help absorb the repetitive high impacts of distance running and lessen strain, allowing you to run comfortably longer. Again, decide what's important to you, then make your buying choice based on your priorities.

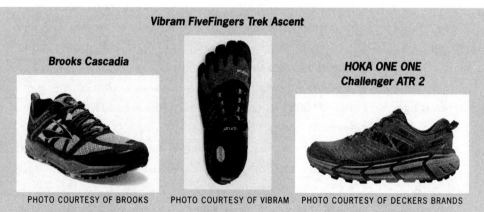

Trail runners have a wide variety of options when it comes to shoes: minimalist, maximalist, and in between.

Along with the right footwear, comfortable clothing makes for a more comfortable run. Choose lightweight fabrics that are breathable and nonbinding and that wick sweat away from your body to help keep you dry. As a general rule of thumb, choose technical materials such as polyester or merino wool over cotton garments (including socks). In colder seasons, wear a moisture-wicking base layer, a breathable midlayer for extra warmth, and a water-repellent outer layer to protect from the elements. Many lightweight running jackets now weigh in at less than 10 ounces and pack down to the size of a billfold, so they're easy to stow when not in use. A hat or running cap and a lightweight pair of gloves are also essential protection against sun, rain, or a quick change in temperature. When it comes to clothing, it's better to bring it and not need it than to need it and be without it!

When buying running gear, consult the experts at your local running shop. (In Bend, **Footzone** [842 NW Wall St.; 541-317-3568, **footzonebend.com**] and **Fleet Feet** [1320 NW Galveston Ave., #1; 541-389-1601, **fleetfeetbend.com**] are among the best.) They not only know the trails but can also advise you on the best clothing for the local environment and how best to match a shoe to your gait, interests, and more. Running stores often put on events with major gear manufacturers for demo purposes, too—this can be a great way to test out shoes on more than just a lap around the block.

Fees and Regulations

Several of the running routes in this book require a **Northwest Forest Pass** to park at the trailhead. At this printing, daily permits cost $5, weekend permits $10, and annual permits $30. All can be purchased at sporting-goods and outdoor stores across the state (see **tinyurl.com/nfpvendors** for a searchable database), as well as at most US Forest Service ranger stations; to buy the annual pass online, go to **store.usgs.gov** and enter **216089** in the search box. Permits must be displayed from April 1 until November 1.

Oregon State Parks day-use fees are as follows for the runs in this book: The Cove Palisades State Park and Smith Rock State Park, $5 each; LaPine State Park, free.

Central Oregon is also home to the **Newberry National Volcanic Monument,** where two routes in this book are located. Admission is $5 for a single day or $10 for a three-day Monument Pass.

Along with a Northwest Forest Pass or other federal recreation pass, the Obsidian Trail (see page 151) requires a special permit to complete the full loop. The **Obsidian Limited Entry Area Permit** costs $6 and can be obtained by phone at 877-444-6777 or online at **recreation.gov** (search for "Obsidian Limited Entry Area" on the home page; you must sign up for a Recreation.gov account to reserve online). Reservations are taken starting on the Friday before Memorial Day.

Access to **Bureau of Land Management** areas is free.

How to Use This Book

Each run opens with a hit list of information about the route, including distance, difficulty, scenery, crowds, season, net elevation gain and loss, user access, contacts, fees and permits, recommendations for supplementary maps, and whether dogs are allowed on the particular route.

Distance

I tracked the distance for each route using a combination of maps and Garmin GPS data collected during my many outings on the chosen route. In the few cases where my GPS data didn't align with my map data, I chose to default to the map distances. The distance reflected in each entry is tallied from the starting trailhead back to, in most cases, the same trailhead via a loop of several connecting trails. In the case of the only point-to-point run in the book, McKenzie River (page 83), distance was calculated from the starting trailhead to the ending trailhead. Many of the runs mention side trips worth checking out—unless noted, however, these are not reflected in the total mileage.

GPS Trailhead Coordinates

These are provided as latitude and longitude, in degree–decimal minute format.

Difficulty

Each run is rated from 1 to 10 for difficulty, with 1 being the easiest and 10 being the most strenuous. Ratings were assigned according to my own interpretation of the run and were influenced by a number of factors, including total distance, elevation, terrain, and navigability. The ratings are an aggregate of the overall route, so some sections may be harder than others. In any case, note that these ratings are totally subjective and were also influenced by the day on which I assigned the rating—as all runners know, you feel better on some days than others.

Scenery

The scenery scale assesses the natural beauty of an area and points of interest along the route. A rating of 1 indicates little beauty or interest, while a rating of 10 indicates an absolutely gorgeous and spectacular experience. Like the difficulty scale, the scenery scale is by no means scientific and is totally subjective. I should probably mention here that I love most all terrain and find it hard to discriminate between the beauty of the mountains and the deserts.

Crowds

One of the great aspects of running in the wilderness is the tranquility and solitude it provides. Jogging along a beautiful river or through a pine-scented mountain forest can elicit a meditative state in many runners and a real connection to nature. But nothing pops that euphoric bubble quicker than a crowd. The crowds rating is designed to help you suss out how likely you'll be to encounter other people. A rating of 1 means you'll encounter few to no people on the trail, while a 10 means you're likely to find people around nearly every bend. Though Central Oregon has a number of popular trails, we count ourselves lucky to enjoy relatively low overall traffic compared with many other running destinations elsewhere.

Season

This section indicates the months (and operating hours) during which the route is typically open or recommended in an average year. Depending on many factors—snow levels, temperatures, and so on—accessibility to mountain trails can vary considerably from year to year. For this reason, I've chosen to organize the book according to seasons instead of by region as typical guidebooks do. With the runs organized by season, you'll know the best time to hit a particular run. Desert runs, for example, are always better in the winter, not only because there's less likelihood of snow but also because the sandy surface is hard-packed and makes an excellent running surface when frozen. Likewise, some runs are recommended in the spring or fall because of wildflowers or foliage, while others are best experienced in summer simply because of accessibility.

Elevation

This section lists the cumulative gains and losses in elevation throughout the run. I recorded this data with my Garmin Forerunner 405, a GPS-enabled sport watch that uses a barometric altimeter to help ensure accurate elevation numbers. While recording the elevation data for each run, I also had the watch's

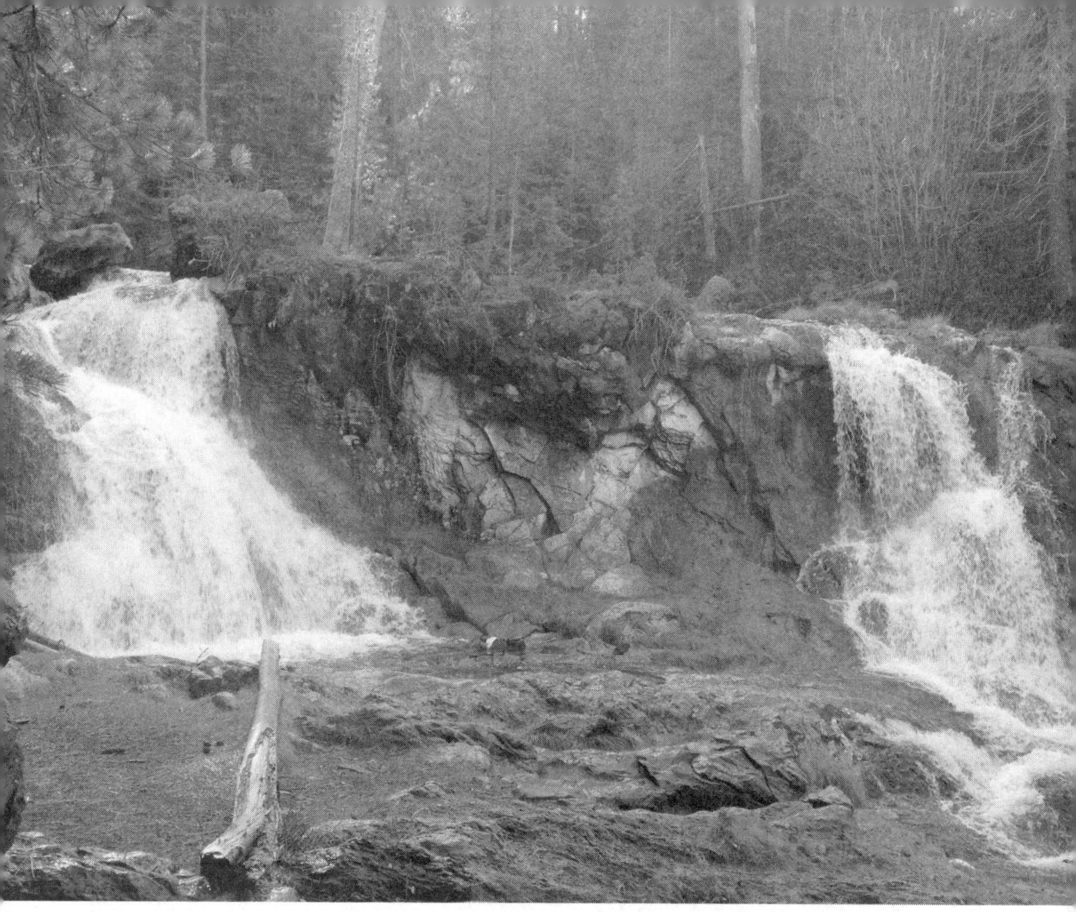

One of the many unnamed waterfalls along Paulina Creek (see pages 116 and 208)

elevation-correction functionality enabled; this pulls data from professional surveys (where available) to ensure the most accurate reading possible.

Users

Notes who is permitted to use a particular section of trail. Some trails are open to hikers only and runners, while others are open to mountain bikers and equestrians.

Contact

Lists the managing agency to get in touch with for additional information before you hit the trail. Also see page 216 for a consolidated list of managing agencies.

Permits/Fees

Lists any associated parking fees, pass requirements, and user restrictions by the governing agencies that you may encounter at the trailhead or on the trail itself.

Recommended Map

Lists a supplementary map that covers a particular trail. I highly recommend bringing along a map (and compass) in addition to your phone/GPS and the maps in this book.

Dogs

Notes whether or not your canine companion is allowed on a particular route. Please note that where dogs are allowed, most wilderness areas require that you leash your dog between July 15 and September 15. Several routes closer to urban areas, such as Shevlin Park, Pilot Butte State Park, Archie Briggs Canyon, the Deschutes River Trail, and the Old Mill, require that dogs be leashed beginning May 15.

Maps and Elevation Profiles

Trail maps are provided for each run, along with a separate diagram illustrating elevation gain/loss for trails with an elevation gain/loss of at least 100 feet. These maps include points of interest along the way and any notable restrictions or

The author runs through the Radlands with the Cascades on the horizon (see page 75).

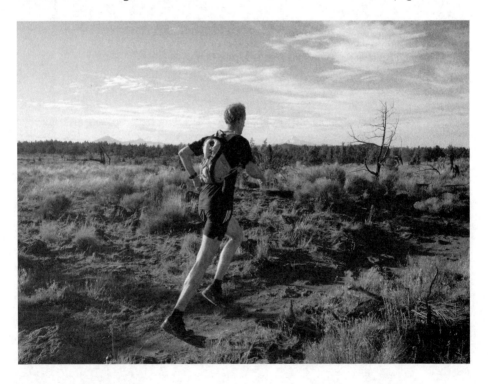

entry points. Please note that these maps are no substitute for a topographic map (see "Recommended Map," opposite)—I strongly recommend that you bring along an up-to-date topo map for the wilderness areas in which you'll be running. The elevation profiles were created from GPS data accumulated during each run to give you an idea of terrain and difficulty.

An overview map showing the locations of all 50 trails is on the inside front cover, and a legend explaining the symbols used is on the inside back cover.

Running Time

I've intentionally left time estimates out of this book. In my personal experience of using guidebooks, these estimates tend to fall into one of two categories. The first is running times that don't square with your actual times at all. This discrepancy arises simply because the author of the guidebook is most likely going to run/hike/backpack and so on at a completely different pace than yours. Essentially, this means that either you're struggling to keep up with the author's pace and then leave feeling inadequate or you cover the route much faster and then never trust the time calculations again. The second type of time estimate is a range. In my opinion, this is even worse—most readers look to these estimates to determine if they can run the route before dark, before or after work, and so on, and giving a range does absolutely nothing to answer these questions.

In the end, everyone has a different pace. Some people like to stop and take side trips or rest breaks along a beautiful alpine lake. There's no wrong way to run a trail and, likewise, no perfect formula for estimating times for a plethora of different runners. In a nutshell: Know yourself, your pace, and how your body handles terrain and mileage. If you're a fast runner but you struggle on steep terrain, know that your normal trail pace will suffer considerably if you're running a trail rated higher on my difficulty scale.

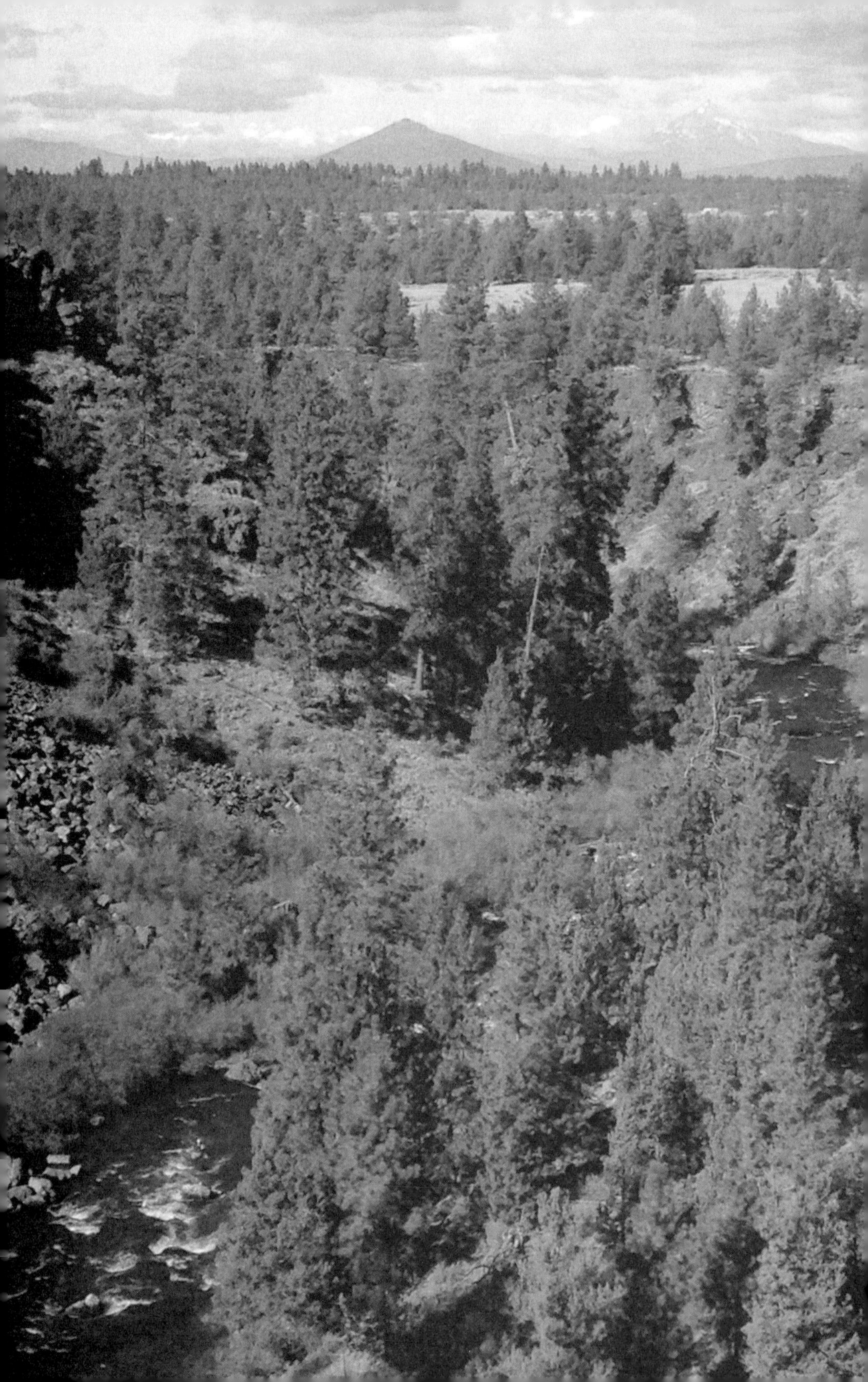

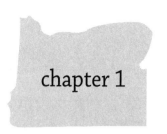

chapter 1

YEAR-ROUND RUNS

YEAR-ROUND TRAIL LIST

OPPOSITE: *The Deschutes River runs through Archie Briggs Canyon as Black Butte and Mount Jefferson rise in the background.* (See Archie Briggs Canyon, page 30.)

1 Old Mill Loop

TRAIL DETAILS AT A GLANCE

- **DISTANCE** 4.3-mile to 5.5-mile loop
- **GPS TRAILHEAD COORDINATES** N44° 2.549' W121° 19.244'
- **DIFFICULTY** 2 • **SCENERY** 4 • **CROWDS** 9
- **SEASON** Year-round; Bend city parks are open daily, 5 a.m.–10 p.m.
- **ELEVATION** Negligible • **USERS** Hikers, runners, mountain bikers (limited access)
- **CONTACT** Bend Park and Recreation, 541-389-7275, **bendparksandrec.org**
- **PERMITS/FEES** None • **RECOMMENDED MAP** PDF map at **tinyurl.com/oldmillloop**
- **DOGS** Yes (leashed only)

THOUGH THIS BOOK FOCUSES MAINLY on running in the wilderness, sometimes it's nice to have a trail run right outside your front door. The Old Mill Loop on the Deschutes River Trail offers myriad distance options and is a great combination of quintessential Central Oregon trail running and the beauty of what makes Bend one of the premier places in the country to live.

There's no trailhead per se for this loop—you can start in many places—but one place I like to begin is at Riverbend Park, off SW Columbia Street and Shevlin Hixon Drive. There's plenty of parking, and this spot tends to be less crowded than some of the others. Plus, the Bend Park and Recreation District is housed in the building adjacent to the park, so I like to think of it as paying homage to all the hard work its employees do to make Bend's parks and trails wonderful.

From the park, head south along the river on a paved pathway that takes you away from the Old Mill District. As you near the first footbridge over the Deschutes River, stay straight, exiting off the pavement onto a wide dirt path—the famed Deschutes River Trail (DRT). In a short distance, you'll run under the Bill Healy Memorial Bridge and through a fenced gate before descending back down to the river's edge.

At this point, the Deschutes River picks up speed, and you'll see the end of the stand-up paddleboarders and the beginning of the river rapids. It's also here that you'll begin to run up and down a few rolling hills to match the increased pitch of the river. Stay left at the next junction to avoid going uphill toward

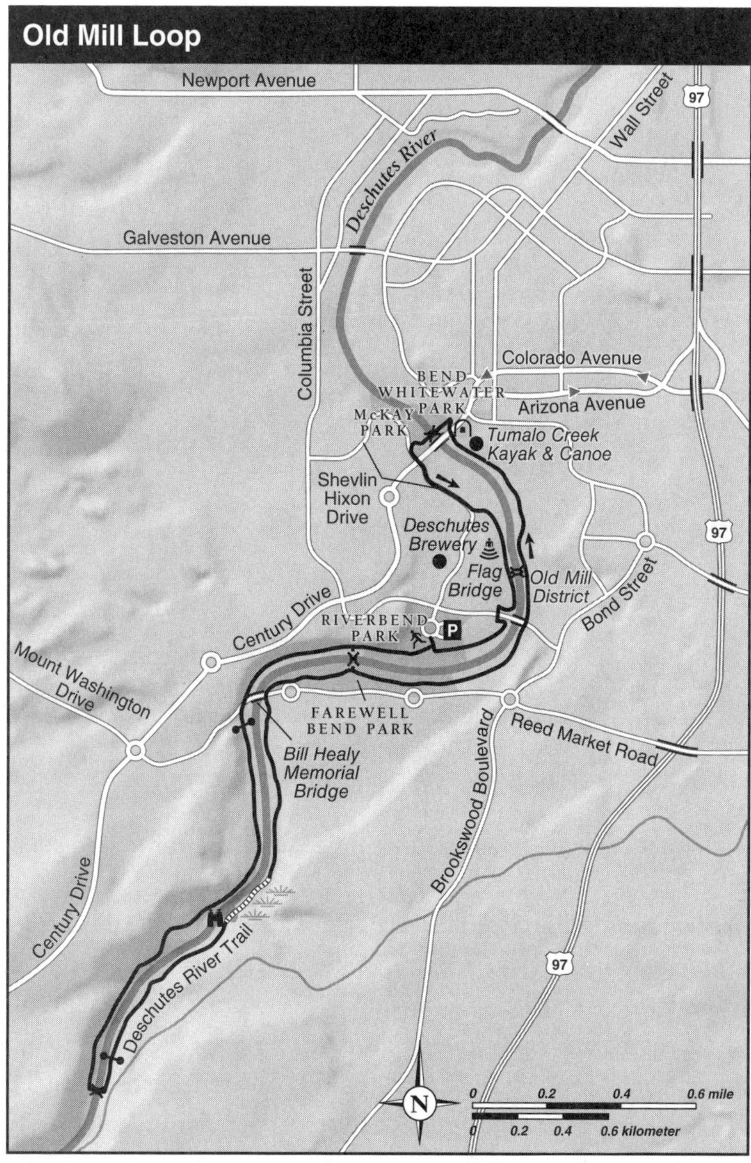

Century Drive, and at 1.6 miles along the DRT you'll reach the second footbridge and southernmost point on the trail.

After admiring the rapids under the footbridge, head back north along the river and pass through another fenced gate. This side of the river is more closed in by the forest, but still allows for spectacular views of the river. A short climb

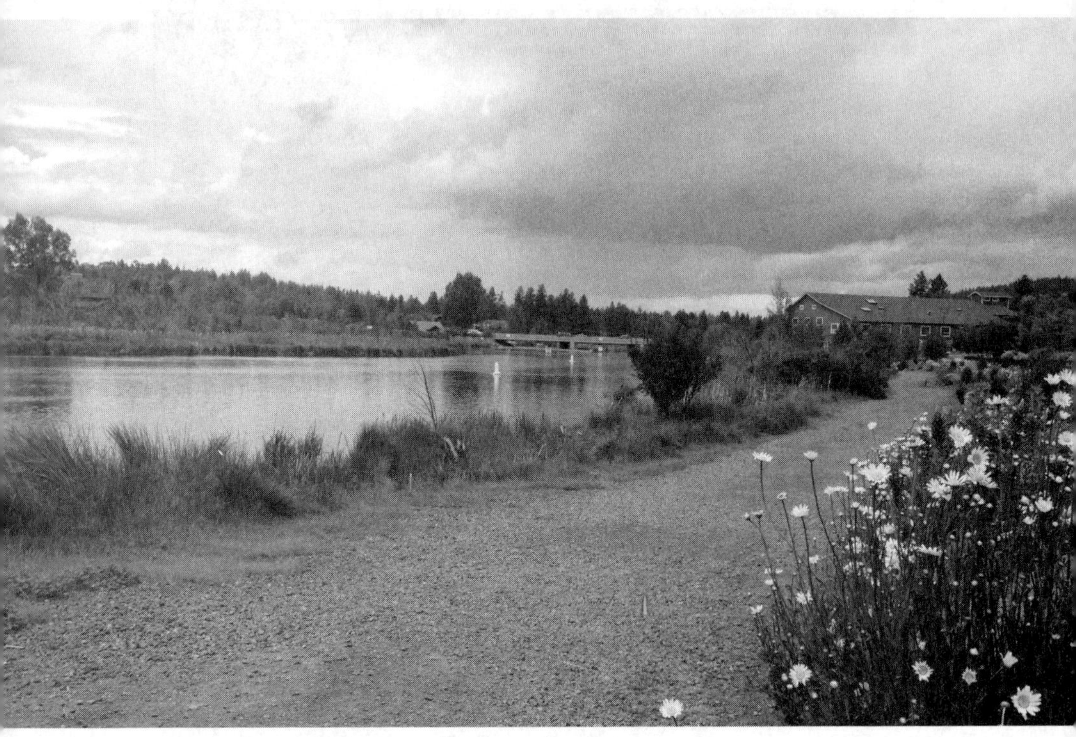

Seeded wildflowers line the pathway along the Deschutes River.

brings you to a viewpoint, where you then descend back down to a spillway and boardwalk before crossing over a marshy area.

Once you pass under the Bill Healy Bridge a second time, the dirt path converts back to sidewalk and you're now in Farewell Bend Park. Continue along the paved pathway where you'll pass by an impressive bronze horse sculpture—a nod to the area's logging and mill working days. Keep right to remain along the east side of the river, and soon you'll enter the Old Mill District, where you'll see firsthand one of the reasons the area is one of the most popular shopping destinations in Bend. *Note:* Be careful of pedestrians and children as you run past the shops and restaurants.

The Flag Bridge offers the first opportunity for a good turnaround spot if you're looking for a shorter run at approximately 4.3 miles. If not, continue along the east side of the river and past Tumalo Creek Kayak & Canoe (a great spot to rent inner tubes or boats for a float on the river) where the dirt path leads you through a newly constructed pedestrian tunnel under the Colorado Avenue bridge.

After exiting the tunnel, turn left to cross the river on the footbridge overlooking Bend Whitewater Park, a state-of-the-art river recreation area built in 2015. If you're not in a hurry, take a moment to watch the surfers, kayakers, and floaters as each navigates through the three channels of the park. Once done, continue on and hang another left at McKay Park onto Shevlin Hixon Drive to round the final corner of the 5.5-mile loop.

It's here where you'll often smell the brewing of Deschutes Brewery before you see it. Follow the sidewalk until the Les Schwab Amphitheater, a summer concert and events space that's hosted everyone from Bob Dylan to Jack Johnson. A left turn puts you back on the paved pathway, and a few curves later you'll be back at your starting point.

DIRECTIONS

From downtown Bend, drive south on NW Wall Street and turn right onto NW Colorado Avenue, following it about 0.5 mile across the Deschutes River. At the roundabout, take the third right onto SW Simpson Avenue and then take another right a block later onto Shevlin Hixon Drive. Follow Shevlin Hixon south about 0.4 mile past SW Columbia Street until you reach the Bend Park and Recreation office, on your left.

The Flag Bridge connects the Old Mill District with the trail and Westside parking.

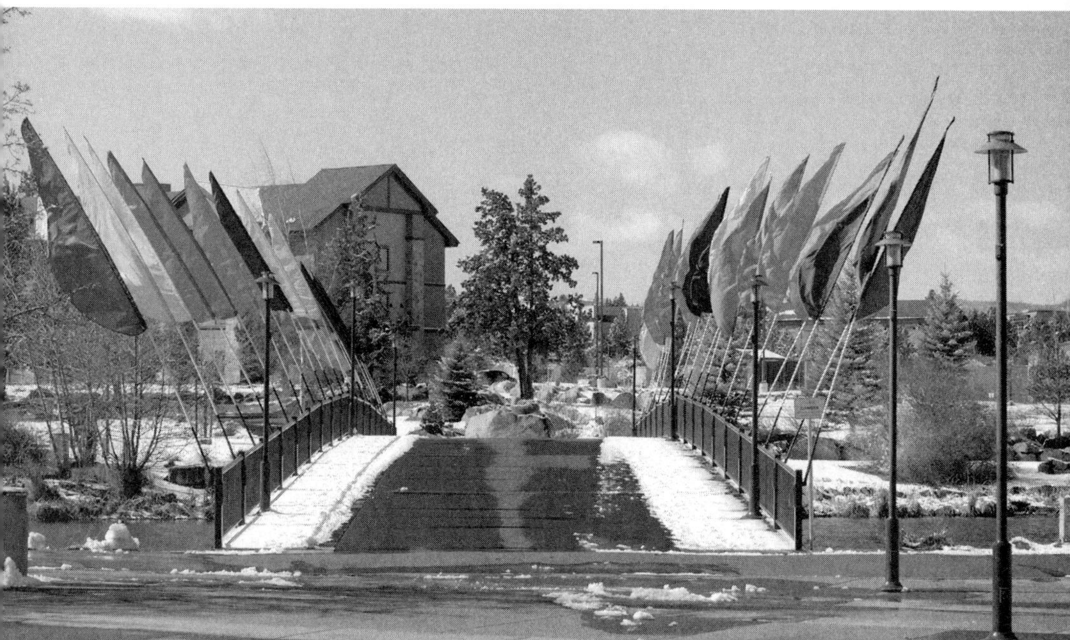

2 Pilot Butte State Park

TRAIL DETAILS AT A GLANCE

- **DISTANCE** 3.5-mile loop + out-and-back
- **GPS TRAILHEAD COORDINATES** N44° 3.476' W121° 16.714'
- **DIFFICULTY** 7 • **SCENERY** 6 • **CROWDS** 7 • **SEASON** Year-round, sunrise–sunset
- **ELEVATION** +/–611' • **USERS** Hikers, walkers
- **CONTACT** Oregon State Parks, 541-388-6055, **tinyurl.com/pilotbuttestatepark**
- **PERMITS/FEES** None • **RECOMMENDED MAP** PDF map at **tinyurl.com/pilotbutte**
- **DOGS** Yes (leashed only)

PILOT BUTTE STATE PARK looms over the city of Bend like a castle turret. It's an iconic landmark and is used by many locals to orient themselves around town. With its trails up, down, and around the butte, not only does it serve as a popular spot for a quick walk, run, or bike, but the 360-degree views at the top make it a popular spot to watch the sunrise and sunset. Each year, Pilot Butte puts on its own show July 4, when it serves as the launchpad for the city's annual Independence Day fireworks display.

This run combines two trails: the Base Trail around the butte and the out-and-back (or up-and-down, depending on how you look at it) Summit Trail, which spirals its way steeply up to the top. The recommended starting point is the parking lot on the southeast side of the butte's base. Since the park is centrally located, expect to see crowds, including dogs, strollers, and families, on the trails. Facilities are available at the parking lot.

Start up the paved walkway and immediately look to your left for the BASE TRAIL sign. Follow the Base Trail clockwise as it gently rolls up and down the side of the butte, first heading back toward the highway side and then on to the (north) back side of the butte, where you'll enjoy views of the Cascades along the western horizon. On the northeast side, you'll come up next to a fence and a school as you start down a set of steep stairs. Once past the school track, look for the singletrack through the trees and begin up several switchbacks on the butte's eastern flanks.

At 1.7 miles, connect with the main Summit Trail where you'll turn right and begin the steep climb up and around the butte (this time counterclockwise) and to the summit parking area. Cars are allowed to drive to the summit starting

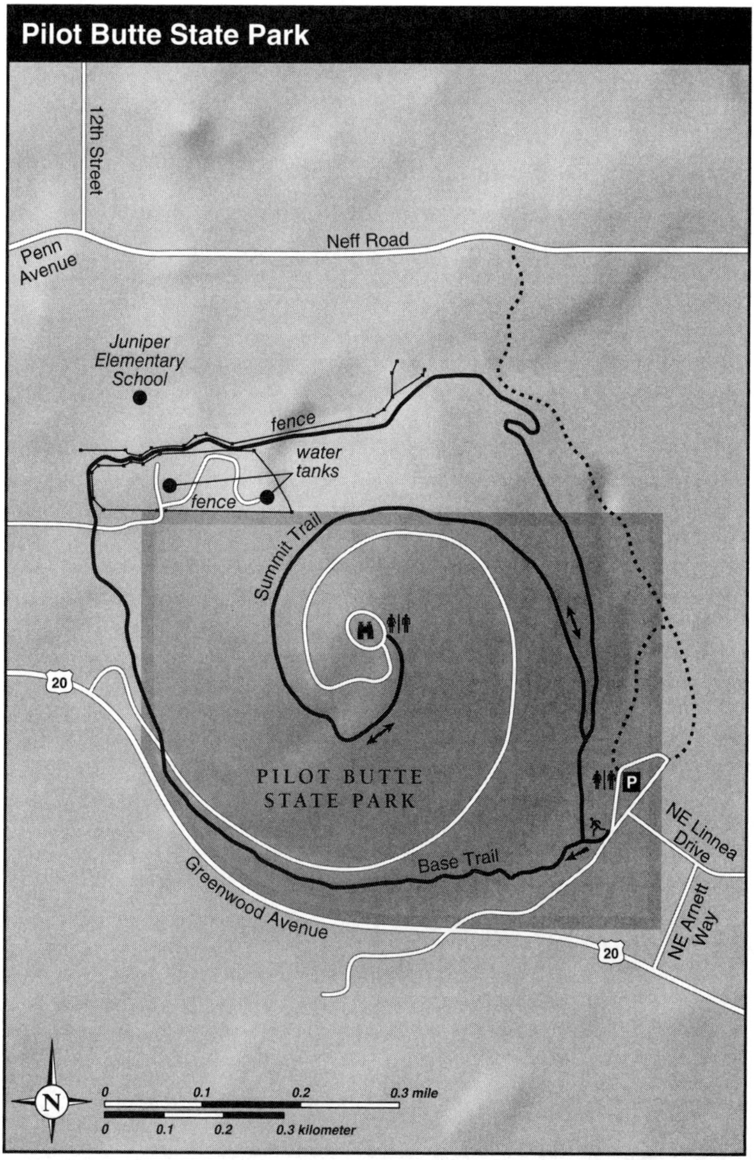

Pilot Butte State Park
12th Street
Penn Avenue
Neff Road
Juniper Elementary School
fence
water tanks
fence
Summit Trail
20
PILOT BUTTE STATE PARK
P
NE Linnea Drive
Base Trail
Greenwood Avenue
NE Arnett Way
20
N
0 0.1 0.2 0.3 mile
0 0.1 0.2 0.3 kilometer

4,200 ft.
4,100 ft.
4,000 ft.
3,900 ft.
3,800 ft.
3,700 ft.
3,600 ft.
0.5 mi.
1 mi.
1.5 mi.
2 mi.
2.5 mi.
3 mi.
3.5 mi.

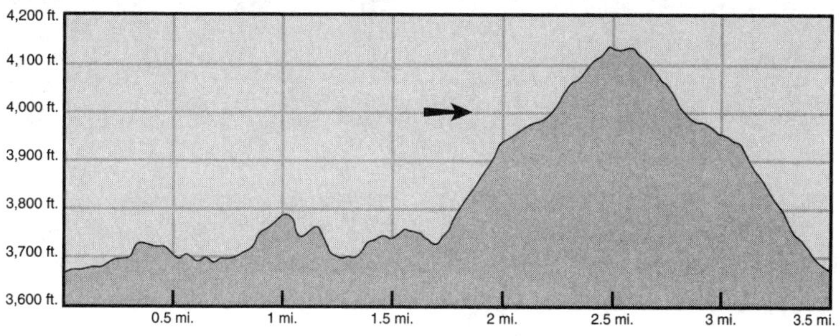

in midspring and typically until November, depending on weather. Be sure to take a moment and take in the scenery at the top. Signs point out the various Cascade peaks, and on clear days, you can see as far north as Washington's Mount Adams and even Mount Rainier.

On the return, head back down the steep summit trail or, in the winter months, take the carless road down for an alternate route where you can rejoin the base trail and head back around to the parking lot.

DIRECTIONS

From downtown Bend, drive east on Greenwood Avenue (US 20). In about 2 miles, look for the signs to the Pilot Butte State Park trailhead and take a left on NE Arnett Way toward the park. At the T, another left on NE Linnea Drive takes you to the parking lot and trailhead.

A view from the summit of Pilot Butte overlooks Bend in the foreground, with snowcapped Mount Bachelor on the horizon.

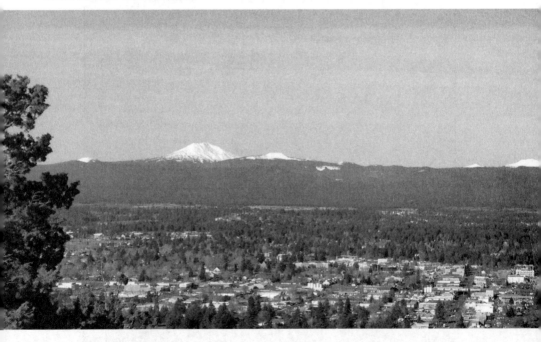

3 Entrada River Loop

TRAIL DETAILS AT A GLANCE

- **DISTANCE** 5.3-mile loop • **GPS TRAILHEAD COORDINATES** N44° 1.385' W121° 21.552'
- **DIFFICULTY** 3 • **SCENERY** 6
- **SEASON** Year-round; Bend city parks are open daily, 5 a.m.–10 p.m.
- **ELEVATION** +/–366' • **USERS** Runners, hikers, mountain bikers
- **CONTACT** Bend Park and Recreation, 541-389-7275, **bendparksandrec.org**
- **PERMITS/FEES** None • **RECOMMENDED MAP** *Bend, Oregon, Trail Map* by Adventure Maps, Inc. ($12, **adventuremaps.net**) • **DOGS** Yes (leashed only)

THE ENTRADA LODGE sits right at the western edge of Bend and is a popular hotel for the hordes of tourists who visit Mount Bachelor in the wintertime. It's also the starting point for this run, made up of parts of the Deschutes River Trail and a second loop, aptly named the Entrada Loop.

To start out, park at the dirt pullout on the north side of the Cascade Lakes Scenic Byway, opposite the main entrance to the Entrada Lodge (19221 SW Century Drive). After carefully crossing the busy highway, begin the run near the Deschutes River Trail (DRT) sign just to the west of the lodge entryway. Within 50 yards, take a sharp left on the doubletrack and then a sharp right to remain on the DRT. Meander your way another quarter-mile until you reach a junction. Veer left up the hill, following signs for the River Loop—*not* a hard left for the Entrada Loop.

At 0.7 mile, turn left at the viewpoint marker and in 100 yards take in the views of the spectacular Deschutes River, your companion for much of this run. When satisfied, return to the trail and continue downhill to the river itself. Stay close to the bank as you head upstream and pay attention to avoid a few scattered, false trails. At roughly 1.6 miles, you'll see the junction—and return route—for the River Loop and the DRT. For now, continue straight, up a rocky section and onto a nice steep overlook above the Deschutes.

At 2.2 miles, you'll come out into the first of several parking areas for the Meadow Camp Trailhead on the DRT. Continue along the path near the bank and make your way in and out of the trailheads to the final picnic area just before the trail steepens. If it's a hot day, this is also a great spot to hop in the river for a quick swim or cool-down midrun.

Entrada River Loop

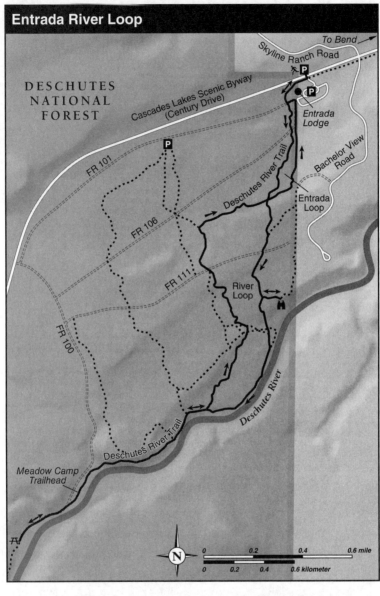

To Bend
Skyline Ranch Road
DESCHUTES NATIONAL FOREST
Cascades Lakes Scenic Byway (Century Drive)
Entrada Lodge
Bachelor View Road
FR 101
Deschutes River Trail
Entrada Loop
FR 106
FR 111
River Loop
FR 100
Deschutes River
Meadow Camp Trailhead
0 0.2 0.4 0.6 mile
0 0.2 0.4 0.6 kilometer

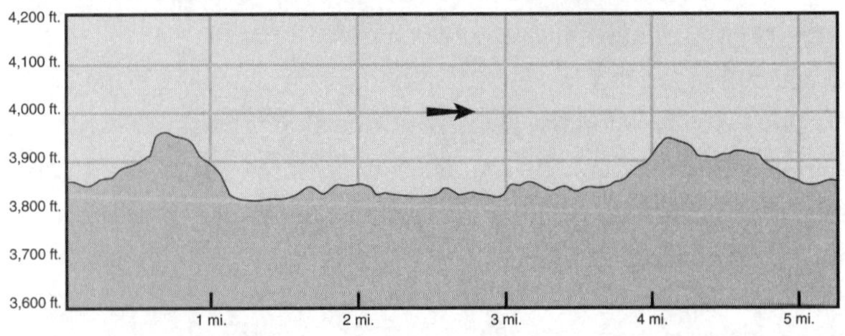

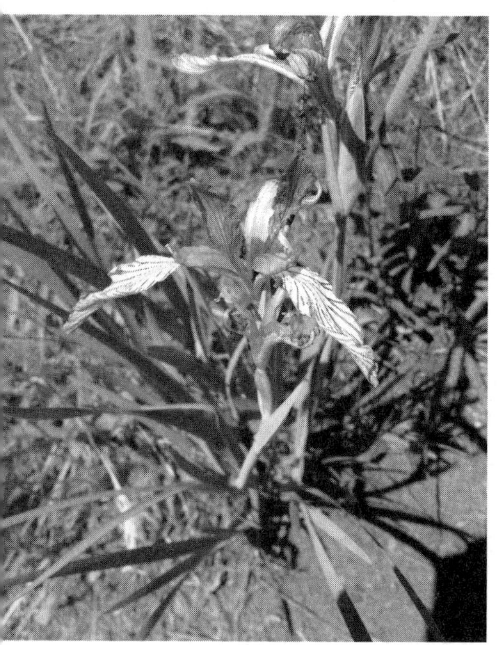

Rocky Mountain iris

For now use this as the turnaround spot, at approximately 2.5 miles, and continue back along the DRT to the junction with the River Loop at 3.5 miles. From here, the DRT veers away from the river and begins a gradual uphill into the pines and past a small rock formation on the hill. Stay straight at 3.8 miles at the unmarked junction and, shortly after, stay right at another unmarked junction to continue up the hill. When cresting the hill, cross the rough logging road to continue on the DRT as the trail drops and veer right back along the rocky ridge.

At mile 4.7, you'll reach a familiar junction, but this time continue straight to stay on the Entrada Loop, which circles back along the Entrada Lodge property. Follow the trail back toward the highway to the DRT trailhead and your starting point.

DIRECTIONS

From Bend, take SW Century Drive (the Cascade Lakes Scenic Byway) south and west toward Mount Hood. Just beyond the city limits, pass the intersection of SW Century Drive and Bachelor View Road (also signed as Skyline Ranch Road to the north) and look for the dirt pullout opposite the Entrada Lodge. Carefully cross the highway and look for the signed Deschutes River Trail just to the right of the lodge.

4 Archie Briggs Canyon

TRAIL DETAILS AT A GLANCE

- **DISTANCE** 7.6-mile out-and-back
- **GPS TRAILHEAD COORDINATES** N44° 4.043' W121° 18.832'
- **DIFFICULTY** 3 • **SCENERY** 6 • **CROWDS** 7
- **SEASON** Year-round; Bend city parks are open daily, 5 a.m.–10 p.m.
- **ELEVATION** +/– 95' • **USERS** Runners, hikers, mountain bikers
- **CONTACT** Bend Park and Recreation, 541-389-7275, **bendparksandrec.org**
- **PERMITS/FEES** None • **RECOMMENDED MAP** PDF map at **tinyurl.com/archiebriggs**
- **DOGS** Yes (leashed only)

BEND RESIDENTS ARE FORTUNATE to have hundreds of miles of fabulous winding singletrack in the nearby lands managed by state parks, national monuments, the national forest, and the Bureau of Land Management. What is even more fortunate is that we also have a multitude of spectacular trails right in the heart of the city. The Deschutes River Trail (DRT) through Archie Briggs Canyon is a prime example.

Featuring waterside running next to the Deschutes River and cliffside running far above it, this section of the Deschutes River Trail provides a variety of scenery on well-marked and well-graded trail through spectacular Archie Briggs Canyon. Though this is an out-and-back, several options exist for those wanting to add a smaller loop segment as well as some challenging hill work.

Start the run at First Street Rapids Park, adjacent to the quaint northwest Bend neighborhood at the end of First Street. A new bridge, built in the fall of 2014, also allows runners to start at Pioneer Park just north of downtown by connecting a paved trail for a brief quarter-mile.

The wide dirt trail begins at a set of rapids just above the bridge, a popular playground for urban kayakers. For the first half-mile, the trail follows the contours of the Deschutes River before a short but steep uphill at 0.6 mile that takes runners up—and then down—alongside Mount Washington Drive. At the bottom of the hill, carefully cross the road and reconnect with the trail as it sneaks its way between holes at the River's Edge Golf Course. At 1.1 miles, pay close attention to any golfers above and to your left on the No. 3 tee box, as the trail goes directly under the intended flight path.

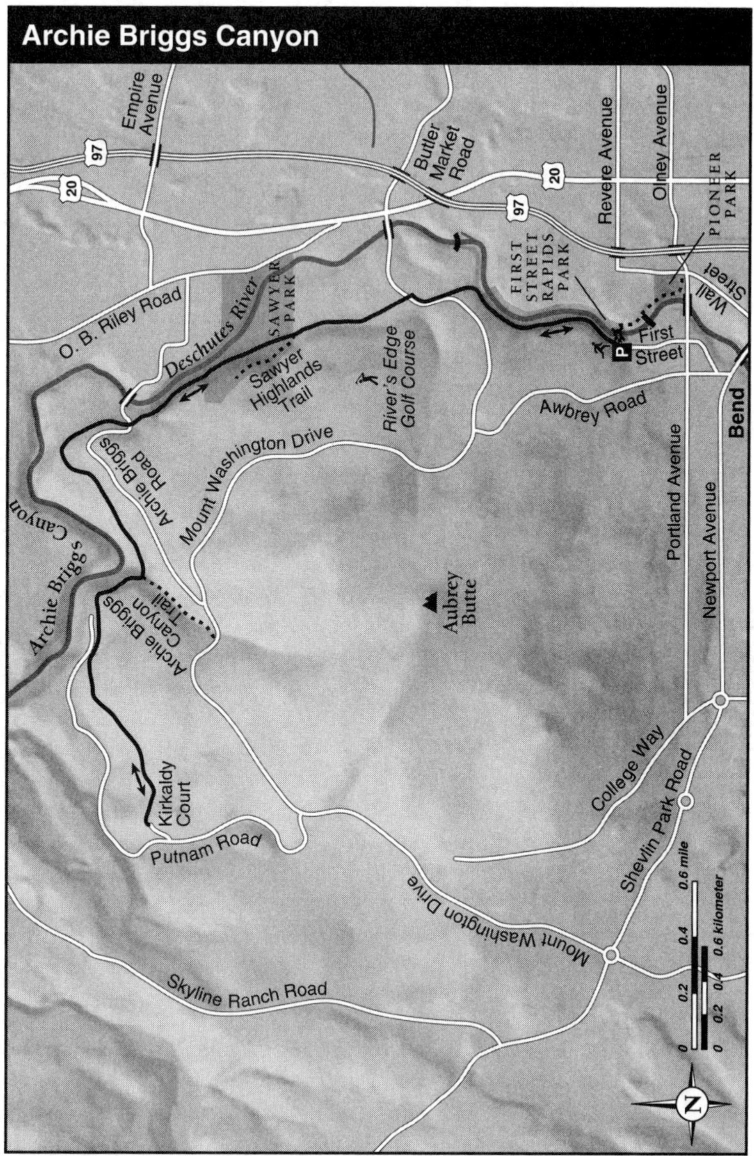

Once safely past the golf course, the trail enters the fringes of Sawyer Park, a popular spot for fly-fishermen and picnickers. Ignore a side junction at 1.25 miles for the Sawyer Highlands Trail and keep straight past any smaller junctions to the right into Sawyer Park. From here, the trail begins to climb gently away from the river. Cross a couple of roads at 1.9 and 2.3 miles before settling into a nice pace and some spectacular views as you enter Archie Briggs Canyon.

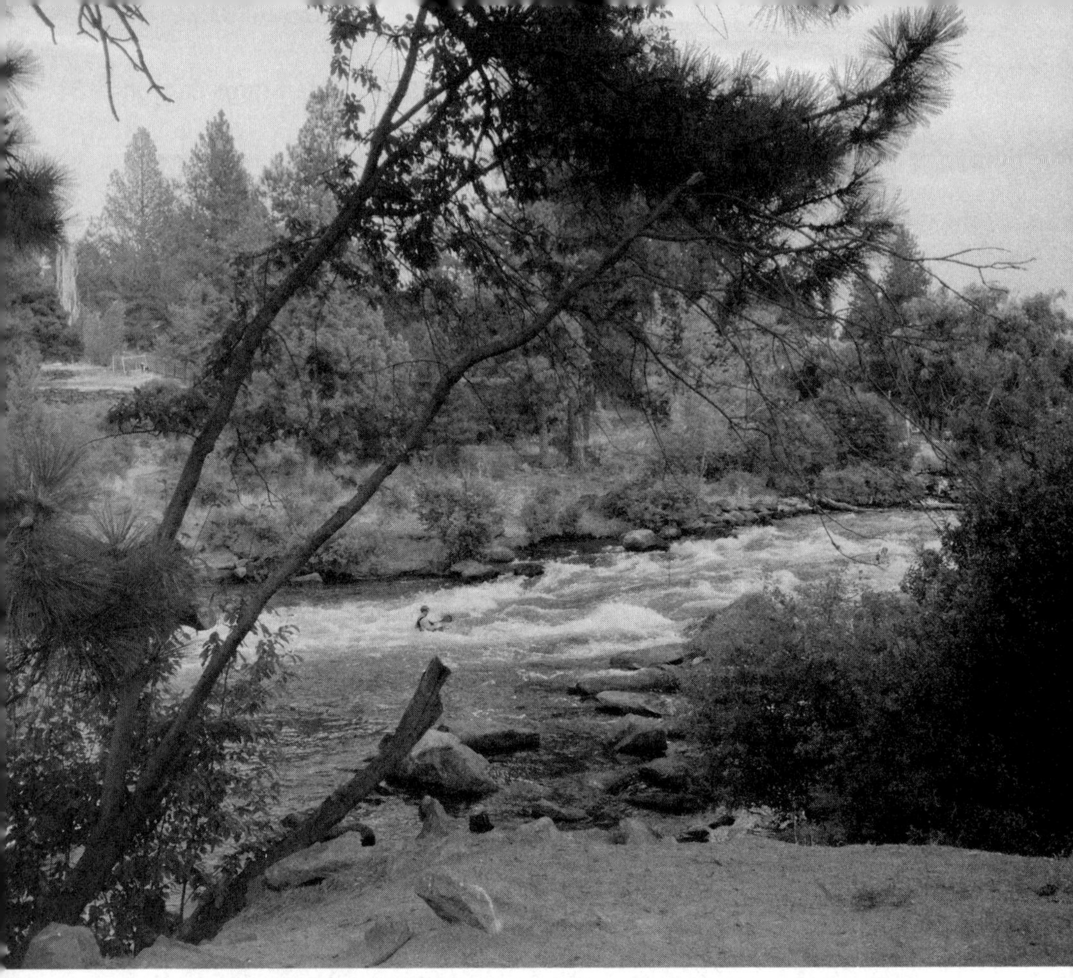

A kayaker tests his skills on the Deschutes River near First Street Rapids Park.

Soon, the Cascades begin to line themselves up on the horizon in front of you, and the rushing Deschutes River reappears far below the canyon walls. Several placards describe the history of the area at intermittent locations along the trail, and a few park benches tempt you for a rest and to take in the views.

If you're looking to add hills to your running regimen, at 2.75 miles look for the junction with the Archie Briggs Canyon Trail—a steep singletrack trail that creeps its way up through the gully and away from the larger Archie Briggs Canyon. *Note:* It's possible to make a short loop here by connecting several paved roads back to the terminus of the DRT off NW Kirkaldy Court.

For those who opt out of the hill work, keep straight and climb briefly back up to the DRT as it turns a corner and once again veers out of sight from the river below. From here, the next mile to the trail's end at Kirkaldy Court is relatively flat and viewless. When you reach the terminus at 3.8 miles, simply turn around and retrace your steps to the start.

DIRECTIONS

From downtown Bend, drive north and east on NW Wall Street and turn left onto NW Portland Avenue. Shortly after the bridge, turn right on NW First Street, which dead-ends after several blocks. Look for a small dirt parking area for the First Street Rapids Trailhead.

Swan sightings are common along this stretch of the Deschutes.

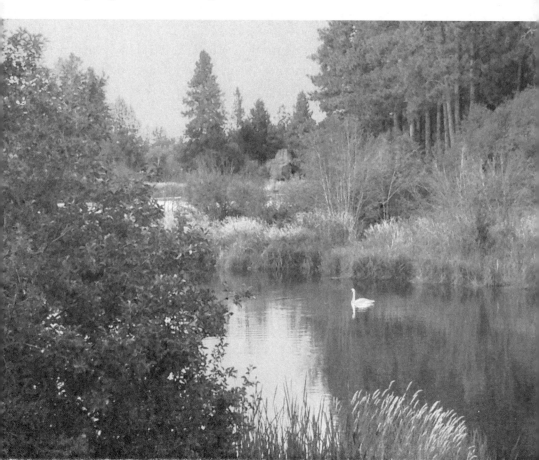

5 Shevlin Park Loop Trail

TRAIL DETAILS AT A GLANCE

- **DISTANCE** 4.5-mile loop
- **GPS TRAILHEAD COORDINATES** N44° 4.898' W121° 22.704'
- **DIFFICULTY** 3
- **SCENERY** 6
- **CROWDS** 7
- **SEASON** Year-round; Bend city parks are open daily, 5 a.m.–10 p.m.
- **ELEVATION** +/– 232'
- **USERS** Hikers, runners, mountain bikers
- **CONTACT** Bend Park and Recreation, 541-389-7275, **bendparksandrec.org**
- **PERMITS/FEES** None
- **RECOMMENDED MAP** *Bend, Oregon, Trail Map* by Adventure Maps, Inc. ($12, **adventuremaps.net**)
- **DOGS** Yes (leashed only)

SHEVLIN PARK IS ONE OF THOSE PLACES that make trail runners like me feel lucky to live in Central Oregon. The park is right on the edge of town and is a quick drive from almost anywhere in Bend, but it provides a wilderness-like experience, as if you were much farther from civilization. It's a favorite of many locals, and for good reason.

This classic Central Oregon park on the west side of Bend has a large network of trails with a variety of distances and scenic options. One of the best places to start is the Shevlin Park Loop Trail, which circles the park on forested pine slopes to the west and high desert landscape to the east. Though the loop can be run in any direction, I prefer to start on the west side and run counterclockwise. The trail begins next to the main parking lot, across from the restrooms next to the gate (locked seasonally during winter months).

The run starts by snaking its way up into the ponderosa pines along the ridge. Within a half-mile, you'll veer slightly left on the singletrack at your first of many intersections on this run. Shortly after, another junction marks the historic Shevlin Railway and the start of what was once an impressive trestle spanning Shevlin Park; a keen eye can also spot the popular covered bridge below and to the east. Keep left at both this and the subsequent intersection, which appears shortly.

The trail flattens for the next 1.5 miles. Around mile 2, a trail to the left leads down to the Fremont Meadow area—a popular spot for summer youth camps. Continue straight until the trail descends to a doubletrack road marked by numerous junctions and signs. Keep straight for approximately 100 yards, and keep an eye out for the Shevlin Loop Trail marker pointing toward the river and your return route.

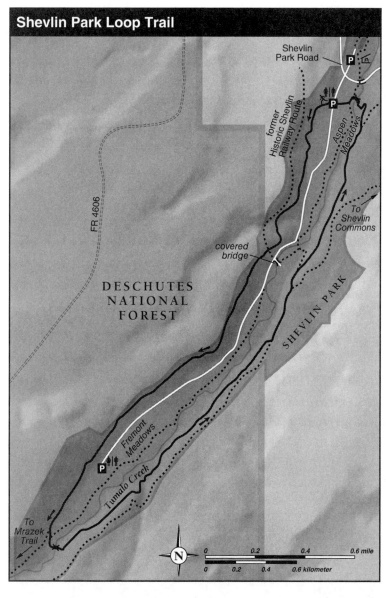

Shevlin Park Loop Trail

Shevlin Park Road
former Historic Shevlin Railway Route
Aspen Meadows
FR 4606
To Shevlin Commons
covered bridge
DESCHUTES NATIONAL FOREST
SHEVLIN PARK
Fremont Meadows
Tumalo Creek
To Mrazek Trail
N
0 0.2 0.4 0.6 mile
0 0.2 0.4 0.6 kilometer

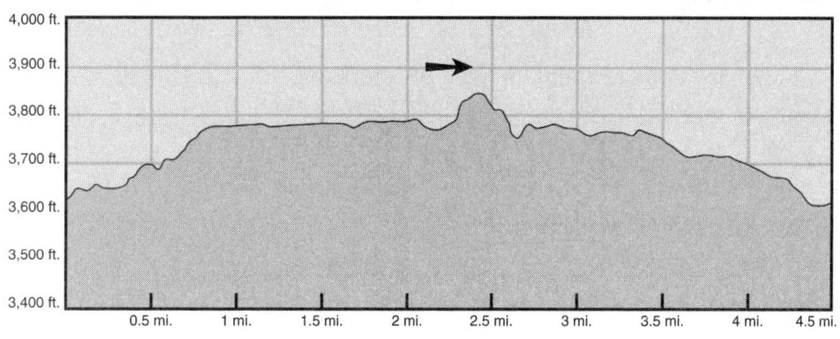

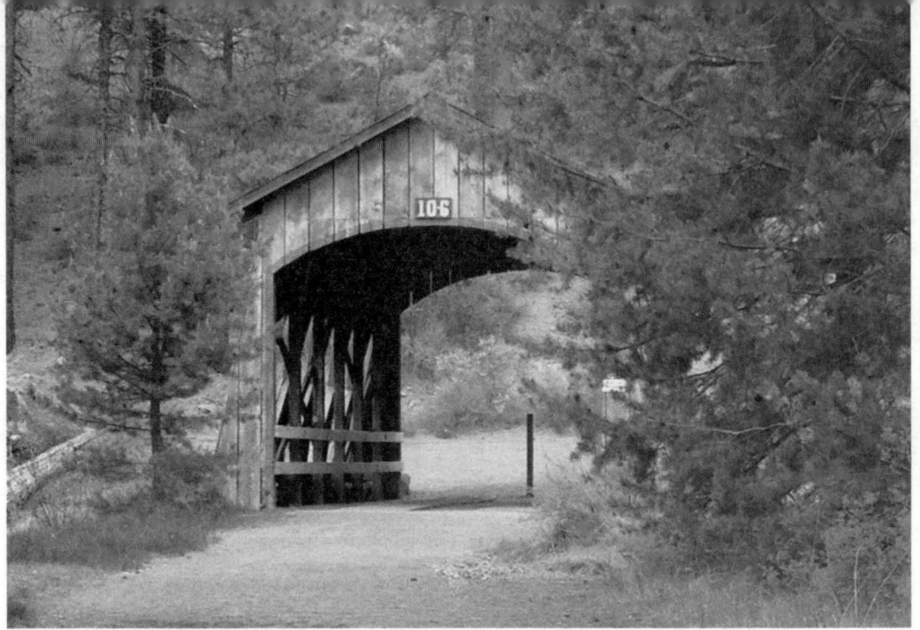

A historic covered bridge along the trail

After crossing the pristine Tumalo Creek, the trail steeply ascends back up the ridge before again plummeting, this time to cross a small stream feeding into Tumalo Creek. Once across the small but sturdy log bridge, make your way back up the singletrack, taking a left at each junction you encounter. Eventually, you'll emerge from the trees to the open eastern ridge, which was devastated by the Awbrey Hall fire in the 1990s.

Here along the ridge, you have great views of the river below as well as the Cascade Mountains to the west. As you get nearer to the road, keep left at the final junction to a couple of short switchbacks taking you back over the river. From the bridge, stay straight to finish your run through a lovely grove of aspen trees, just a short walk from the parking lot and the start.

DIRECTIONS

From downtown Bend, drive south on NW Wall Street and turn right (west) on NW Newport Avenue, which turns into NW Shevlin Park Road after about 1.3 miles. Follow this road about 2.5 miles until you see signs for Shevlin Park at the bottom of a large hill. Enter the park on the south side of the road after crossing Tumalo Creek, and continue about 100 yards to the parking area near the restrooms.

6 Ben's Trail

TRAIL DETAILS AT A GLANCE

- **DISTANCE** 4.3-mile loop • **GPS TRAILHEAD COORDINATES** N44° 2.593' W121° 23.163'
- **DIFFICULTY** 2 • **SCENERY** 3 • **CROWDS** 8 • **SEASON** Year-round, sunrise–sunset
- **ELEVATION** +/–262' • **USERS** Hikers, runners, mountain bikers
- **CONTACT** Bend–Fort Rock Ranger District, Deschutes National Forest; 541-383-4000, **www.fs.usda.gov/deschutes**
- **PERMITS/FEES** None • **RECOMMENDED MAP** *Bend, Oregon, Trail Map* by Adventure Maps, Inc. ($12, **adventuremaps.net**) • **DOGS** Yes (leashed only)

THE PHIL'S TRAIL NETWORK IN BEND is one of the most well-known and well-loved trail systems for mountain bikers in the state of Oregon. The superbly designed trails provide the perfect fast, sweeping flow of riding that off-road bikers love. Plus, the sheer number of trails, variety of terrain, and loop possibilities keep riders entertained all year long.

Though built originally for mountain biking, the trails are open to runners and hikers as well. It should be noted that the trails stemming from the main Phil's Trailhead are arguably some of the best for mountain biking but not necessarily the best for trail running. The continuous S-curve singletrack paths, along with a lack of vistas and the popularity of the network, mean that for runners, Phil's is probably not the most ideal. If you're in a pinch, however, or you're new to town and you simply want to run in a place your friends have told you about, Phil's works just fine.

This quick loop, perfect for a lunchtime run, combines Ben's, MTB, and Kent's Trails. Starting from the main parking lot, look for the signs for Ben's Trail at the far end. Because of its popularity, Ben's was converted to a one-way trail in 2014 to help with traffic flow and reduce accidents. The first half-mile of trail weaves in and out of ponderosa pines on the edge of the network. Look to your right and you may see some of the more daring freeride bikers careening off 20-foot-high jumps at the bike park that butts against the northern edge of the area.

At mile 1.25, the trail takes a short uphill climb to the junction with the MTB. Turn left here to continue the loop. Around the second mile, the trees open up slightly to reveal a few mountainous views above the pines as you zigzag through the tight curves and begin a short descent through a couple of dusty switchbacks.

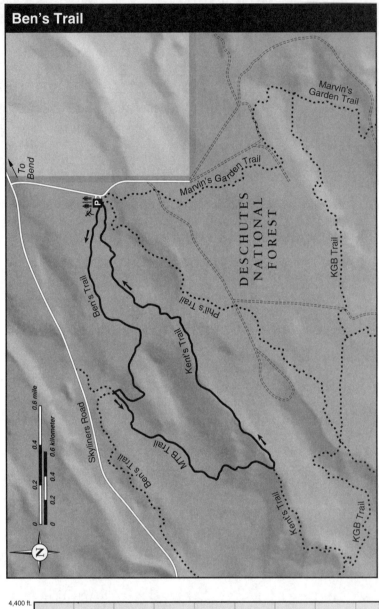

Ben's Trail

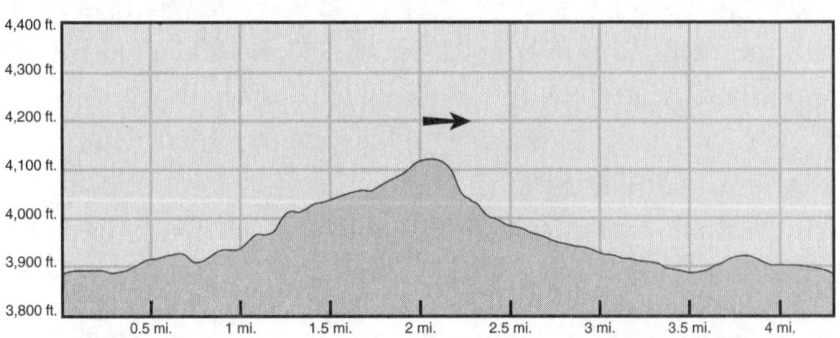
4,400 ft.
4,300 ft.
4,200 ft.
4,100 ft.
4,000 ft.
3,900 ft.
3,800 ft.
0.5 mi.
1 mi.
1.5 mi.
2 mi.
2.5 mi.
3 mi.
3.5 mi.
4 mi.

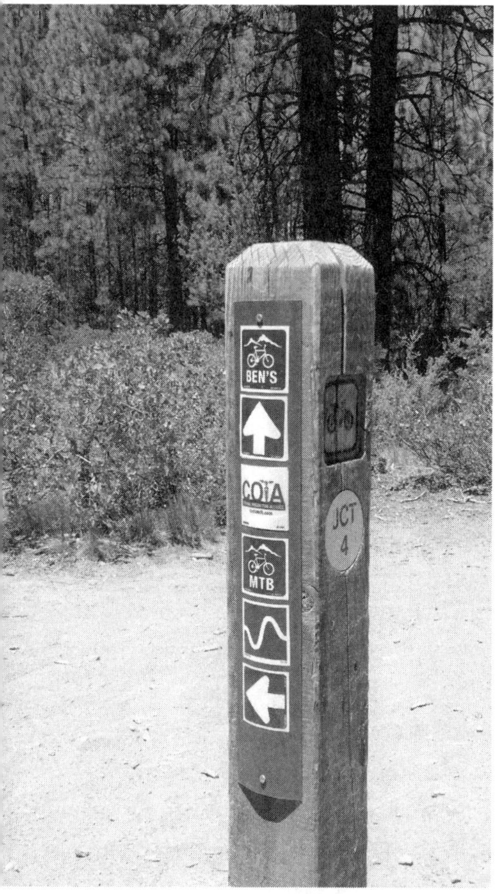

Well-signed posts mark each junction through the Phil's Trail network.

A quick half-mile later, you reach the marked intersection of Kent's Trail, the final corner of the loop. Turn left to continue the run and head back the roughly 2 miles through the dotted pine forest to reach the parking lot and trailhead.

DIRECTIONS

From downtown Bend, drive west on NW Tumalo Avenue, which becomes NW Galveston Avenue after it crosses the river. At Flagline Drive (about 0.8 mile), Galveston turns into NW Skyliners Road. Continue about 0.7 mile through the roundabout at NW Mount Washington Drive; after another 1.5 miles, look for the signs for Phil's Trailhead. Turn left (south) and drive another 0.5 mile to the parking lot and trailheads.

7 Phil's Trail

TRAIL DETAILS AT A GLANCE

- **DISTANCE** 5.6-mile loop
- **GPS TRAILHEAD COORDINATES** N44° 2.593' W121° 23.163'
- **DIFFICULTY** 3
- **SCENERY** 4
- **CROWDS** 8
- **SEASON** Year-round, sunrise–sunset
- **ELEVATION** +/–213'
- **USERS** Hikers, runners, mountain bikers
- **CONTACT** Bend–Fort Rock Ranger District, Deschutes National Forest; 541-383-4000, **www.fs.usda.gov/deschutes**
- **PERMITS/FEES** None
- **RECOMMENDED MAP** *Bend, Oregon, Trail Map* by Adventure Maps, Inc. ($12, **adventuremaps.net**)
- **DOGS** Yes (leashed only)

THE PHIL'S TRAIL NETWORK was pioneered in the early 1980s by a handful of die-hard outdoor-loving Bendites. Local legends Phil Meglasson (the network's namesake), Bob Woodward, Jim Terhaar, and former Olympian Ben Husaby gradually converted the game trails and rogue trails west of Bend into legitimate mountain biking trails. Over the years, the network has grown exponentially, as has the popularity of what many national publications call a mountain biking Mecca.

Though originally built for knobby tires, the Phil's Trail network also offers a wide variety of loop options that are great for trail runners. With over hundreds of miles of singletrack accessible from the main trailhead, and sitting just on the edge of town, the network is a perfect running spot for those who prefer to be out on the trails instead of behind the wheel. The Marvin's Garden/Phil's Loop highlights two of the more popular trails in the network and includes a few open views of the Cascades on the western horizon—something that is not often present on the lower trails of the network.

Begin the run at the main trailhead parking lot and zigzag your way through the pine trees on Marvin's Garden. Be especially careful of (and courteous to) others on the trail—including walkers, hikers, dogs, and, of course, mountain bikers. After quickly crossing a forest road, the trail begins to settle into the network's famous flowy singletrack, weaving gently back and forth through the trees. Just over a mile into the run, the trail crosses a second forest road (and popular summer camp spot for those who simply have to ride 24/7) before curving back east.

At 1.75 miles, turn right at the junction with the KGB Trail. Take KGB back west, slightly climbing and then leveling out over the next 2.0 miles until reaching

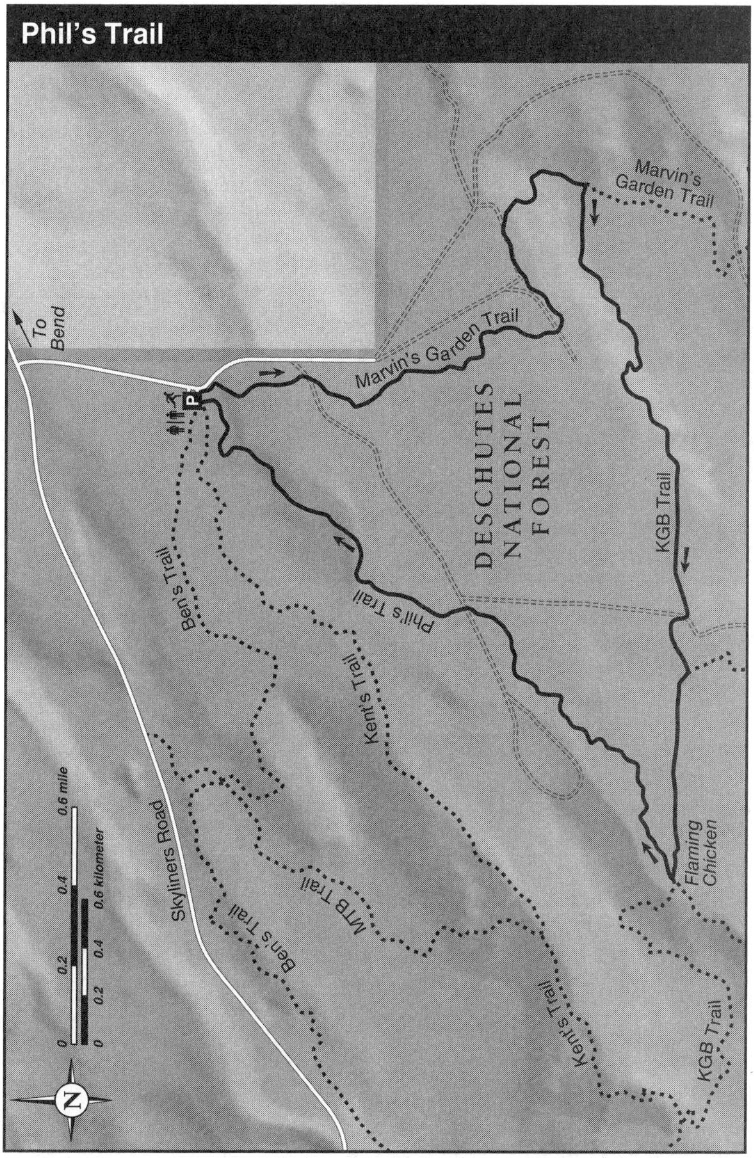

Phil's Trail
To Bend
Marvin's Garden Trail
Marvin's Garden Trail
DESCHUTES NATIONAL FOREST
KGB Trail
Phil's Trail
Ben's Trail
Kent's Trail
Skyliners Road
MTB Trail
Ben's Trail
Kent's Trail
Flaming Chicken
KGB Trail
0 0.2 0.4 0.6 mile
0 0.2 0.4 0.6 kilometer
N

4,200 ft.
4,100 ft.
4,000 ft.
3,900 ft.
3,800 ft.
3,700 ft.
3,600 ft.
1 mi.
2 mi.
3 mi.
4 mi.
5 mi.

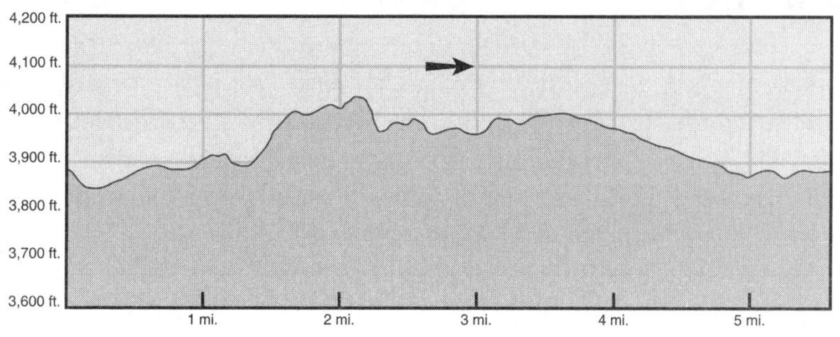

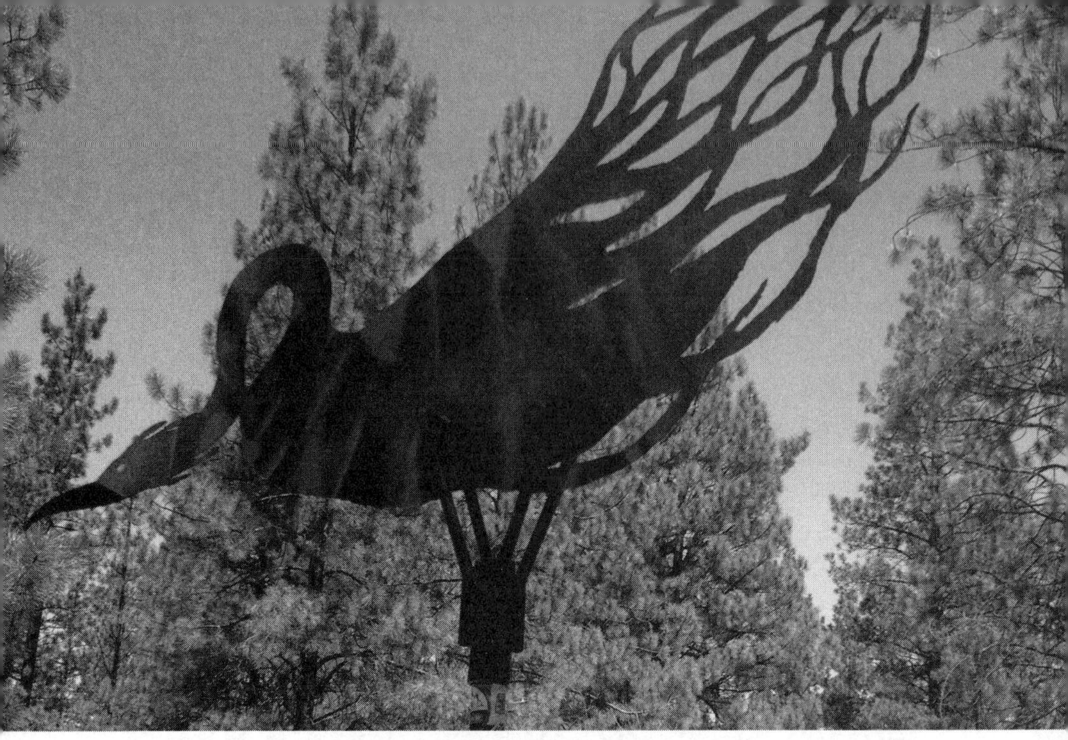

The "Flaming Chicken" stands sentry at a six-way junction.

the six-way junction at the famous "Flaming Chicken" marker. The sign, based on a roundabout sculpture at Galveston Avenue and Century Drive in Bend, represents the mythical phoenix rising from the flames. Most locals in Central Oregon, however, prefer to call it by its more endearing nickname.

From the Flaming Chicken, turn right on the namesake Phil's Trail to return to the parking lot and complete your loop. *Note:* This section of Phil's Trail is one-way only to help maintain the flow of traffic on the trail. Keep alert for mountain bikers coming up behind you. The remaining 2.0 miles of singletrack are fast and smooth, with some unique rock formations around 4.5 miles to keep you interested.

DIRECTIONS

From downtown Bend, drive west on NW Tumalo Avenue, which becomes NW Galveston Avenue after it crosses the river. At Flagline Drive (about 0.8 mile), Galveston turns into NW Skyliners Road. Continue about 0.7 mile through the roundabout at NW Mount Washington Drive; after another 1.5 miles, look for the signs for Phil's Trailhead. Turn left (south) and drive another 0.5 mile to the parking lot and trailheads.

8 Lower Peterson Ridge Trail

TRAIL DETAILS AT A GLANCE

- **DISTANCE** 7-mile loop
- **GPS TRAILHEAD COORDINATES** N44° 17.050' W121° 32.984'
- **DIFFICULTY** 2
- **SCENERY** 3
- **CROWDS** 6
- **SEASON** Year-round, sunrise–sunset
- **ELEVATION** +/–232'
- **USERS** Hikers, runners, mountain bikers
- **CONTACT** Sisters Trail Alliance, 541-719-8822, **sisterstrails.com**
- **PERMITS/FEES** None
- **RECOMMENDED MAP** *Sisters & Redmond High Desert Trail Map* by Adventure Maps, Inc. ($12, **adventuremaps.net**)
- **DOGS** Yes (leashed only)

WHAT PHIL'S TRAIL IS TO BEND, the Peterson Ridge Trail (PRT) is to Sisters. Originally built in 1989 with major additions in 2008, the PRT network is maintained by the hardworking and dedicated volunteers of the Sisters Trail Alliance. The 501(c)3 believes strongly that trails are an indispensable and necessary part of the vibrancy and high quality of life in Sisters Country. The PRT is physical proof of these beliefs and one of the most well-maintained and organized trail networks in the state.

The PRT contains more than 30 miles of meticulously marked singletrack with loop options to satisfy any desired distance. Designed as a ladder system, the PRT features two linear trails—the PRT West and the PRT East—along with a number of connector trails between the two. Well-stocked map boxes are located at the main trailhead and upper trailhead (described in the Upper Peterson Ridge run on page 198).

The Lower Peterson Ridge Trail is a mostly flat, fast stretch of trail weaving in and out of ponderosa pines, sagebrush, and juniper. Originally designed as a mountain biking network, the PRT also makes for some great trail running for runners of all levels. Unlike the Phil's Trail Network, the PRT sees far fewer people by comparison. The recommended loop here takes runners on a tour of the lower network up the PRT West to the Running Elk connector trail and back down to the trailhead via the PRT East.

From the lower trailhead, run a quick 20 yards to the first marked intersection. Take a right here to continue along PRT West. Within the first mile, you'll quickly realize why the area is so popular with mountain bikers, with its flowy singletrack and smooth, banked turns. Continue past the odd-numbered trail

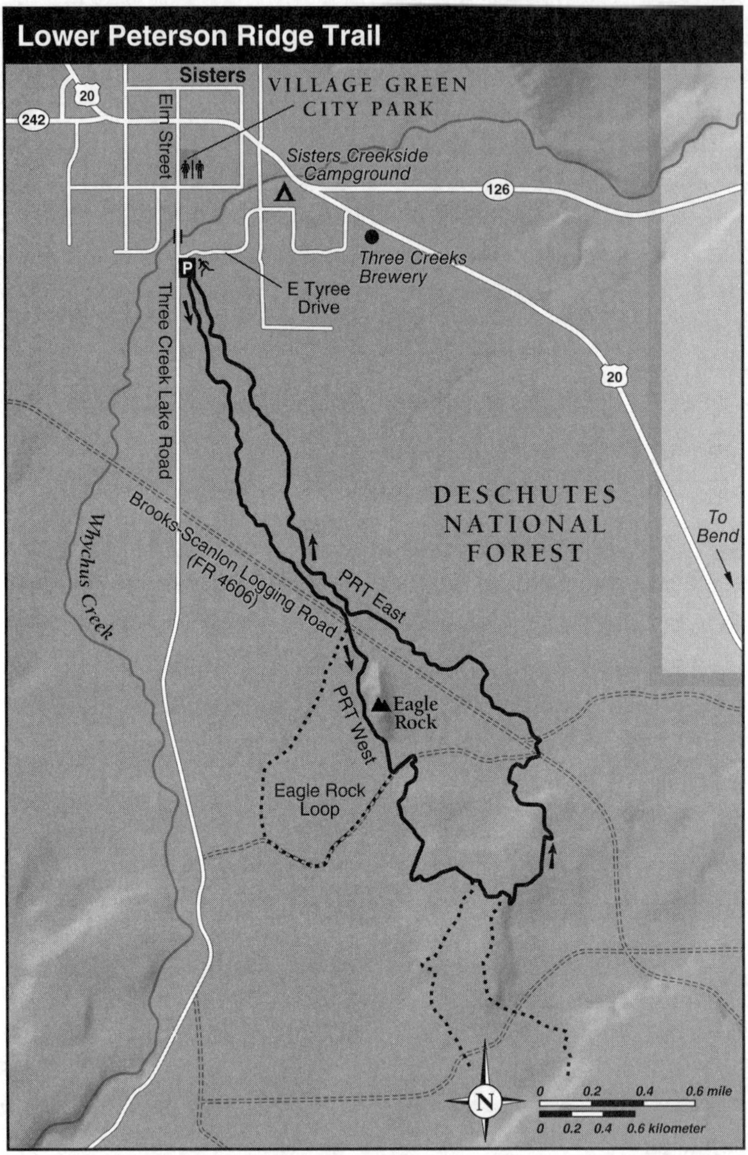

Lower Peterson Ridge Trail

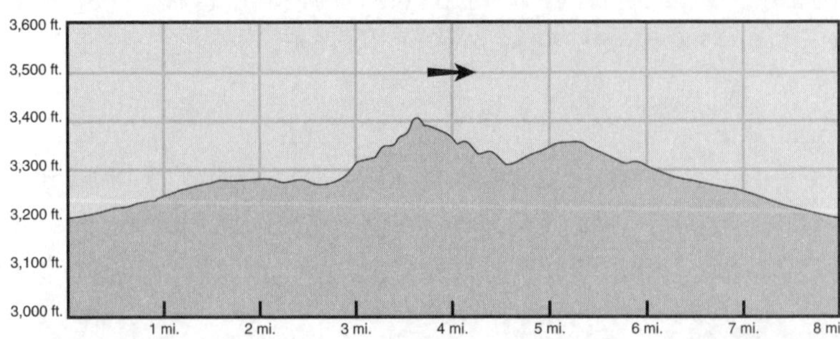

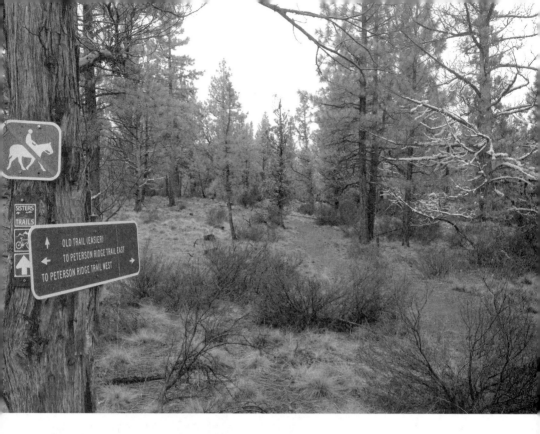

Informative signs are posted near each trail junction.

markers until Signpost 11, which stands just before the Brooks-Scanlon Logging Road (Forest Road 4606). Cross the road and look for the signs pointing toward the continuation of PRT West. Though you may be tempted, ignore the signs for the Eagle Rock Loop, as much of the trail is on old logging roads.

Weave your way through the trees, and soon you'll start to see the rocky outcropping of Eagle Rock ahead in the distance, jutting above the pines. If you're looking to add elevation to your run, this is your opportunity. If not, continue straight on PRT West, passing the Eagle Rock Pass trail at mile 1.8 and continuing along the base of the rocky outcropping. A short half-mile later, keep left at an unmarked intersection and run alongside a large clearing where underground pipe was laid years ago. Soon you'll reach Signpost 13 (appropriately dubbed PIPELINE), where you'll follow the signed pointers to stay on PRT West.

At this point, you'll begin your short and gentle climb—the only one along the route. Quickly pass by Signpost 15 (and the horse trail), and begin running through one of several interesting low-lying volcanic rock formations. As you carefully pick your footing through the rock, enjoy the stark contrast of the bright mosses and lichens clinging to the muted colors of the rock and trees.

Shortly after you pass Signpost 17, look for indicators on the trees pointing toward PRT East. Follow the clues and veer left (away from the "Old Trail") to climb a short distance over rocky terrain until you reach Signpost 18, the high point of the Lower Peterson Ridge Trail loop.

Turn left for your return on PRT East and wind your way down the sweeping curves back to lower ground, passing Signpost 16 and the east side of Eagle Rock. Cross several logging roads, including the Brooks-Scanlon Logging Road once again, and at 5.4 miles, continue straight across a small wooden bridge to Signpost 12. From here, enjoy the flat, fast return back on smooth singletrack to the trailhead and your car.

DIRECTIONS

From Bend, drive 21.8 miles northwest on US 20 toward Sisters. In downtown Sisters, turn left (south) on Elm Street and drive 0.5 mile. Just after the bridge crossing for Whychus Creek, you'll find the trailhead on your left.

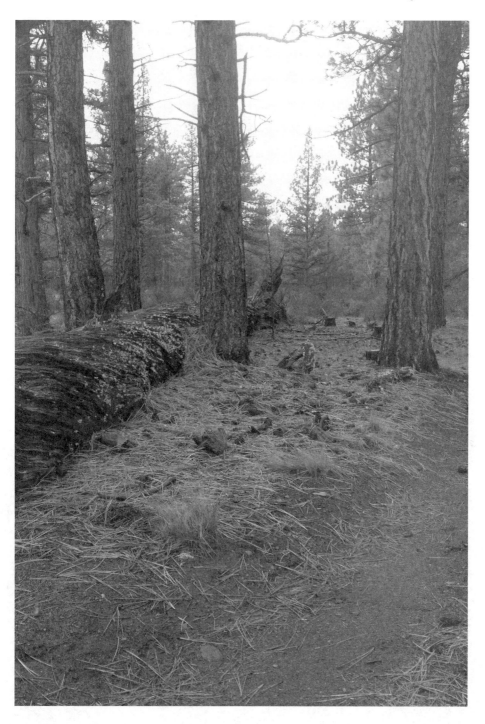

Singletrack runs through mature pine forest.

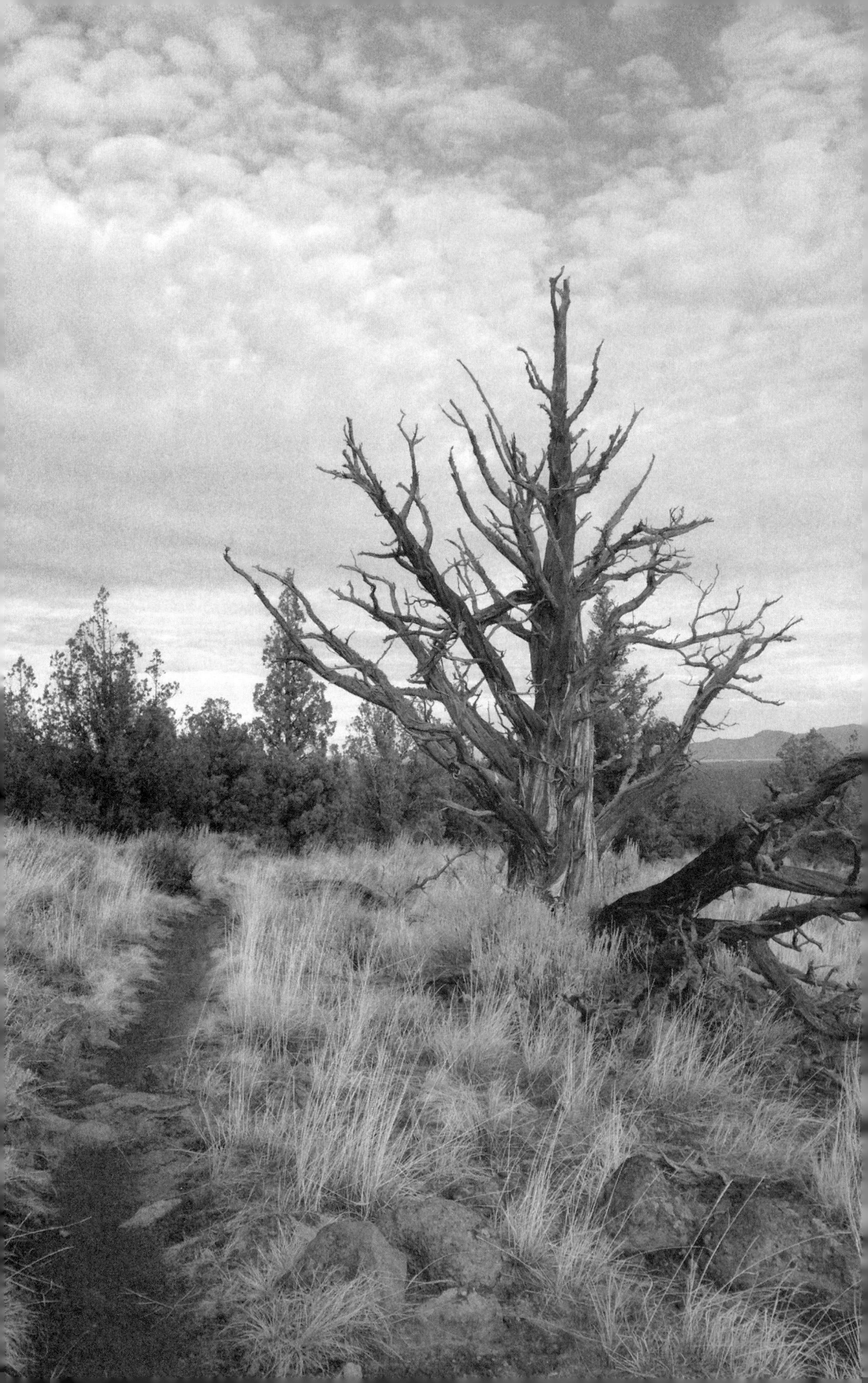

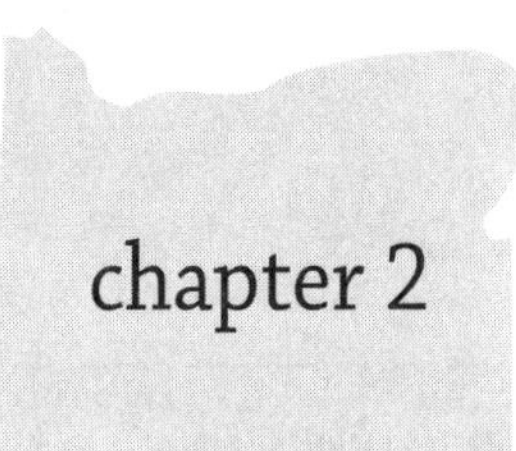

WINTER RUNS

WINTER TRAIL LIST

OPPOSITE: *An old juniper tree stands alongside singletrack near the Horse Ridge Research Natural Area.* (See Horse Ridge, page 54.)

9 Horse Butte

TRAIL DETAILS AT A GLANCE

- **DISTANCE** 10-mile loop
- **GPS TRAILHEAD COORDINATES** N43° 58.641' W121° 14.062'
- **DIFFICULTY** 4
- **SCENERY** 6
- **CROWDS** 5
- **SEASON** Year-round, sunrise–sunset
- **ELEVATION** +/–551'
- **USERS** Hikers, runners, mountain bikers, horses
- **CONTACT** Bend–Fort Rock Ranger District, Deschutes National Forest; 541-383-4000, **www.fs.usda.gov/deschutes**
- **PERMITS/FEES** None
- **RECOMMENDED MAP** *Bend, Oregon, Trail Map* by Adventure Maps, Inc. ($12, **adventuremaps.net**)
- **DOGS** Yes (leashed only)

THE HORSE BUTTE LOOP is known in Central Oregon as a great spot for winter riding, running, and hiking. The attractive loop also makes up the Horse Butte 10-Miler, which has become known to local runners as the unofficial spring kickoff to trail racing. The run is a good one any time of year, though it can get very hot and dusty in the summer. Regardless of the season, however, you'll be guaranteed gorgeous, open views of the Cascade Mountains and closeup views of the area's namesake butte—a reddish-tinted structure that's striking in and of itself. The run can be undertaken clockwise or counterclockwise; I prefer the latter.

From the parking lot, look for the SWAMP WELLS TRAIL 61 sign just to the opposite side of the road. Quickly run up and around a short, rocky section before crossing a jeep road and encountering your first junction 0.5 mile into the run. Turn left, following the signs toward the Boyd Cave Trail, and meander your way through the ponderosa pines. At this point, you'll likely hear gunfire as local gun enthusiasts target-shoot at several nearby buttes. Though this can be unnerving at first, you'll grow accustomed to it and you can rest easier knowing that you're never in the line of fire.

Just beyond 1.25 miles, emerge from the forest and into the High Desert. From this point on, the vast majority of the remaining loop is out of the trees thanks to a past forest fire, providing wonderful views but little shade. Early-morning and late-evening runs are especially rewarding due to the "golden hour" of light on the mountains in the background and the lovely High Desert landscape in the foreground.

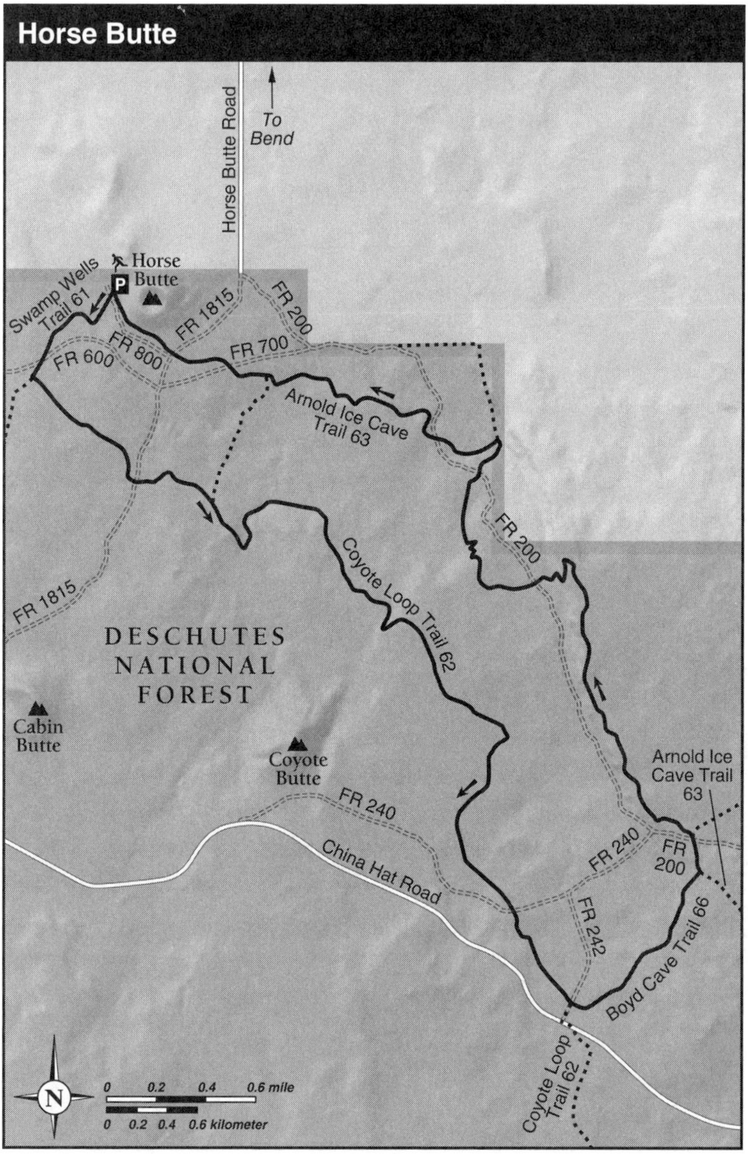

Horse Butte
Horse Butte Road
To Bend
Horse Butte
Swamp Wells Trail 61
FR 1815
FR 200
FR 600
FR 800
FR 700
Arnold Ice Cave Trail 63
FR 200
Coyote Loop Trail 62
FR 1815
DESCHUTES NATIONAL FOREST
Cabin Butte
Coyote Butte
FR 240
Arnold Ice Cave Trail 63
FR 240
FR 200
China Hat Road
FR 242
Boyd Cave Trail 66
Coyote Loop Trail 62
N
0 0.2 0.4 0.6 mile
0 0.2 0.4 0.6 kilometer

4,400 ft.
4,300 ft.
4,200 ft.
4,100 ft.
4,000 ft.
3,900 ft.
3,800 ft.
1 mi.
2 mi.
3 mi.
4 mi.
5 mi.
6 mi.
7 mi.
8 mi.
9 mi.
10 mi.

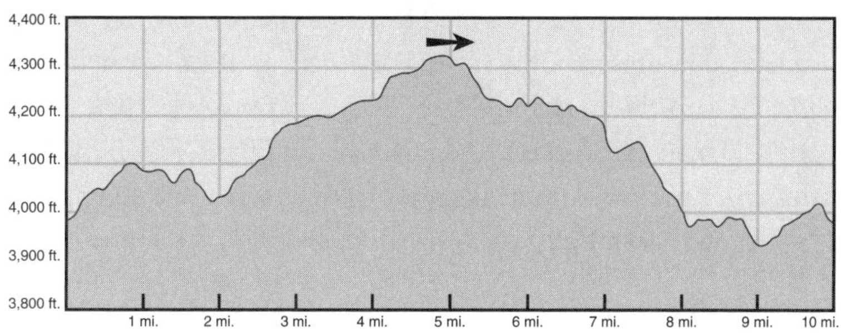

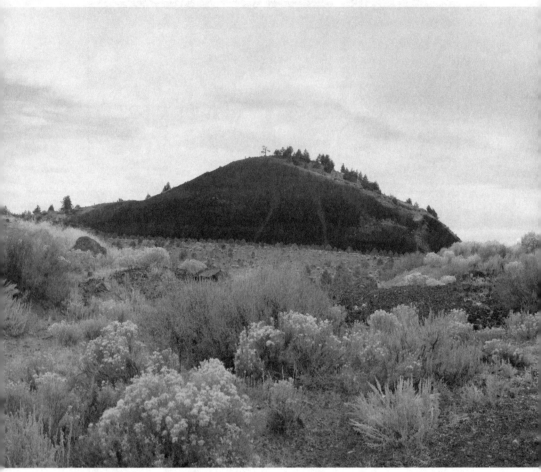

The distinctive reddish-tinted Horse Butte

At 4.6 miles, cross Forest Road 242, the southernmost point on the loop. (You may also use this as a starting point if you wish, as paved China Hat Road/ FR 18 is only a quarter-mile up FR 242). For adventure seekers, this is also a good point to explore a few of the nearby caves. For others, continue straight onto Boyd Cave Trail 66 toward the Arnold Ice Cave Trail junction. Less than a mile later, turn left at the signed junction for Skeleton Cave and the Horse Butte Trailhead. Shortly after this turn, pay careful attention to keep left at an unmarked fork in the trail just beyond a jeep trail.

The next mile provides wonderful views of the cascades as you run along a ridge overlooking the first part of your loop. Horse Butte begins to pop into view in the distance as well, reeling you in with progress. Just under 7 miles, drop from the ridge via a series of short, rocky switchbacks that turn into a gradual descent as you work your way back to your starting point. You may encounter a few unmarked forks over the remaining couple of miles, but keep left at each one and you'll be in good shape.

Before long, you'll reach the gravel road you drove in on. A quick half-mile later brings you back to the base of Horse Butte and your starting point.

DIRECTIONS

From Bend, drive east on Greenwood Avenue (US 20). After about 2 miles, turn right (south) onto 27th Street; then, after about 3 miles, take a left onto Rickard Road, just past Deschutes Recycling. In less than 2 miles, turn right (south) onto Billadeau Road, which turns into Horse Butte Road. Continue straight about 2 miles as the pavement ends, following the signs for the Horse Butte Trailhead. Turn right onto Forest Road 800 and drive to a large parking area near the base of Horse Butte.

A signpost along the Horse Butte loop

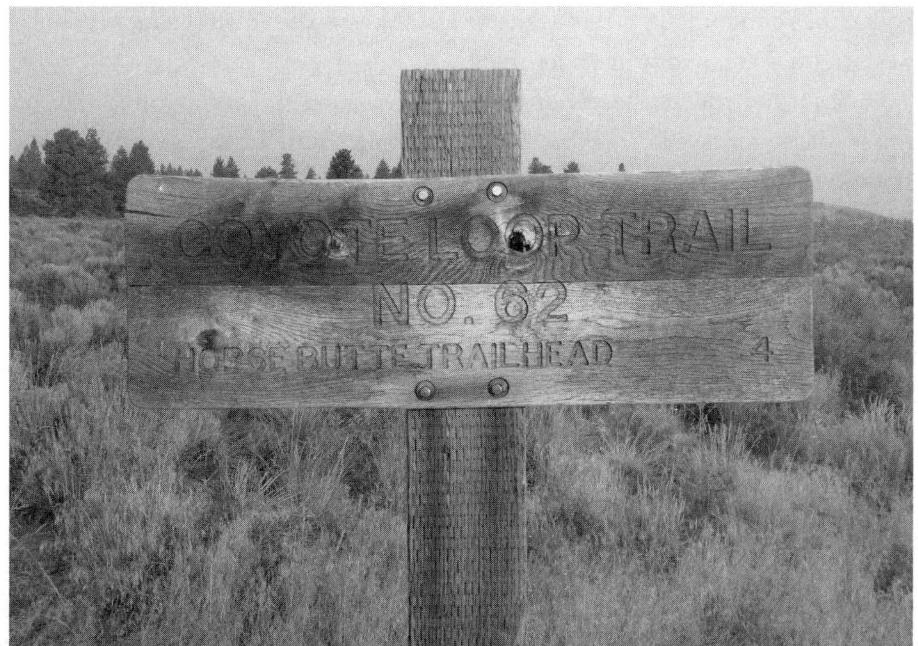

10 Horse Ridge

TRAIL DETAILS AT A GLANCE

- **DISTANCE** 4.6-mile to 7.4-mile loop
- **GPS TRAILHEAD COORDINATES** N43° 56.752' W121° 2.595'
- **DIFFICULTY** 5 • **SCENERY** 6 • **CROWDS** 5 • **SEASON** Year-round, sunrise–sunset
- **ELEVATION** +/–1,084' • **USERS** Hikers, runners, mountain bikers
- **CONTACT** BLM Prineville District, 541-416-6700, **blm.gov/or/districts/prineville**
- **PERMITS/FEES** None • **RECOMMENDED MAP** PDF map at **tinyurl.com/horseridgemap**
- **DOGS** Yes (leashed only)

NOT TO BE CONFUSED WITH HORSE BUTTE (see previous trail), Horse Ridge lies farther out of Bend, approximately 15 miles east of town. A great destination in the winter months, the area rarely sees snow and has wide-open western views of the Cascades. During summer months, sections of the trail network can get very sandy, while spring brings desert wildflowers along the singletrack near the crest of the ridge.

Myriad trails wind through this area run by the Bureau of Land Management (BLM), but a couple of loops are especially tempting for trail runners. As with most BLM land, the trails here are unmarked, though most are easy to follow and distinguish. Be sure to bring a map just in case. During the winter months, be cautious of mountain bikers as the area sees heavy use when the more popular western trails are muddy or under snow.

Begin the run at the parking area located about 0.75 mile off US 20 on Horse Ridge Frontage Road. From the trailhead sign, turn left onto a well-defined, smooth, singletrack path as it weaves its way through mature juniper and sagebrush. The trail parallels the road as you head back east toward the highway. At 0.6 mile, keep straight past an unmarked junction, and soon the trail begins to curve along US 20 and begin its long, gradual climb. As you gain elevation, views of the Oregon Badlands Wilderness to the north open up and are visible for miles.

Turn right at an unmarked junction at 1.8 miles and continue slightly uphill while enjoying sporadic views of the Cascades along the horizon. At 2.5 miles, turn left at an unmarked T-junction to continue on the longer loop. For a shorter run, turn right here and take the fast and rocky downhill back to the junction you

Horse Ridge

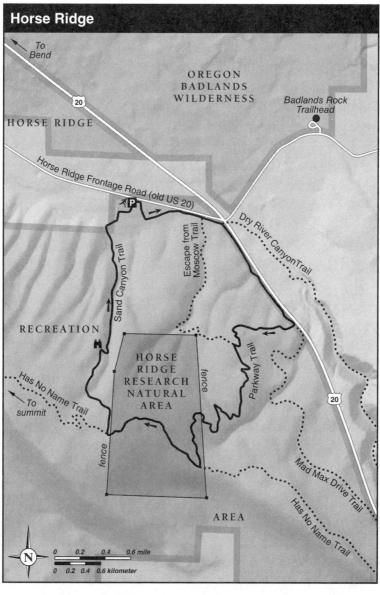

To Bend
OREGON BADLANDS WILDERNESS
Badlands Rock Trailhead
20
HORSE RIDGE
Horse Ridge Frontage Road (old US 20)
P
Dry River Canyon Trail
Escape from Moscow Trail
Sand Canyon Trail
RECREATION
HORSE RIDGE RESEARCH NATURAL AREA
fence
Parkway Trail
20
Has No Name Trail
To summit
fence
Mad Max Drive Trail
Has No Name Trail
AREA
N
0 0.2 0.4 0.6 mile
0 0.2 0.4 0.6 kilometer

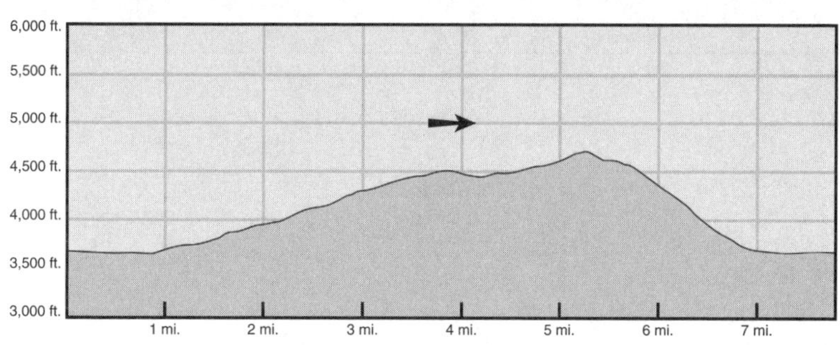

passed at 0.6 mile. From there, simply retrace your steps back to the trailhead for a 4.6-mile loop.

For the longer route, a left-hand turn means more climbing, this time through several stretches of technical lava rock. Choose your steps wisely and remember to pick up your feet as it's likely you'll be tired and out of breath by now from the 3-mile climb.

Just shy of 4 miles, the singletrack leads to a fence crossing, which serves as the border for the BLM's Horse Ridge Research Natural Area (RNA). Established in 1967, the area serves as a research and study plot for Western juniper, big sagebrush, and threadleaf sedge. Recreationalists should always be respectful of work in progress and stay on existing trails. Be sure to leave gates as you found them, whether open or closed.

Now on the other side of the fence, enjoy the relatively flat trail as it winds its way through volcanic rock and classic High Desert scenery. Turn right at another T-intersection at 4.4 miles and, just under a mile later, cross through the fence to leave the Horse Ridge RNA. Immediately after, ignore the trail jutting to the left—a one-way singletrack to the ridge's summit—and instead turn right to complete the loop. Within a quarter-mile, views once again begin to open, and soon you can see the Three Sisters, along with Mount Jefferson, standing proudly on the horizon.

The next 1.5 miles is a fast downhill through Sand Canyon—aptly named, with wide, sandy singletrack. The trail levels out at 7.0 miles and quickly widens into a doubletrack trail. Ignore the singletrack side trail at 7.2 miles and keep straight on the more established doubletrack, which curves around and back toward the trailhead. A short 0.25 mile later, arrive back at the trailhead and your car.

DIRECTIONS

Drive east out of Bend on US 20. About 15 miles from the edge of town, turn right on Horse Ridge Frontage Road (Old US 20). The trailhead is about 0.75 mile from the main highway, on your left.

11 Badlands Rock

TRAIL DETAILS AT A GLANCE

- **DISTANCE** 10.6-mile loop
- **GPS TRAILHEAD COORDINATES** N43° 57.451' W121° 3.073' (Flatiron Rock Trailhead), N43° 57.232' W121° 0.885' (Badlands Rock Trailhead)
- **DIFFICULTY** 5
- **SCENERY** 6
- **CROWDS** 3
- **SEASON** November–April, sunrise–sunset
- **ELEVATION** +/–345'
- **USERS** Hikers, runners, horses
- **CONTACT** BLM Prineville District, 541-416-6700, **blm.gov/or/districts/prineville**
- **PERMITS/FEES** None
- **RECOMMENDED MAP** *Bend, Oregon, Trail Map* by Adventure Maps, Inc. ($12, **adventuremaps.net**)
- **DOGS** Yes (leashed only)

IT TAKES A SPECIAL PERSON TO LOVE THE DESERT. The dry heat, the sand, and the barren landscape tend to shoo away all but the hardy. The Oregon Badlands Wilderness is no exception. A large swath of land southeast of Bend, the Badlands is an inhospitable but beautiful place. Ancient juniper trees dot the landscape among unique outcroppings of volcanic rock and sagebrush. And though the miles of trails can be challenging due to the rough terrain, the solitude and desert beauty you'll find in the Badlands make it well worth exploring.

The Badlands Rock loop is a great run with several distance options and starting points. I like to start at the Flatiron Rock Trailhead, which sees fewer people (but is a bit rougher) than the Badlands Rock Trailhead.

From the parking lot, start out on the Ancient Juniper Trail, a 1.9-mile section highlighting some of the area's oldest and gnarliest juniper trees. Don't be alarmed at the small hills, as this is the only section on the entire run where you'll encounter slight elevation.

At the trail junction with the Flatiron Rock Trail, turn left and continue north on a wide, sandy path. Soon you'll reach Flatiron Rock, a castlelike formation of circular volcanic rock. If you have a few minutes and aren't in a hurry, be sure to run up, into, and around the formation, which resembles a fortress overlooking the desert.

After your exploration is done, exit off of the Flatiron Rock Trail and onto the Castle Trail, whose beginning starts at a junction just on the north side of Flatiron Rock. The Castle Trail winds its way past Castle Rock, another labyrinthine

Badlands Rock

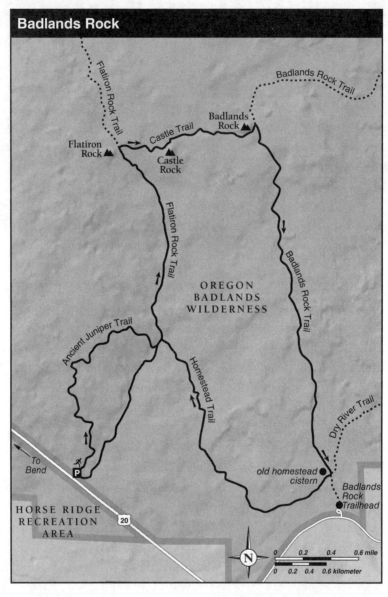

Flatiron Rock Trail
Badlands Rock Trail
Badlands Rock
Castle Trail
Flatiron Rock
Castle Rock
Flatiron Rock Trail
Badlands Rock Trail
OREGON BADLANDS WILDERNESS
Ancient Juniper Trail
Homestead Trail
Dry River Trail
To Bend
old homestead cistern
Badlands Rock Trailhead
HORSE RIDGE RECREATION AREA
20
N
0 0.2 0.4 0.6 mile
0 0.2 0.4 0.6 kilometer

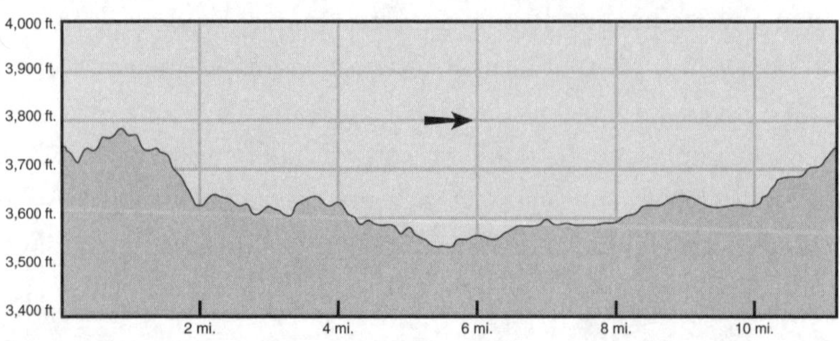

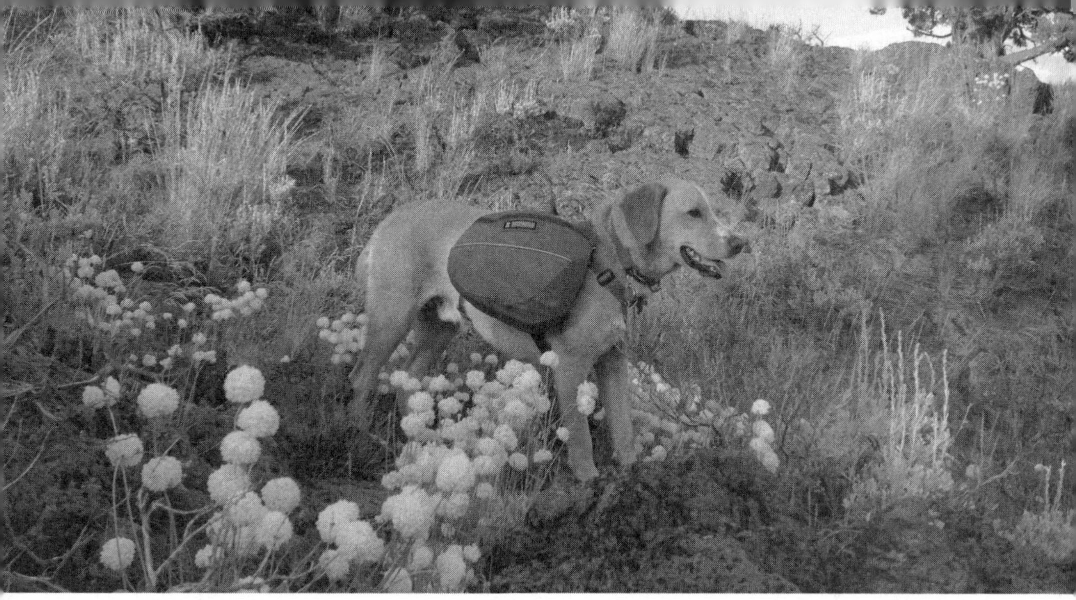

Dogs can make great trail-running partners.

fortress worth checking out, and soon you'll see Badlands Rock itself jutting up out of the desert. From the west, the rock formation resembles an ancient volcano, with steep walls and a jagged crater. The trail continues around the front of Badlands Rock, where it connects with the Badlands Rock Trail.

From here, turn right to begin the journey back on the sandy, winding Badlands Rock Trail. After 2.7 miles, just shy of the Badlands Rock Trailhead (another option for parking), you'll encounter a junction with the Homestead Trail, named for people who settled in the area in the early 1900s. Though there's not much remaining in the way of evidence, you can check out an old cistern just off the trail marked by the wire fencing around it.

At the junction, turn right onto the Homestead Trail for 2.2 miles to return to the initial junction with the Flatiron Rock Trail. At the junction, turn left to complete the loop and run the remaining 1.3 miles to return to the trailhead and your car.

DIRECTIONS

From Bend, take US 20 East toward Burns. About 18 miles from the edge of town, look for the Flatiron Rock Trailhead signs and parking lot, on the north side of the highway around Milepost 16. To reach the Badlands Rock Trailhead, continue east on US 20 another 1.5 miles and, at the bottom of the hill, turn left onto a gravel road. Continue another mile on a paved road to the trailhead parking lot, on the left.

12 Larry Chitwood Trail

TRAIL DETAILS AT A GLANCE

- **DISTANCE** 7.25-mile loop
- **GPS TRAILHEAD COORDINATES** N44° 1.262' W121° 4.647'
- **DIFFICULTY** 4
- **SCENERY** 4
- **CROWDS** 2
- **SEASON** November–April, sunrise–sunset
- **ELEVATION** +/–149'
- **USERS** Hikers, runners, horses
- **CONTACT** BLM Prineville District, 541-416-6700, **blm.gov/or/districts/prineville**
- **PERMITS/FEES** None
- **RECOMMENDED MAP** *Bend, Oregon, Trail Map* by Adventure Maps, Inc. ($12, **adventuremaps.net**)
- **DOGS** Yes (leashed only)

THE BADLANDS WILDERNESS CONSISTS of more than 29,000 acres of land just to the east of Bend on US 20. Known as a shield volcano, the land exemplifies desolate High Desert beauty, filled with sagebrush, lava rock, and—you guessed it—a whole lot of sand. Though the southern trail network (see the previous trail) can get busy on the weekends, the northern trails off of Dodds Road see considerably less traffic. Lacking the impressive rock formations in the southern Badlands, the Larry Chitwood Trail is less scenic but still worth checking out—especially if you're in need of a quick trail run from town but you want to avoid the crowds.

From the trailhead, run a quarter-mile to the intersection of the loop. Follow the signs to the East Loop (left) and begin your clockwise loop. At a half-mile in, take a hard right and begin running south. Carefully make your way through sand and worn lava rock, and over the course of the next 1.5 miles you'll gradually reel in the slight elevation the run has to offer. At just under 3 miles, reach the apex of your loop and a sign indicating your direction on the trail. In another 100 feet, a second sign marks the junction for the Center Trail and the West Loop, to your left.

Keep left for the loop and run on the former jeep road through the sand. At mile 3.75, you'll see BLM boundary markers and a fence marking private property. Here, the trail turns sharply north, where you'll continue along the fence for a while before gradually veering back into the Badlands Wilderness.

After rounding the fourth corner of the run near 5.3 miles, follow the marked trail sign and continue on the doubletrack. The trail begins to get more interesting about a mile later as you hit the home stretch. You'll begin to notice some greener grass alongside the path, and soon enough you're running parallel

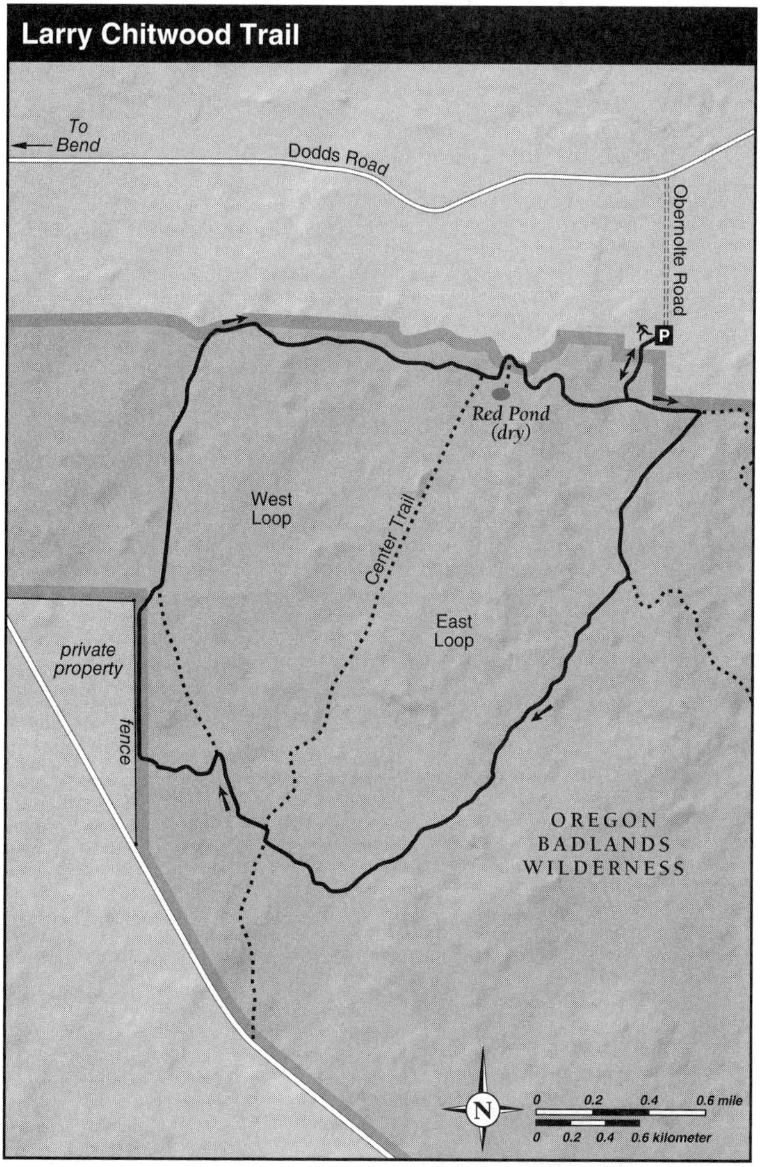

Larry Chitwood Trail
To Bend
Dodds Road
Obernolte Road
P
Red Pond (dry)
West Loop
Center Trail
East Loop
private property
fence
OREGON BADLANDS WILDERNESS
N
0 0.2 0.4 0.6 mile
0 0.2 0.4 0.6 kilometer

3,800 ft.
3,700 ft.
3,600 ft.
3,500 ft.
3,400 ft.
3,300 ft.
3,200 ft.
1 mi.
2 mi.
3 mi.
4 mi.
5 mi.
6 mi.
7 mi.

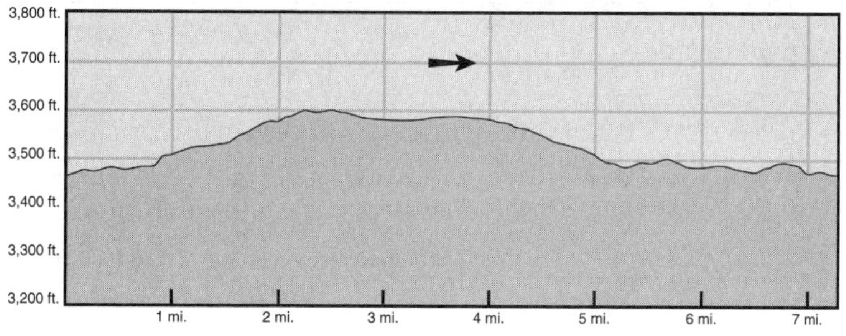

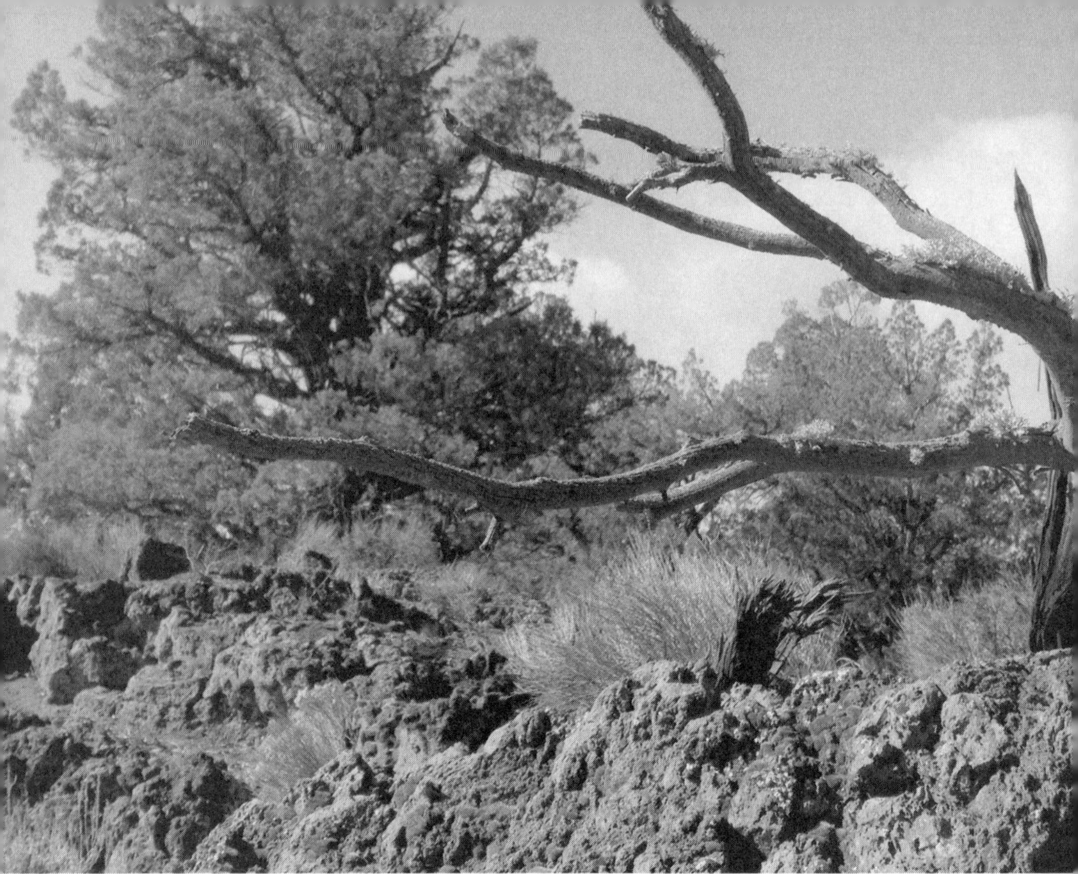

Groupings of tumuli are a prominent feature of the Badlands Wilderness.

to a smoothly flowing irrigation stream, which seems out of place in the desert. A few strides later, you'll encounter a couple of short ups and downs through some jagged, raised rock formations among twisted junipers.

After the much needed scenery, you'll pass the signs pointing to the Center Trail and, shortly after, the initial junction to the trailhead, where you'll take a left and return the 0.25 mile to your car.

DIRECTIONS

From Bend, take US 20 east toward Burns. About 7 miles from the edge of town, around Mile Marker 9, turn left (east) onto Dodds Road. After about 4 miles, turn right (south) on Obernolte Road. Follow this gravel road about a half-mile until you reach the Larry Chitwood Trailhead.

13 Tumulus Trail

TRAIL DETAILS AT A GLANCE

- **DISTANCE** 4.4-mile to 6.75-mile loop
- **GPS TRAILHEAD COORDINATES** N44° 2.751' W121° 2.281'
- **DIFFICULTY** 4 • **SCENERY** 5 • **CROWDS** 2
- **SEASON** November–April, sunrise–sunset • **ELEVATION** +/–119'
- **USERS** Hikers, runners, horses
- **CONTACT** BLM Prineville District, 541-416-6700, **blm.gov/or/districts/prineville**
- **PERMITS/FEES** None • **RECOMMENDED MAP** *Bend, Oregon, Trail Map* by Adventure Maps, Inc. ($12, **adventuremaps.net**) • **DOGS** Yes (leashed only)

THE OREGON BADLANDS WILDERNESS formed in a unique way. The main lava tube that supplied lava flow to the Badlands ruptured, and eventually the errant lava built up the giant shield volcano that today we call the Badlands. The landscape consists of inflated lava, volcanic ash, and pumice, and sagebrush dotted with mature juniper trees. High Desert flora and ancient volcanic geology combine to create an otherworldly feel in a beautiful but desolate area just a quick drive from Bend.

At the very heart of the Badlands is the Tumulus Trail. Named after tumuli—cracked pressure ridges throughout the shield volcano—the Tumulus Trail is probably the most remote of all trails in the Badlands. It's on the northern side of the wilderness area run by the Bureau of Land Management. Those who venture to the area are rewarded with solitude and desert beauty and will likely be alone for their journey.

From the parking area, cross the main canal on a metal footbridge above the canal lock. Once on the other side, keep right of the side canal where the TUMULUS TRAIL sign marks your starting point. There is also a map box here, though I've never actually seen it stocked. Run the first half-mile down the wide, sandy path of light-colored volcanic ash. At 0.5 mile, keep straight at the junction to remain on the Tumulus Trail. The side trail—the Black Lava Trail—will be your return loop.

The trail follows the canal for a brief period before curving to your right. After a short incline and the rounding of a second corner, the trail meets up with the junction for the Basalt Trail at 2.0 miles. Follow this short 0.6-mile connector trail and enjoy the views of the Three Sisters mountains as the skyline begins to open up. During

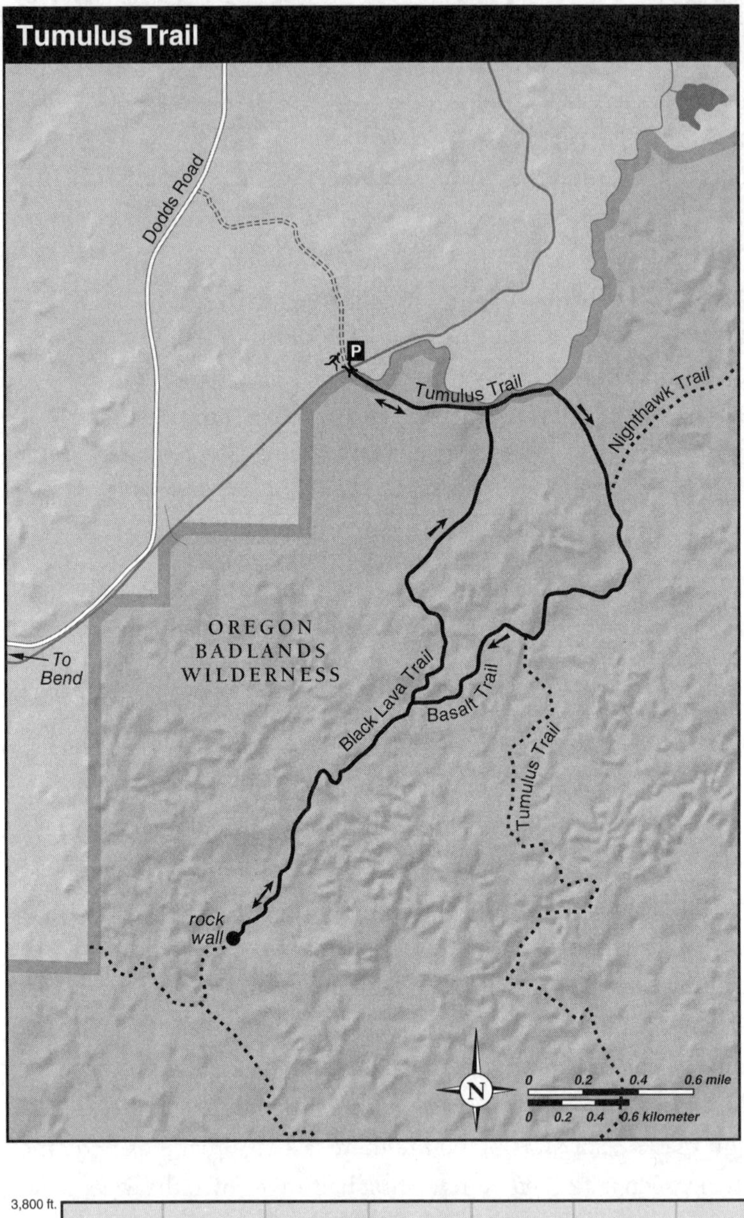

Tumulus Trail
Dodds Road
P
Tumulus Trail
Nighthawk Trail
OREGON
BADLANDS
WILDERNESS
To
Bend
Black Lava Trail
Basalt Trail
Tumulus Trail
rock
wall
N
0 0.2 0.4 0.6 mile
0 0.2 0.4 0.6 kilometer

3,800 ft.
3,700 ft.
3,600 ft.
3,500 ft.
3,400 ft.
3,300 ft.
3,200 ft.
1 mi.
2 mi.
3 mi.
4 mi.
5 mi.
6 mi.

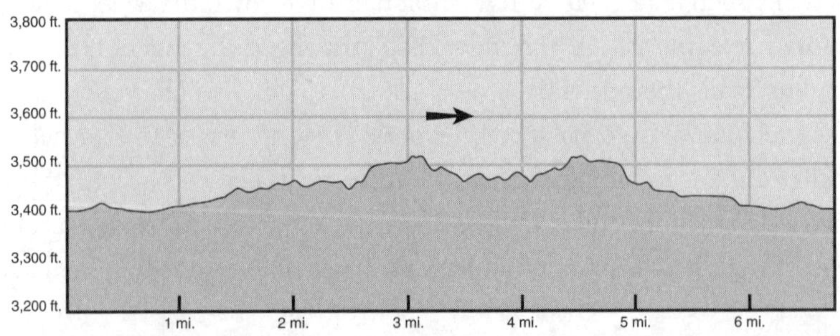

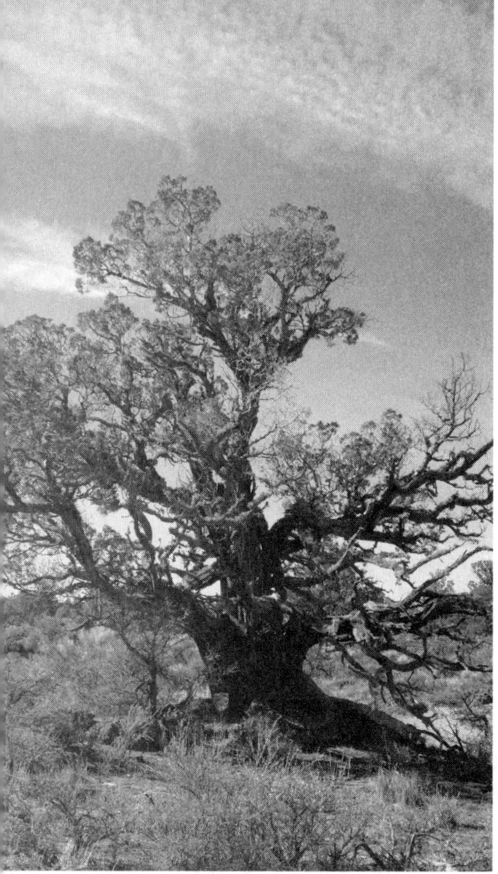

A twisted juniper tree along the trail

spring months, keep your eyes trained on the desert floor for wildflowers, including star-of-Bethlehem, yellow sanddune wallflower, and desert sand lilies.

At 2.6 miles, the Basalt Trail intersects the Black Lava Trail. Here, you have a decision to make: If you'd like to make a shorter 4.4-mile loop, turn right to make the return, but if you'd like to extend the loop a bit, keep straight.

Those who push on will soon be rewarded with some interesting scenery. At 3.3 miles, you'll encounter the remnants of a fenced-in corral built into a natural enclosure within the volcanic rock, along with unique rock formations along the way. The grand views of the western horizon are the biggest draw, with views of nearly all of the Oregon Cascades from Mount Jefferson, Mount Hood, the Three Sisters, and more. A natural turnaround spot for the extension comes at 3.8 miles, where a small rock wall blocks the path.

After returning to the junction, continue along the Black Lava Trail by veering left at the trail sign. From there, the trail winds its way among scenic junipers and in and out of gullies in the landscape. Once you're back at the junction with the Tumulus Trail and the canal, turn left to retrace your steps the 0.5 mile back to your car.

DIRECTIONS

Take US 20 East from Bend toward Burns. About 7 miles from the edge of town, around Mile Marker 9, turn left (east) onto Dodds Road. At Mile Marker 6 on Dodds Road, turn right onto a dirt road, keeping right at any intersections until you reach the trailhead after 1 mile. The trail begins on the opposite side of the canal and can be accessed via a catwalk.

14 Maston

TRAIL DETAILS AT A GLANCE

- **DISTANCE** 12-mile loop
- **GPS TRAILHEAD COORDINATES** N44° 12.710› W121° 18.181'
- **DIFFICULTY** 6
- **SCENERY** 6
- **CROWDS** 5
- **SEASON** October–June, sunrise–sunset
- **ELEVATION** +/–416'
- **USERS** Hikers, runners, mountain bikers, horses
- **CONTACT** BLM Prineville District, 541-416-6700, **blm.gov/or/districts/prineville**
- **PERMITS/FEES** None
- **RECOMMENDED MAP** *Sisters & Redmond High Desert Trail Map* by Adventure Maps, Inc. ($12, **adventuremaps.net**)
- **DOGS** Yes (leashed only)

THE MASTON AREA IS A PRIME EXAMPLE of how thought and planning can churn out an outstanding trail system. During 2012–13, the Prineville Bureau of Land Management built out the network to allow a variety of recreation users to peacefully coexist in one area. Primarily known as a hot spot for winter mountain biking, Maston also contains hiker-only trails, in addition to a great network of horse trails interspersed throughout its many acres.

Maybe what Maston is most well known for, however, is the distinction of being the lowest in elevation of Central Oregon's High Desert trails. This means you can expect the trails to be (a) very dusty and very hot in the summertime and (b) open and snow-free nearly all year long. Though not the most scenic of all routes, this network offers some variety to keep things interesting and, at less than 15 minutes from downtown Bend, is a quick getaway to some great trails.

To begin the perimeter loop, start at the main Maston Trailhead on Newcomb Road. This trailhead, finished in 2013, has ample parking, picnic areas, and nice restroom facilities for changing. A few trails lead to picnic tables—take the first dirt path to your right off the paved path from the restrooms. Within 20 yards, you'll pass through a gated fence and into the trail system proper.

At a half-mile, cross through an old rock wall and shortly after encounter your first marker on the trail. *Note:* It's important to point out here that all Maston junctions are marked by numbered signs. Running the perimeter in the recommended counterclockwise direction will have you passing the markers in ascending order.

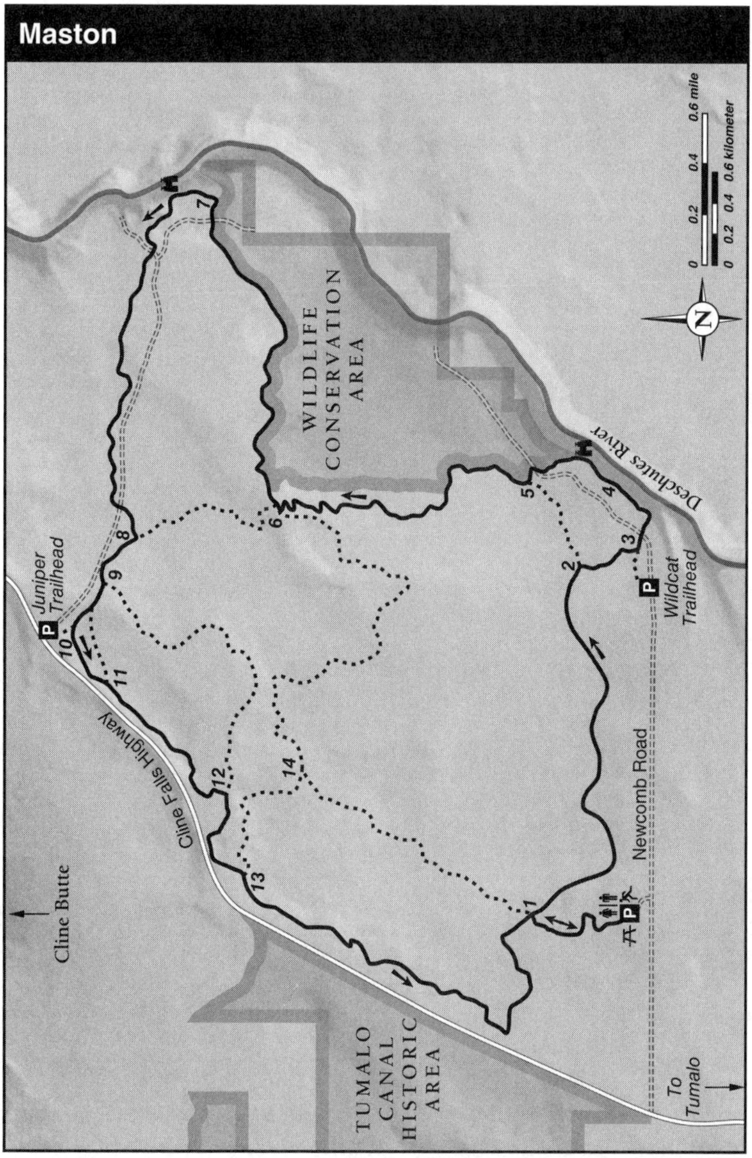

Maston
Juniper Trailhead
Cline Butte
Cline Falls Highway
TUMALO CANAL HISTORIC AREA
WILDLIFE CONSERVATION AREA
Deschutes River
Wildcat Trailhead
Newcomb Road
To Tumalo
0 0.2 0.4 0.6 mile
0 0.2 0.4 0.6 kilometer
N
1
2
3
4
5
6
7
8
9
10
11
12
13
14

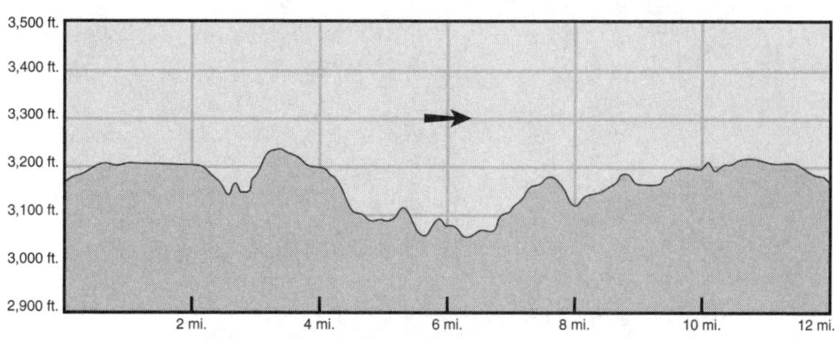

3,500 ft.
3,400 ft.
3,300 ft.
3,200 ft.
3,100 ft.
3,000 ft.
2,900 ft.
2 mi.
4 mi.
6 mi.
8 mi.
10 mi.
12 mi.

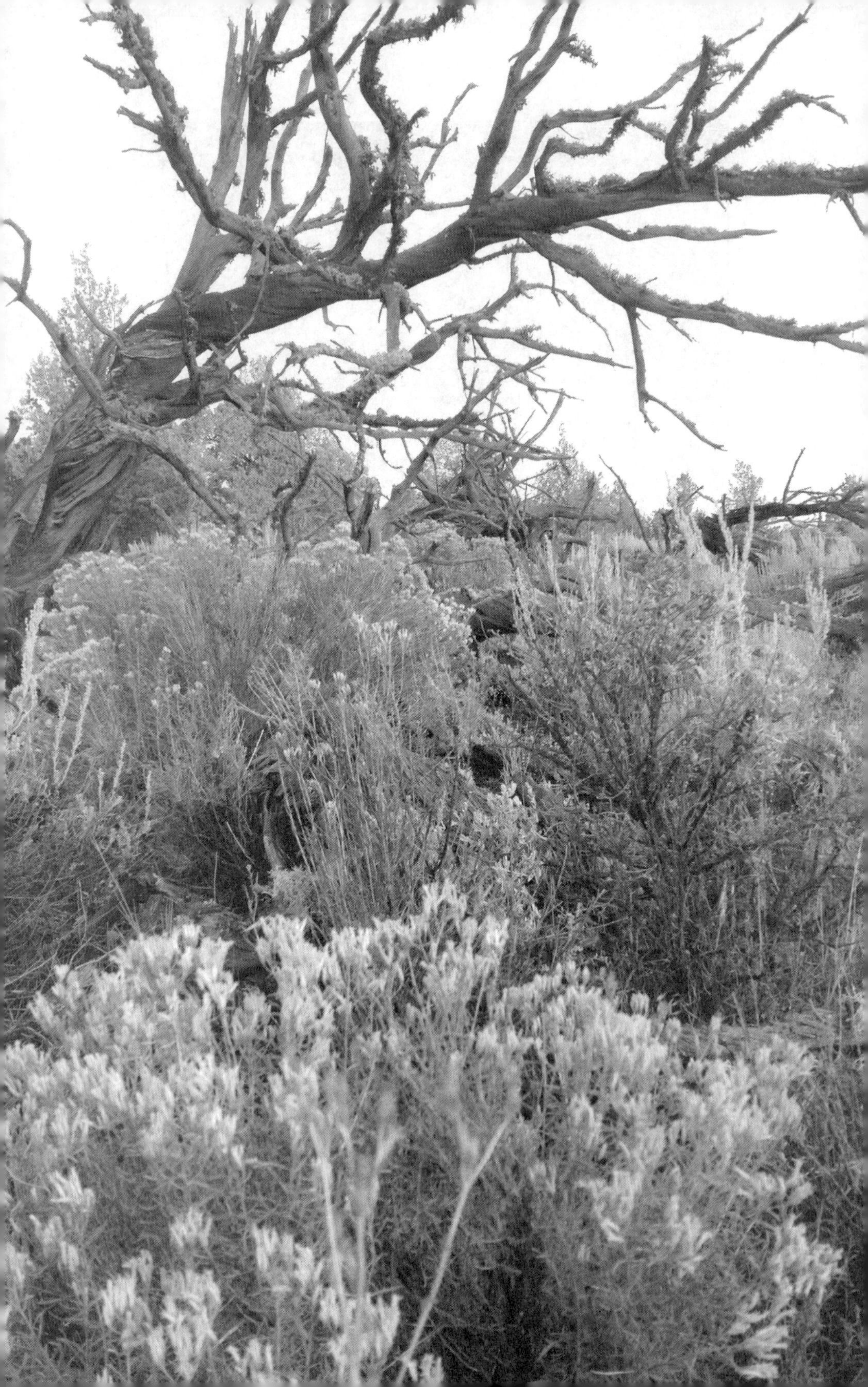

Keep straight at Signpost 1, and soon the trail begins to curve to the right through slightly bermed sides—a reminder of the old irrigation canals that once gave life to long-forgotten farms. At 2.2 miles, turn right at the signed Marker 2 for the full perimeter loop. Shortly after, ignore the side trail for Wildcat Trailhead at 2.3 miles and continue straight, crossing a dirt road and running up to the canyon's rim, overlooking the Deschutes River far below. Here, the trail gets a little technical and rocky, which adds a bit of variety to the terrain. Be sure to look up every now and then—the scenery here is spectacular.

Just beyond 3 miles, cross the same dirt road and reconnect with the thinner, firmer singletrack to the right (not to be confused with the wider horse trail straight across). Within a quarter-mile, hit Signpost 5 and turn right to keep on the loop. Over the next several miles, the trail meanders over a fairly even terrain of juniper and sagebrush, with the occasional peek of Cline Butte off to the west. Keep right at all junctions and ignore any jeep roads.

After mile 6, the trail again abuts the canyon rim and provides great views of the river below and, this time around, the snowcapped cascades along the horizon. Several houses sit on the opposite side of the canyon and one can't help but be a bit envious of their views every evening. From here, the trail turns a corner and begins to head back inland away from the river. Ignore several old roads and continue straight at each interruption.

At 7.7 miles (Signpost 8), take a right toward Juniper Trailhead. A quarter-mile later, repeat this action at Signpost 9. At 8.1 miles, look for Signpost 10 just to the right of the trail and veer left at the jutting singletrack away from the sign—you'll know you've missed this junction if you hit Juniper Trailhead. The trail here is the newest in the network and slightly rougher than the previous trails, incorporating more curves.

About a mile from the previous junction, veer right at Signpost 12. Ignore any side trails over the next 0.5 mile; those cross the nearby highway and connect to Cline Butte. At 9.6 miles you'll encounter Signpost 13 and—you guessed it—you'll turn right at the T-intersection. A half-mile later, the trail splits but quickly rejoins on the other side of the hill. To stay on the loop, continue straight here or right if you took the right fork before the hill.

OPPOSITE: *Sagebrush blooms at the foot of a gnarled juniper tree.*

Over the next mile, several unmarked intersections present themselves as options. Though all choices will lead you to your final destination, the preferred direction is straight, which will keep you on the true perimeter loop. Finally, at mile 11 (just beyond the last unmarked intersection), you'll follow the former rock-lined canal back to Signpost 1, where you'll take a hard right to complete your loop and return to the trailhead.

DIRECTIONS

Take US 20 northwest toward Sisters; after about 10 miles, turn right (north) on Cook Avenue in the small town of Tumalo. Stay on the road, which becomes Cline Falls Highway, for about 5 miles and look for the MASTON TRAILHEAD sign at the intersection of Newcomb Road. Make a right on Newcomb here—the main trailhead will be on your left, less than a mile down the dirt road.

15 Tumalo Canal Historic Area

TRAIL DETAILS AT A GLANCE

- **DISTANCE** 6.4- to 10-mile loop
- **GPS TRAILHEAD COORDINATES** N44° 13.087' W121° 20.218'
- **DIFFICULTY** 4 • **SCENERY** 6 • **CROWDS** 3
- **SEASON** November–May, sunrise–sunset • **ELEVATION** +/–97'
- **USERS** Hikers, runners • **CONTACT** BLM Prineville District, 541-416-6700, **blm.gov/or/districts/prineville**
- **RECOMMENDED MAP** PDF map at **tinyurl.com/tchamap** • **DOGS** Yes (leashed only)

THE TUMALO CANAL HISTORIC AREA (TCHA) is a recently built trail network developed adjacent to the Maston area, which has quickly become a popular winter mountain biking destination. Whereas Maston welcomes bikers and runners alike, the TCHA is pedestrian-only to help preserve the historic remains of the canals for which it's named.

First developed in the early 1900s for irrigation, these canal remains make up the majority of the TCHA trail system, which lends itself to smooth meandering pathways that are wide enough for two-abreast running. Though it's easy to envision the pathways as canals, sadly the only real remnants of the actual canals are confined to the uppermost northeast portion of the trail system, dubbed the Canal Raceway Structure by the BLM. Don't let that dissuade you, however, as the entire trail system is well worth exploring—especially because it's still fairly new and not yet as well known.

The trail system is well marked by 12 numbered posts throughout the area, and many loop options are possible. Be forewarned, however, that although the canal trails and main outer loop are wide and flowy, the connector trails (specifically 4–5, 6–7, and 11–12) can have many quick and jagged turns, making for an interesting (and possibly slightly disruptive) leg of the run. These trails are best during the winter months as well, as the sandy bottoms of the former canals soften up and make for difficult, sandy runs in the warmer months.

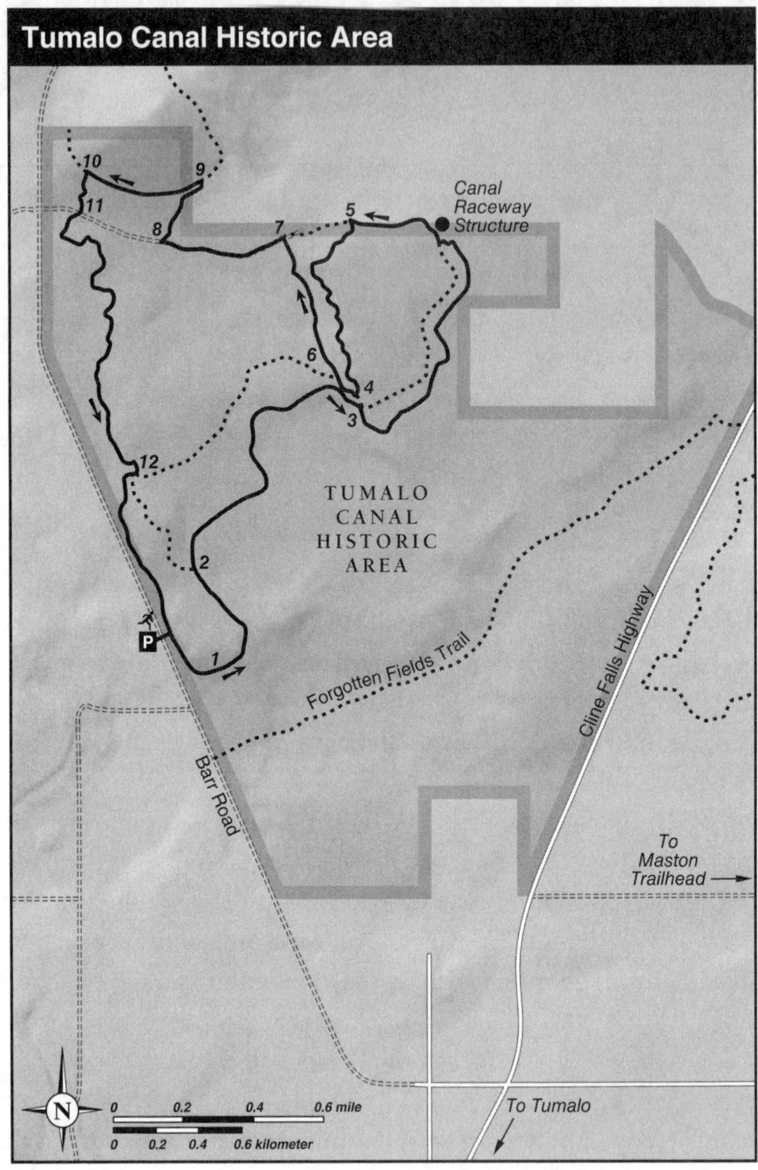

To start the run, follow the signs from the main trailhead parking area through the gate just across Barr Road, then use the short connector trail to join the Lower Laidlaw Loop and turn right once you're on the trail. Follow the numbers up the chain and keep straight at Signposts 1 and 2. When you encounter Signpost 3, keep right to meander your way through the canal depression to the Canal Raceway

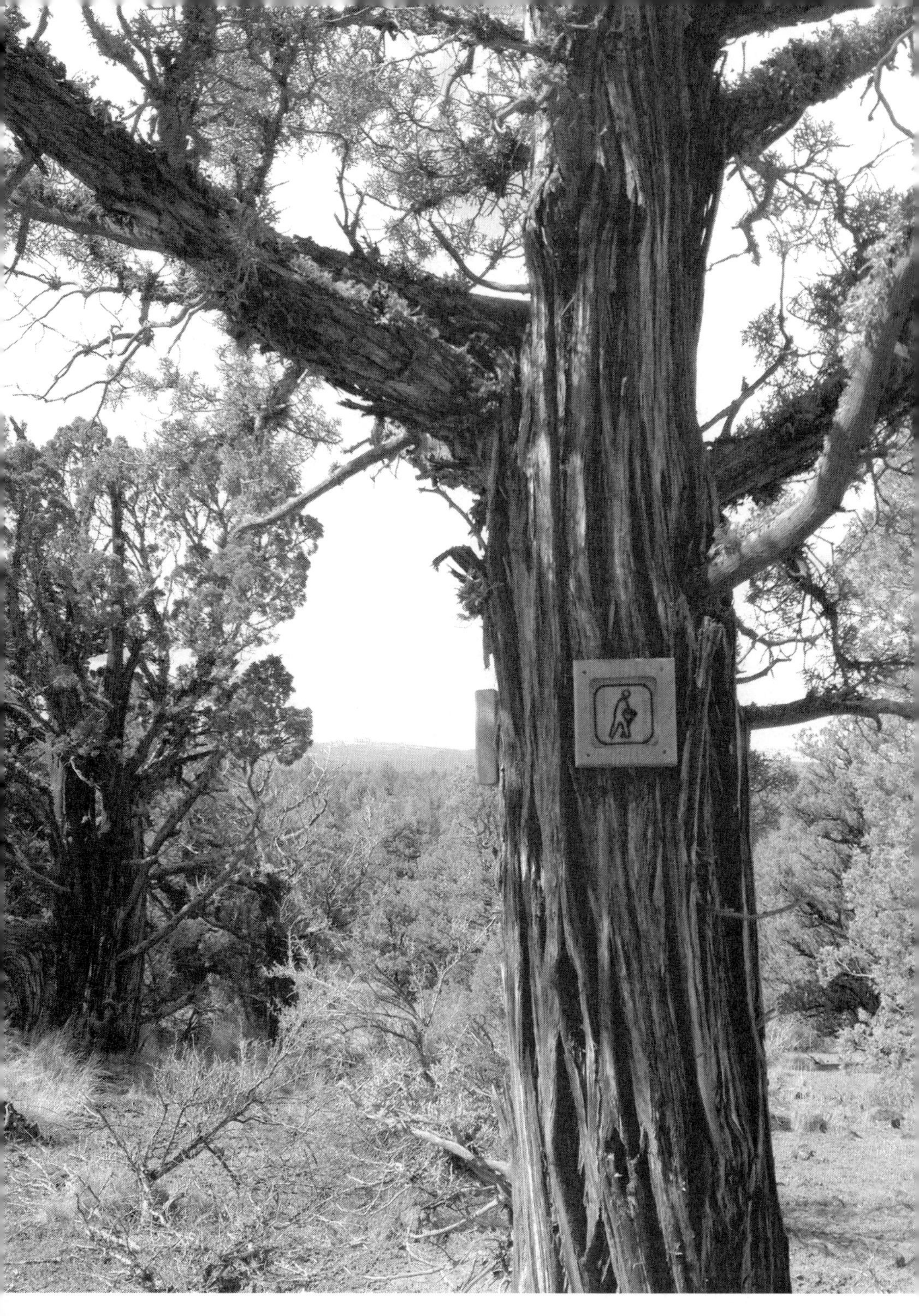

Wooden hiking markers help identify the trail.

Structure for a glimpse of the best-preserved portion of the canals. Though there's no marker at this point, the fence boundary will keep you going left (west) along the TCHA toward Signpost 5. At this point, turn left (south) toward Signpost 4, where you'll run along a ridge with stellar views of the Cascades.

At Signpost 6, take a sharp right (north) toward Signpost 7, where you'll continue along the outer edge of the TCHA past 8 and 9. At Signpost 10, turn left off the wide, sandy path to Signpost 11, where you'll see another parking option a hundred yards off to your right. Continue through Signpost 11 and wind your way uphill through the tight corners to Signpost 12. At this point, a right turn will take you toward Barr Road and back to Signpost 1 and the trailhead for a run of 6.4 miles. If you'd like to extend the run and cover the entire TCHA, you can add the interior loop (12, 6, 4, 3, 2, 12) to push the total closer to 10 miles.

DIRECTIONS

Take US 20 northwest toward Sisters; after about 10 miles, turn right (north) on Cook Avenue in the small town of Tumalo. Stay on the road, which becomes Cline Falls Highway, for about 4.2 miles and turn left on Barr Road—if you see the sign for the Maston Trailhead on your right, you've gone too far. The road shortly turns to dirt and in another mile takes you to the large, spacious TCHA Trailhead parking lot on your left. Follow the signs and start your run on the opposite (east) side of the road to gain entry to the TCHA. *Note:* New trails are being developed west of the main trailhead parking lot.

16 Radlands

TRAIL DETAILS AT A GLANCE

- **DISTANCE** 3.3-mile loop
- **GPS TRAILHEAD COORDINATES** N44° 17.517' W121° 8.771'
- **DIFFICULTY** 2
- **SCENERY** 5
- **CROWDS** 4
- **SEASON** Year-round, sunrise–sunset
- **ELEVATION** +/–61'
- **USERS** Hikers, runners, mountain bikers
- **CONTACT** Redmond Area Park and Recreation District, 541-548-7275, **raprd.org**
- **PERMITS/FEES** None
- **RECOMMENDED MAP** *Sisters & Redmond High Desert Trail Map* by Adventure Maps, Inc. ($12, **adventuremaps.net**)
- **DOGS** Yes (leashed only)

THE RADLANDS IS A BURGEONING NETWORK of trails in northeast Redmond on Deschutes County land. A joint project of the Redmond Area Park and Recreation District and the Central Oregon Trail Alliance, the network comprises more than a dozen miles of twisty singletrack through barren high desert landscape. Plans call for over 30 miles of trail to eventually be built, and hopes are that the Radlands will someday be on par with trail systems such as the Peterson Ridge Trail network near Sisters and the Phil's Trail network in Bend.

Though still in its infancy, the Radlands has much to offer trail enthusiasts. Its close proximity to Redmond and Bend, along with the year-round availability, make it an ideal spot for a quick weekday run before or after work or on a busy weekend day in between activities.

Views of the Cascade Mountains on the western horizon are prevalent throughout the Radlands, and northern glimpses offer runners a chance to see Smith Rock State Park from a distance. Up close, the area's gnarled and ancient junipers dot the landscape off the trails while the countless lava rocks deftly incorporated into the singletrack make for some challenging footwork for trail runners with tired feet.

Start the run at the far end of the parking lot, just beyond the sports complex and opposite the BMX track. From the trailhead sign, run north on singletrack as it skirts a baseball field and winds through sagebrush and over porous lava rock away from the complex. Soon the views of the Cascades open up in earnest, and on clear days you're reminded of the majestic beauty of the area's snowcapped volcanoes.

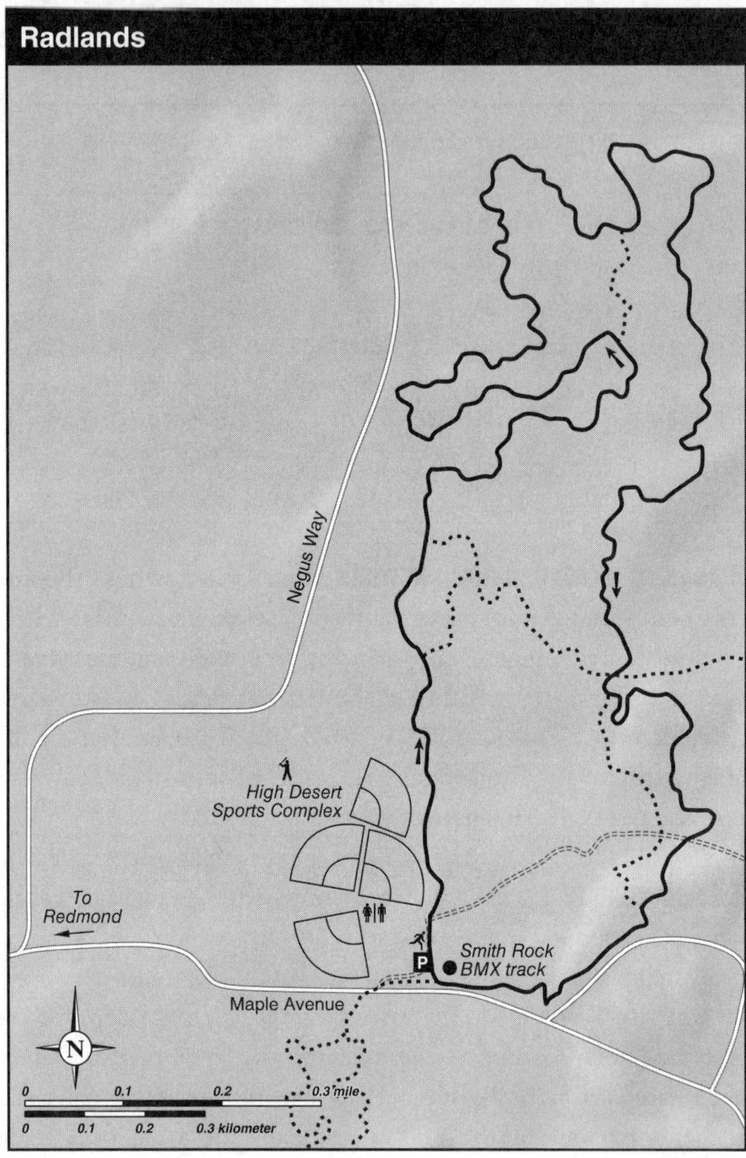

At 0.26 mile, keep straight at the first intersection as views of Smith Rock open up in front of you. Repeat this a short time later, and soon you're up and over your first of several lava rock outcroppings. As a general rule of thumb, or if you're running the Radlands for the first time, keep left at all junctions to circle the perimeter of the northwest section of the network. Most junctions are marked with signs for easy, more difficult, or most difficult trails; unfortunately, the signs don't provide names or distances.

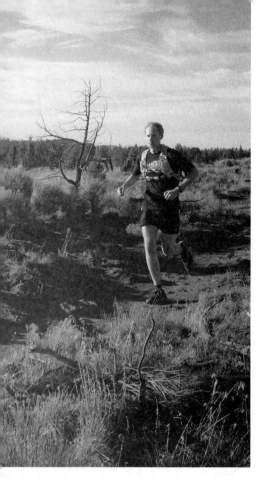

The author runs the Radlands.

Continue zigzagging your way through the singletrack, passing a collection of tires before you start to make the turn back south toward the sports complex. Keep straight at 1.5 miles, ignoring the unmarked and faint side trail veering north. A mile later, run up a short hill to come upon a large hub and multitrail junction. Ignore the first (unmarked) trail on your left—instead, choose the second trail, this one marked with an arrow pointing left.

As you run up the rocky path, pick your way carefully through the lava rock, watching your footing. Cross a faint jeep road; as you emerge onto the rocky shelf, you once again start to see the complex and your starting point. Keep left at the junction at 2.9 miles for the full loop around the perimeter. The trail then begins to parallel a road and shortly after loops around the outer edge of the BMX track before spitting you out at the opposite end of the parking lot from the trailhead. A quick jaunt across the gravel parking lot puts you back at the trailhead for 3.3 miles in total.

DIRECTIONS

Take US 97 north from Bend toward Redmond. About 13 miles from the edge of town, turn right on OR 126/SE Evergreen Avenue toward Prineville. Drive about 0.5 mile, keeping left at the intersection, then turn left on SE Ninth Street. After 1.26 miles, turn right on NE Negus Way. Drive about 0.6 mile, keeping straight on NE Maple Avenue as Negus Way turns north, and turn left into the trailhead parking area, between the High Desert Sports Complex and the Smith Rock BMX track.

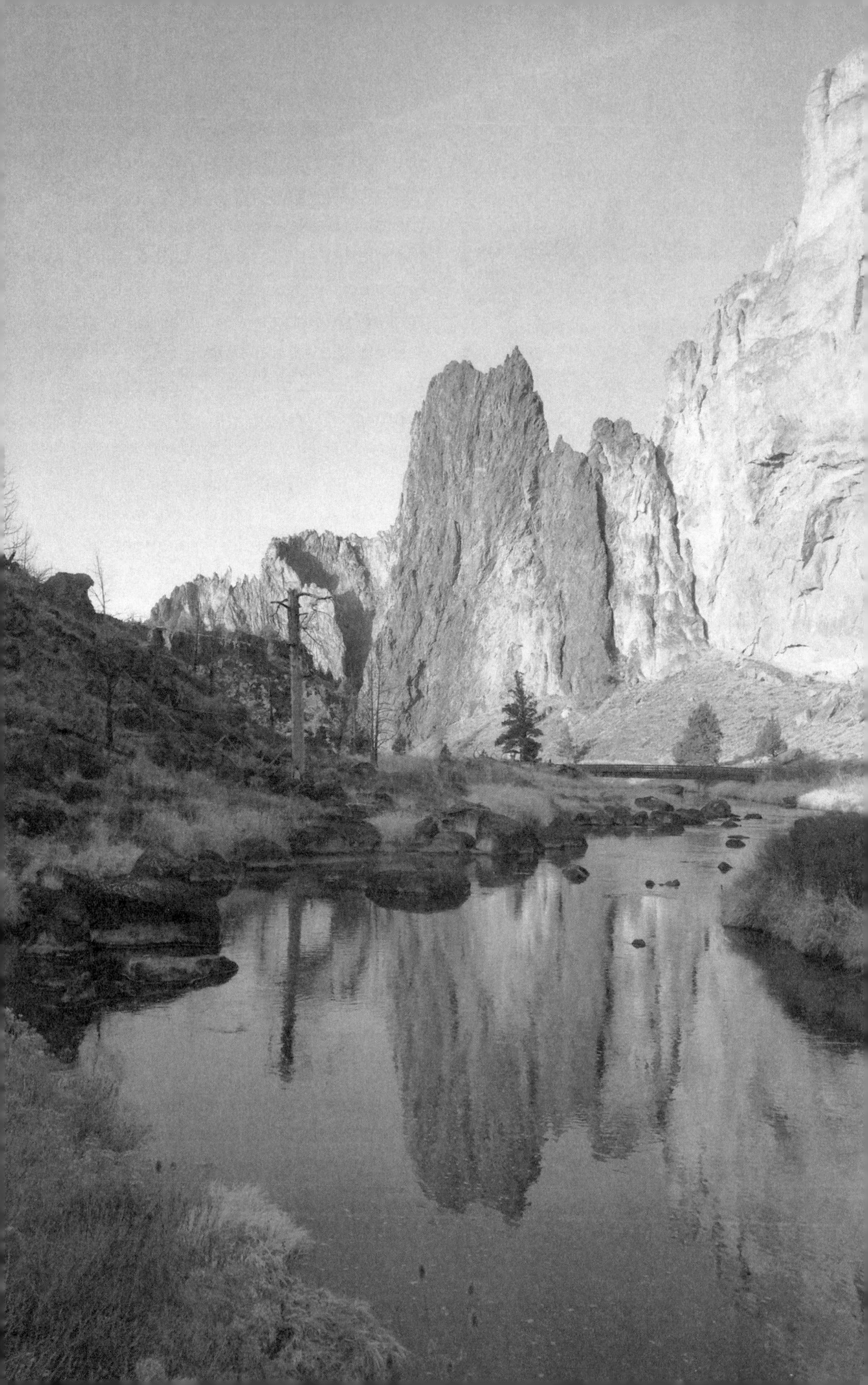

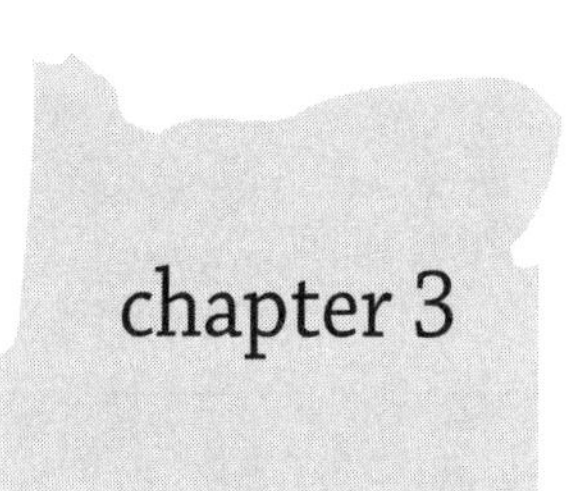

SPRING RUNS

SPRING TRAIL LIST

OPPOSITE: *The vast red expanse of Smith Rock is reflected in a calm stretch of the Crooked River.* (See Smith Rock State Park, page 96.)

17 Suttle Lake

TRAIL DETAILS AT A GLANCE

- **DISTANCE** 3.5-mile loop
- **GPS TRAILHEAD COORDINATES** N44° 25.664' W121° 43.861'
- **DIFFICULTY** 2 • **SCENERY** 4 • **CROWDS** 8 • **SEASON** Year-round, sunrise–sunset
- **ELEVATION** +/–82' • **USERS** Hikers, runners, mountain bikers
- **CONTACT** Sisters Ranger District, Deschutes National Forest; 541-549-7700, **www.fs.usda.gov/deschutes**
- **PERMITS/FEES** None
- **RECOMMENDED MAP** *Sisters & Redmond High Desert Trail Map* by Adventure Maps, Inc. ($12, **adventuremaps.net**)
- **DOGS** Yes (leashed only)

SUTTLE LAKE IS AN IDEAL STOPOVER for a quick run on your way into or out of Central Oregon. Surrounded by mixed conifers, the lake is a deep blue and is well loved by fishermen for its native kokanee and brown trout. During the summer, families flock to the shores for lakeside campsites and great swimming. A resort formerly known as Suttle Lake Lodge offered accommodations and cabin rentals at the east end of the lake until late 2015, when the property changed hands. (At press time, an extensive renovation was being planned, but no reopening date had been announced.)

The Suttle Lake Loop, which circles the lake itself on a gentle grade over the course of 3.5 miles, is suitable for all ages. The ease of access to the trail, however, also means that you won't be finding solitude anywhere on this run. In fact, at times you may feel like a part of the family as you're literally running through the edge of someone's campsite. Expect to encounter many others, and be watchful of children, dogs, and fishing poles. If possible, try to visit Suttle Lake on a weekday or during the shoulder seasons, when camping is not as prevalent.

To start the run, follow the signs for Suttle Lake Lodge and the Suttle Lake Day-Use Area. Here you'll find a nice long beach where you can relax afterward or, on those hot days, take a swim. For now, begin your run in a clockwise direction at the far end of the day-use area. The trail takes you back the way you came and parallels the road for a short while before crossing back on the bridge over Lake Creek, the outlet of Suttle Lake.

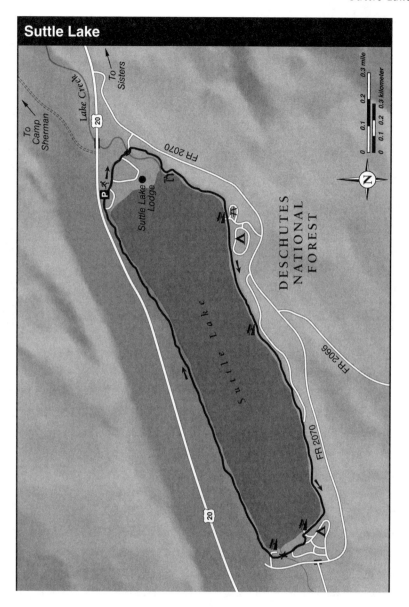

Enjoy a nice, smooth trail under a shaded canopy of green for the first half-mile before the trees open up to a nice view of the lake by a private dock. A short quarter-mile up the trail, you'll encounter your first taste of camp life as the trail edges the lake and numerous campsites.

Shortly after knocking out the first mile, cross a boat ramp and proceed back into the trees along the shore, getting a nice respite from the campgrounds. Take in the lake and scenery here, as you'll soon pop back out into civilization.

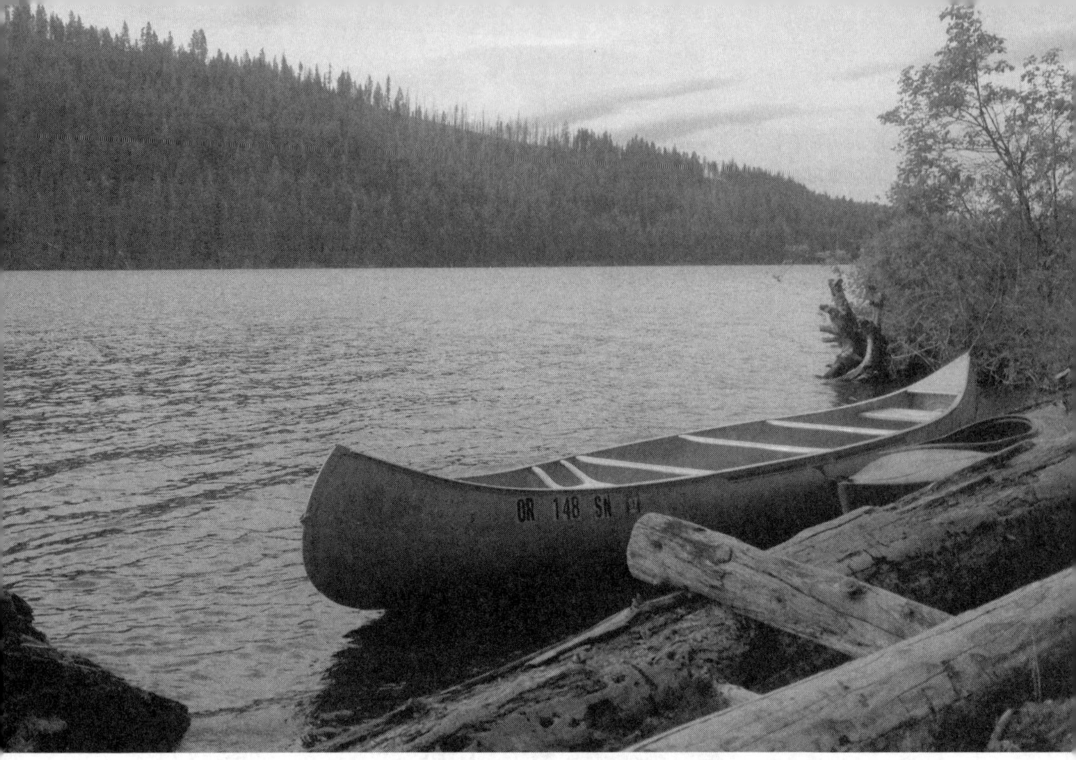

A canoe sits moored along the banks of Suttle Lake.

Around mile 2, cross another boat ramp and follow the pavement up and to the right, looking for a blue diamond marking the trail path. A shortcut through the grass and in between campsites takes you to a road, where you'll turn right for 0.1 mile until a trail marker and footbridge put you back on the path. While on the footbridge, look out across the lake for great views of Black Butte in the distance.

Once across the bridge, stay right and look for the trail pickup on the other side of yet another boat ramp. At this point, you can wipe your brow knowing that your dodging and weaving through the campgrounds is done. For the remainder of the run, the well-maintained trail hugs the shores as it undulates back toward the beach and day-use area. Glance over your shoulder occasionally to take in the views of spectacular Mount Washington over the ridge.

DIRECTIONS

From Sisters, drive west on US 20/OR 126 for about 13 miles, then turn left at the signs for Deschutes National Forest and Suttle Lake Lodge & Resort. Take your first right toward the lodge and keep right to get to the Suttle Lake Day-Use Area.

18 McKenzie River

TRAIL DETAILS AT A GLANCE

- **DISTANCE** 26.5-mile point-to-point with shuttle
- **GPS TRAILHEAD COORDINATES** N44° 10.628' W122° 8.162' (Upper Trailhead), N44° 10.628' W122° 8.156' (Lower Trailhead)
- **DIFFICULTY** 10 • **SCENERY** 10 • **CROWDS** 5
- **SEASON** March–November, sunrise–sunset • **ELEVATION** +903/–2,616'
- **USERS** Hikers, mountain bikers • **CONTACT** McKenzie River Ranger District, Willamette National Forest; 541-822-3381, **www.fs.usda.gov/willamette**
- **PERMITS/FEES** None • **RECOMMENDED MAP** *Sisters & Redmond High Desert Trail Map* by Adventure Maps, Inc. ($12, **adventuremaps.net**)
- **DOGS** Yes (leashed only)

HANDS-DOWN, THE MCKENZIE RIVER NATIONAL RECREATION TRAIL is one of the most spectacular trails in the United States. This may sound like a bold claim, but after running a few miles through the pristine old-growth wilderness, most trail users will agree. The 26.5 miles of singletrack are punctuated by amazingly clear lakes and streams, roaring waterfalls, interesting lava flows, deep and mesmerizing aquamarine pools, and some of Oregon's most breathtaking scenery.

While it makes for a very long and difficult day, running the length of the McKenzie River Trail (MRT) also makes for a very rewarding one. The trail's topography changes dramatically throughout its length, giving runners constantly evolving landscapes and scenic views. The upper portion is more technically challenging due to exposed roots and lava flows, while the middle and lower sections require less concentration on hard-packed singletrack.

Top to bottom, the trail drops more than 2,600 feet, most of it gradual with only a few notable declines. Accordingly, there are very few climbs on the route. Don't let the downhill fool you, however: The sheer distance will have your legs reminding you for several days afterward of the trail's challenging nature.

Numerous access points allow for ample opportunities to run shorter segments, but be aware that any length will require a shuttle. Hitchhiking is possible but not guaranteed, so plan accordingly—or better yet, bring a friend (or two) and shuttle vehicles. If you prefer a shorter run, I recommend the upper two-thirds of the trail over the lower third due to better scenery and distance from the highway.

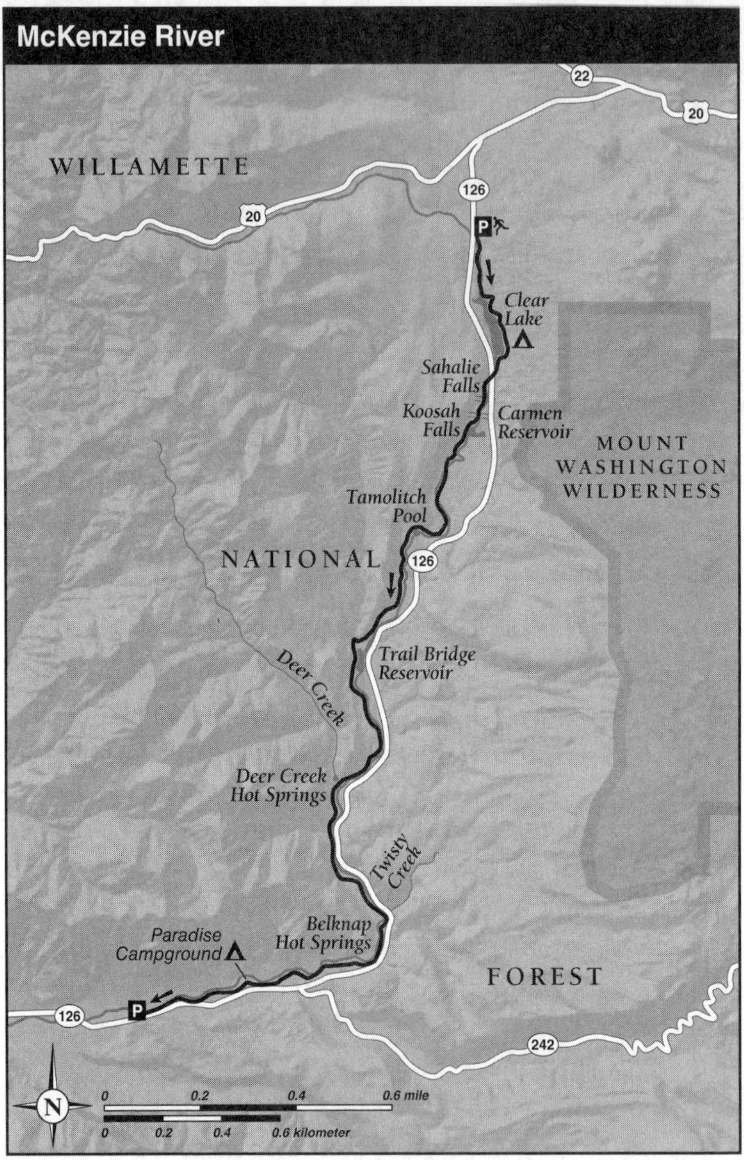

McKenzie River
22
20
WILLAMETTE
126
20
Clear Lake
Sahalie Falls
Koosah Falls
Carmen Reservoir
MOUNT WASHINGTON WILDERNESS
Tamolitch Pool
NATIONAL
126
Trail Bridge Reservoir
Deer Creek
Deer Creek Hot Springs
Twisty Creek
Belknap Hot Springs
Paradise Campground
FOREST
126
242
N
0 0.2 0.4 0.6 mile
0 0.2 0.4 0.6 kilometer

4,000 ft.
3,500 ft.
3,000 ft.
2,500 ft.
2,000 ft.
1,500 ft.
1,000 ft.
5 mi.
10 mi.
15 mi.
20 mi.
25 mi.

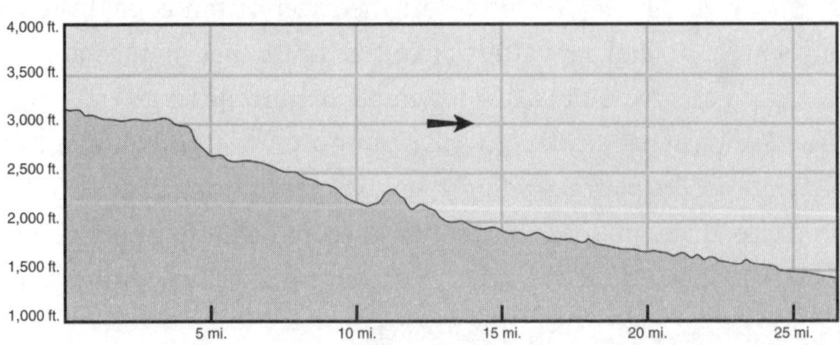

Starting from the northern trailhead, immediately cross the first of many sturdy, well-maintained log footbridges. Run among old-growth Douglas-firs and pines for the first mile before crossing back over Fish Lake Creek just shy of 1 mile. A short 0.25 mile later, you'll pass the remarkably blue and clear Great Spring, the primary source that feeds the aptly named Clear Lake.

Emerge from the forest at 2.2 miles and enter an impressive lava flow on the east side of Clear Lake. Short stints of pavement briefly replace dirt singletrack, and the crystal-clear waters draw you into its depths. Soon enough, you're forced to focus your attention to the rocky terrain and your footing. To twist an ankle this early into the run would simply be a disappointment, so be extra-cautious as you traverse the technical lava flow.

Near the southern end of the lake, keep left at the trail junction to remain on the MRT. Around 3.5 miles, carefully cross McKenzie Highway and settle into a nice rhythm as the music of the McKenzie River propels you alongside its rushing waters. Over the next several miles, pass through beautiful sections of winding, rocky trail and get up-close views of the spectacular 100-foot Sahalie Falls (4.1 miles) and 70-foot Koosah Falls (4.5 miles). The trail zigzags down at each of the falls to match the vertical drops before finally leveling out by Carmen Reservoir.

Beyond the reservoir, the landscape begins to hint at gradual changes as you continue to drop slightly in elevation. Groves of deciduous trees emerge among the evergreens, and the trail distances itself from the river. Though you never see this on the trail, it's around the 6.6-mile point where the river disappears below the surface through a series of ancient lava tubes.

Enjoy the stillness and quiet of the forest for the next 1.6 miles, and soon you run up to one of the most spectacular sights on the MRT: Tamolitch Pool. Simply dubbed the Blue Pool by most, this magical area is where the McKenzie reemerges from the lava tubes back to the surface through a series of springs. Above the Blue Pool is Tamolitch Falls, which remains bone-dry for the majority of the year, though it seems to be the invisible source of the pool itself. The truth is Tamolitch Falls does run sometimes, but the reason it's typically dry is that, since the 1960s, the river above has been diverted to Carmen and Smith Reservoirs to generate hydroelectric power; when the falls does run, it's due to runoff from seasonal snowmelt or water occasionally being diverted back into the riverbed. Those lucky enough to catch Tamolitch Falls wet usually have to plan for early spring, when the water levels are at their high point.

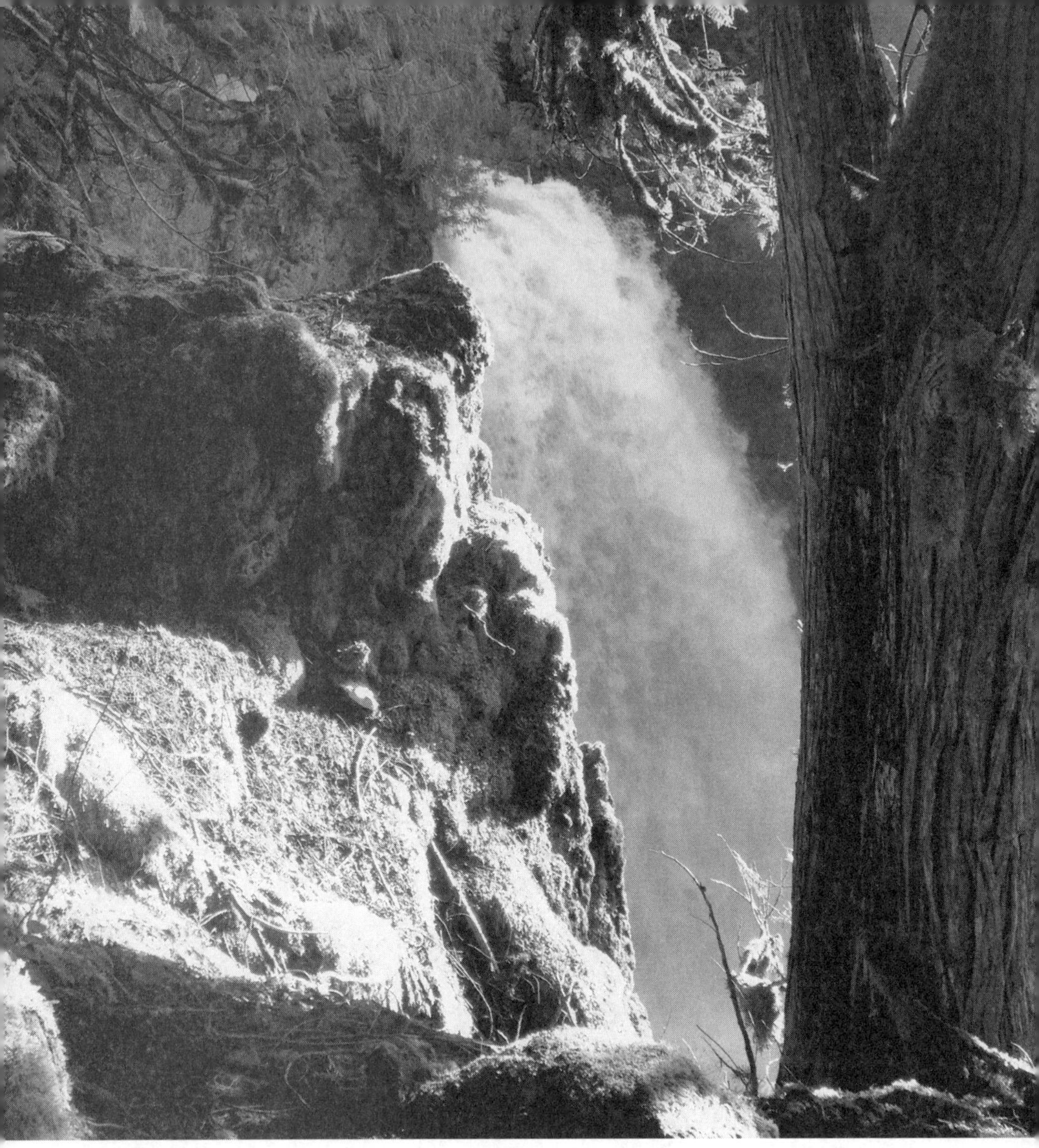

Sahalie Falls

The real treasure, though, is the Blue Pool itself. A vibrant aquamarine in color, the water is so tranquil and clear that from the 80-foot rocky perch above the pool, the deep bottom seems just beneath the surface. The basalt rock surrounding the pool, along with the moss-covered rock and the green ferns lining the shores, boosts the vibrancy of the color and gives the whole area an otherworldly quality. If you're looking for a rest after the first third of your run, this is your place.

From the Blue Pool, continue along the MRT through your last substantial lava flow and pass Trail Bridge Reservoir at 11.6 miles—a good spot to end your run if you're looking for something shorter. Otherwise, continue south and soon settle into your pace on the smooth singletrack. Over the next 8 miles, the trail is fast, flowy, and gentle—allowing a perfect rhythm as you run through the dense, moss-covered trail lined with ferns and classic Western Cascades scenery.

One area worth noting in this segment is at the confluence of Deer Creek, just after you cross Forest Road 2654 around the 15.8-mile mark. An unsigned but obvious singletrack trail juts left toward the river and takes you to the lovely and primitive Deer Creek Hot Springs after a quick 100 yards. Though a midrun soak may be out of the question, this is a nice place to stop on your way back up if you've brought a shuttle. Unlike the more popular and well-known Belknap Springs, Deer Creek Hot Springs is much less crowded, and, best of all, it's free.

Though the MRT is nearly all singletrack, the trail does make a few short connections on roads. The largest is around 16.7 miles, where you'll run for a quarter-mile along an old jeep road before plunging back onto singletrack at a winding section aptly named Twisty Creek.

From Boulder Creek, the trail passes over the paved road to Belknap Hot Springs a short time later and begins to veer in a more westerly direction. Ignore the signed junction back to the highway approximately 0.5 mile later to continue along the MRT, passing the outskirts of the large and popular Paradise Campground. At this point, the trail begins to lose its luster as it skirts the highway at several points and the views become less scenic. You're on the home stretch, however, and before you know it, you've hit the southern terminus of the trail at 26.5 miles.

DIRECTIONS

For the northern trailhead, drive northwest from Sisters on US 20/OR 126 for about 26 miles. At Santiam Junction, bear left at the Y-junction to stay on US 20/OR 126 toward Eugene (straight turns into OR 22 toward Salem). About 3 miles later, US 20 and OR 126 split; turn left (south) to continue on OR 126. Keep your eyes peeled for the MCKENZIE RIVER TRAILHEAD sign on your left, shortly after the turnoff for Fish Lake on your right.

For the southern trailhead, continue south on OR 126 another 20 miles. About 0.5 mile beyond the McKenzie River Ranger Station, look for a large pullout along the right (river) side of the road and the MCKENZIE RIVER TRAIL sign.

19 Whychus Canyon Preserve

TRAIL DETAILS AT A GLANCE

- **DISTANCE** 7.25-mile loop
- **GPS TRAILHEAD COORDINATES** N44° 20.215' W121° 27.185'
- **DIFFICULTY** 6 • **SCENERY** 6 • **CROWDS** 4
- **SEASON** March–December, sunrise–sunset • **ELEVATION** +/–963'
- **USERS** Hikers, runners • **CONTACT** Deschutes Land Trust, 541-330-0017, **deschuteslandtrust.org**
- **PERMITS/FEES** None • **RECOMMENDED MAP** PDF map at **tinyurl.com/whychuscanyonmap**
- **DOGS** Yes (leashed only)

LOCATED BETWEEN SISTERS AND REDMOND, Whychus Canyon Preserve is an area newly developed by the Deschutes Land Trust. With over 7 miles of zigzagging trails up and down the steep canyon, the preserve has ample views of the blue waters of Whychus Creek, the Cascade Mountains, and—during the spring months—great opportunities to see High Desert wildflowers such as balsamroot and many others.

The preserve was established to provide a high-quality habitat for salmon and steelhead in the Upper Deschutes Basin. Historically, the preserve was the most productive steelhead stream feeding into the Upper Deschutes River, and now it plays a major part in efforts to reintroduce the species to the area.

The trails provide a few options depending on your desire for distance and elevation. For the hardy, a nice inner–outer loop covers nearly the entire network without much backtracking. From the trailhead, start by running down the doubletrack, passing both the junction for the canyon trail and the signs pointing to the Santiam Wagon Road. In a quarter-mile, you'll reach a gate and, shortly after, an open meadow where you'll have the option of skirting the meadow on either side (both come out to the same point).

After a mile in, you'll reach another junction, which will be the return point for the Santiam Wagon Road and the final leg of the run. For now, continue along the doubletrack, which starts into a series of S-curves and begins dropping slightly in elevation. In another half-mile, you'll see a singletrack junction off the road to your left, which will be your turn. Before taking this trail, however, it's worth it to

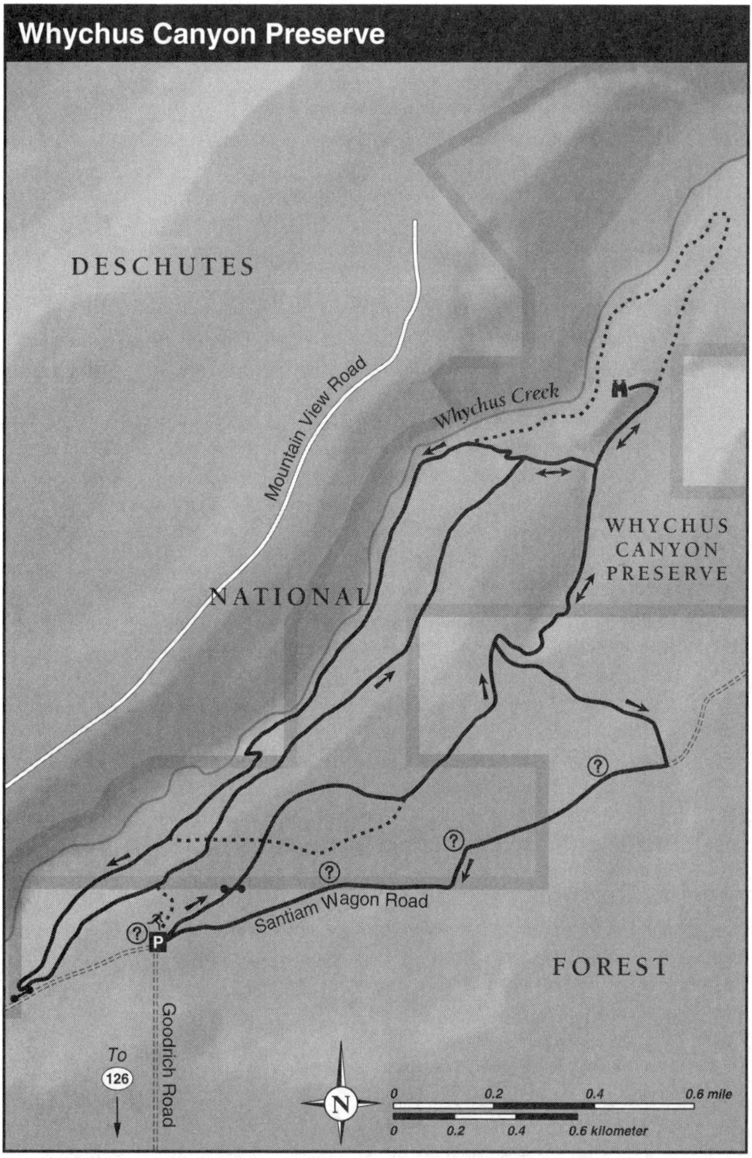

Whychus Canyon Preserve
DESCHUTES
NATIONAL
FOREST
Mountain View Road
Whychus Creek
WHYCHUS
CANYON
PRESERVE
Santiam Wagon Road
Goodrich Road
To
126
N
0
0.2
0.4
0.6 mile
0
0.2
0.4
0.6 kilometer

3,200 ft.
3,100 ft.
3,000 ft.
2,900 ft.
2,800 ft.
2,700 ft.
2,600 ft.
1 mi.
2 mi.
3 mi.
4 mi.
5 mi.
6 mi.
7 mi.

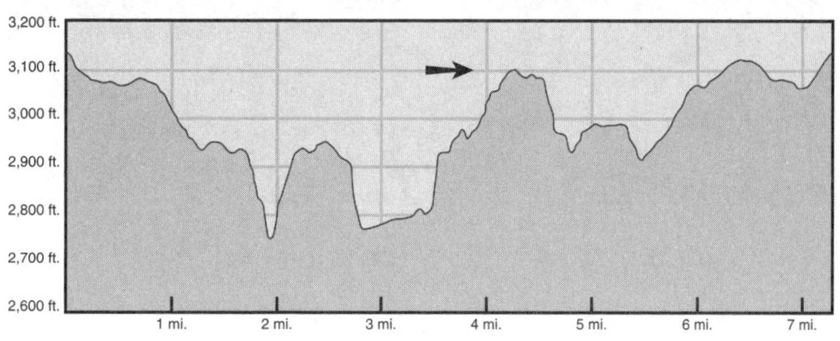

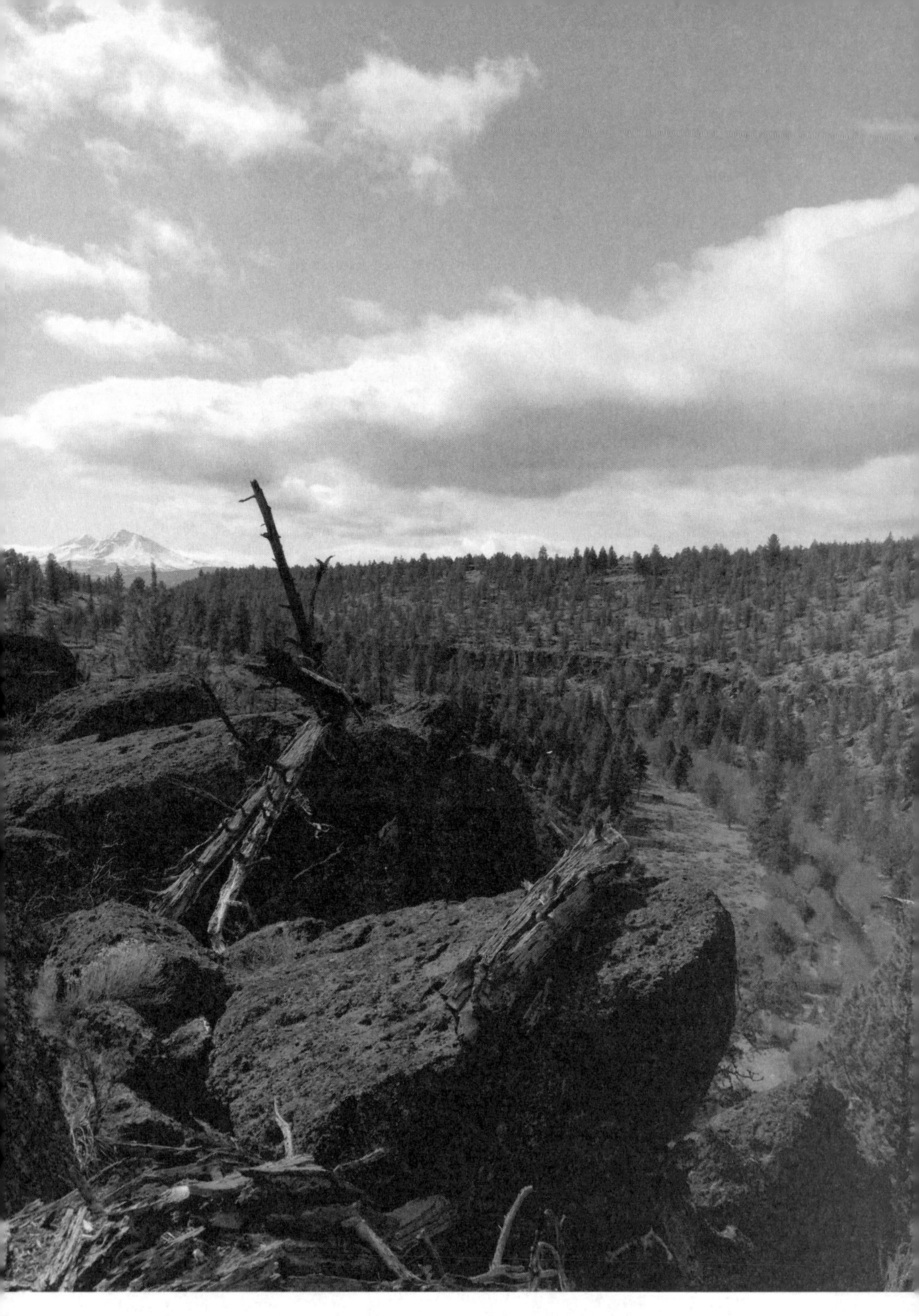

Whychus Creek bends toward the North and Middle Sisters.

continue a quarter-mile to a signed viewpoint. Off in the distance you'll see the snowcapped Cascade peaks on the horizon, as well as an impressive canyon and Whychus Creek far below.

Once you take in the views, return to the junction and take a right down into the canyon. Continue past a junction on the left (your return route) and descend the steep, well-made trail until you reach the creek below. Watch your steps carefully on this descent, which has many rock stairs and short, sharp switchbacks.

Once on the floor of the canyon, continue along Whychus Creek and eventually start ascending back up the canyon wall. When you reach the next junction, stay right and gradually work your way back up while taking in the gorgeous views of the Three Sisters Mountains, along with the perfectly symmetrical Black Butte in the foreground. Within a mile from the junction, you'll reach another gate, which is the westernmost point in the trail network.

Follow this trail over the rolling terrain, passing the gated junction on your right and then descending to another junction, where you'll keep right. From here, a quick 0.75 mile takes you back to a familiar crossing where you'll take a right to begin the loop return. Another right-hand turn takes you back to the doubletrack and back up the curves. This time, instead of returning the same way, take a left at the T and, in another half-mile, look for signs for the Santiam Wagon Road. Follow the arrows 1.1 miles back to the start.

DIRECTIONS

From Bend, drive northwest on US 20 toward Sisters about 13 miles. Turn right (north) on Fryrear Road and, after 5.5 miles, turn left on OR 126. After 1 mile, turn right on Goodrich Road. Around 1.5 miles, the road will curve sharply to the right—continue straight at the curve onto the gravel road, and follow this road until you reach the trailhead 1.7 miles later.

20 The Cove Palisades State Park

TRAIL DETAILS AT A GLANCE

- **DISTANCE** 6.5-mile balloon loop
- **GPS TRAILHEAD COORDINATES** N44° 31.895' W121° 17.416'
- **DIFFICULTY** 6 • **SCENERY** 7 • **CROWDS** 5 • **SEASON** Year-round, sunrise–sunset
- **ELEVATION** +/–1,109' • **USERS** Hikers, runners
- **CONTACT** The Cove Palisades State Park, 541-546-3412, **tinyurl.com/covepalisades**
- **PERMITS/FEES** $5 day-use fee • **RECOMMENDED MAP** PDF map at **tinyurl.com/covepalisadesmap**
- **DOGS** Yes (leashed only)

THE COVE PALISADES STATE PARK is known as a boating paradise, but tucked among the hills overlooking the junctions of three of Central Oregon's most prominent rivers—the Deschutes, the Metolius, and the Crooked—is also one of the region's best High Desert loop trails: the Tam-a-láu Trail.

From atop the section of the park called The Peninsula, Tam-a-láu provides jaw-dropping views of the Crooked and Deschutes River arms of Lake Billy Chinook and transforms the boats on the waters and cars on the road to miniature Matchbox vehicles. Seemingly closer at hand are the stately Cascade peaks of Mount Jefferson, the Three Sisters, and the more faint Mount Hood.

The Tam-a-láu Trail passes through three distinct geological formations on its way up to the plateau. Living up to its name, which means "a place of big rocks on the ground," the trail zigzags through bus-sized boulders that broke off from The Peninsula's edge long ago. Though dodging rocks is no longer a worry, you should be mindful of the time of day when you run this trail—there is little shade, and it can be very hot here in the summer.

To begin the run, park at the Upper Deschutes Day-Use Area, off SW Jordan Road just past The Peninsula (about 6 miles from the park entrance); the trail can also be accessed near Loop B at Deschutes Campground. The trail starts opposite the water and makes its way uphill on a well-defined path through boulders, rocks, and juniper. In a quick 0.5 mile, cross the road and the self-pay kiosk for parking that you drove through earlier. This time, follow the signs and take a right

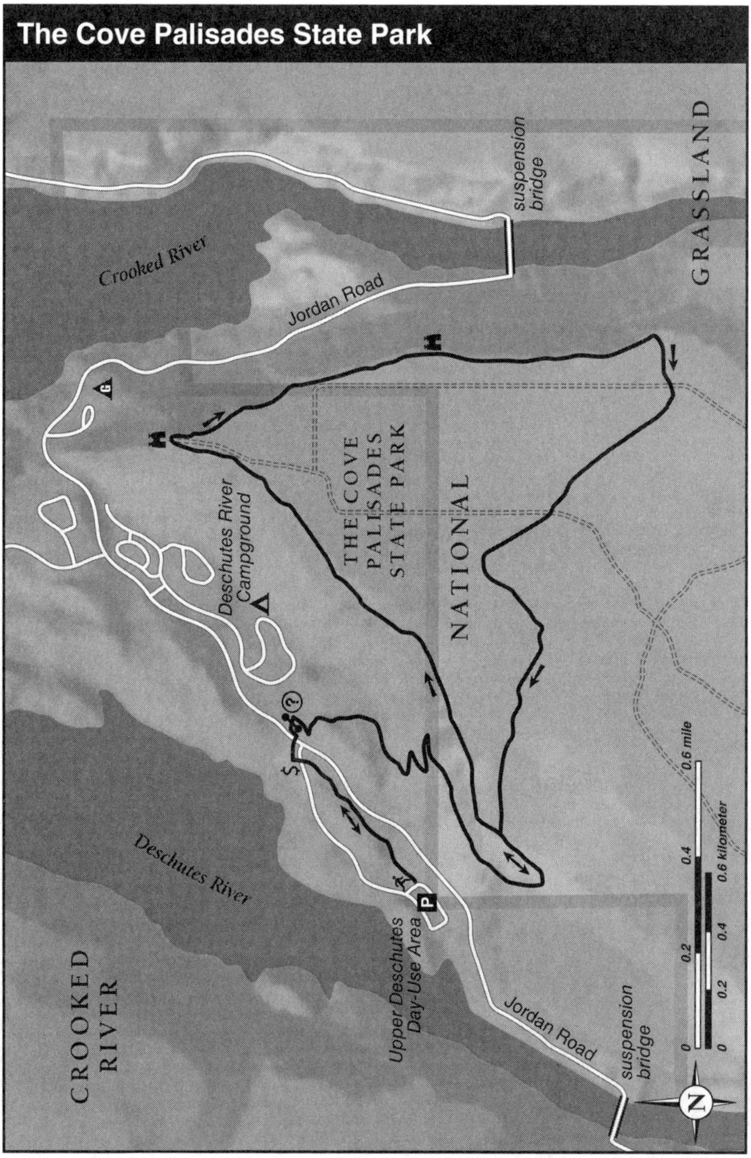

The Cove Palisades State Park

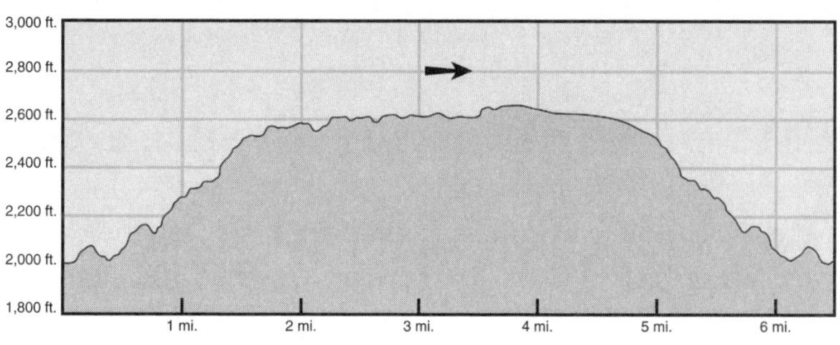

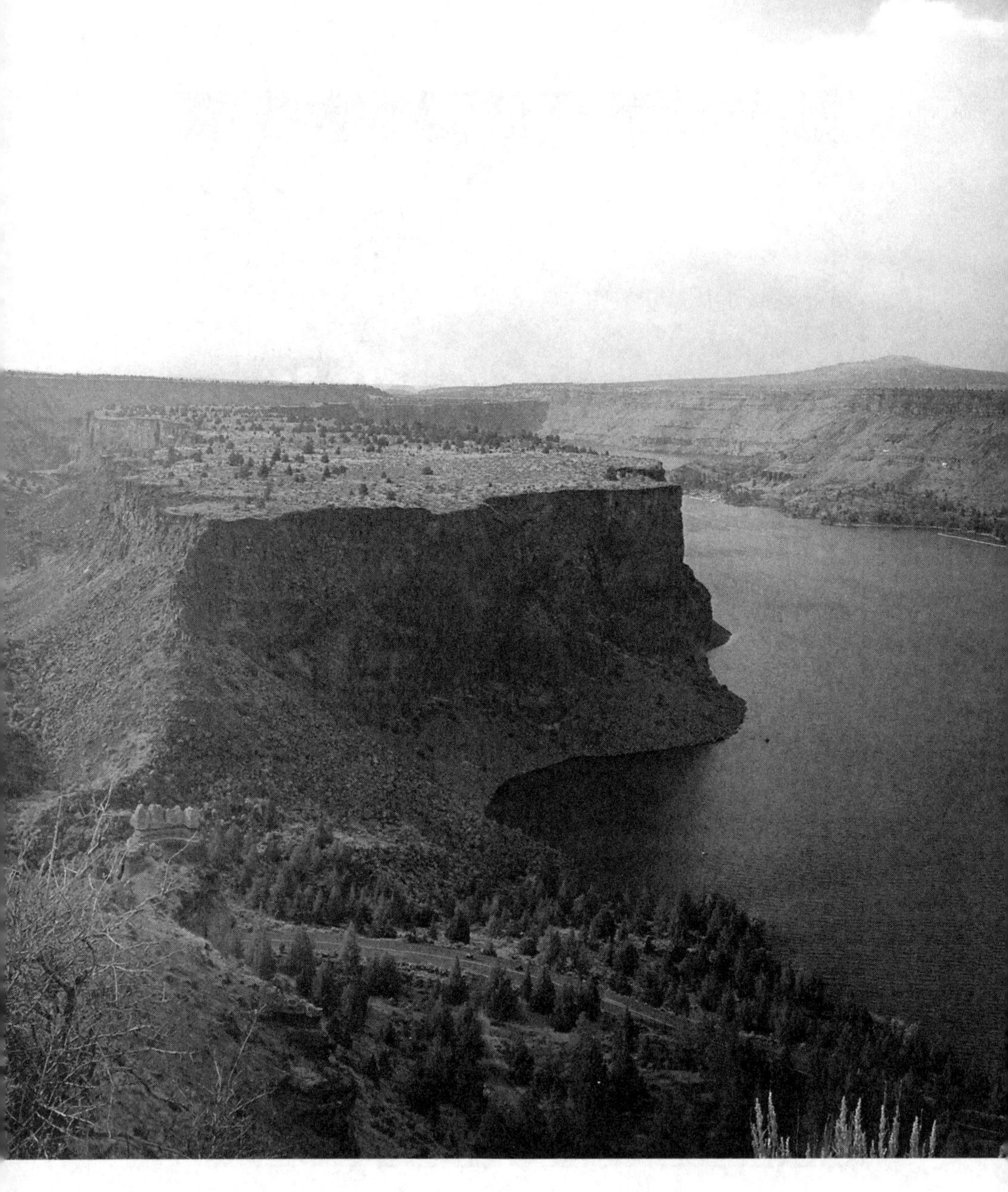

The Island

on the paved pathway before you cross Jordan Road and pass through a gate to the main trailhead at the campground.

You begin your climb in earnest at this point with a series of steep switchbacks up the face of The Peninsula. The trail then hugs the ridgeline and undulates up toward the top. Keep your eyes peeled to the right, where you can see the parking lot and your already shrinking car.

At just over 1.5 miles, you reach the top and the junction for the 3.5-mile plateau loop. Congratulate yourself on making the climb and concentrate on simply enjoying the views over the next few miles. From the junction, turn left and follow the trail as it weaves along the edge overlooking first the Deschutes River and then the Crooked River.

At 2.7 miles, the trail reaches The Peninsula's point, marked by a trail sign noting the first 1.1 miles of the plateau's loop. Take a moment to take in the views of the rivers and The Island, a now-protected 200-acre plateau that is said to be one of the few remnants of pre-settlement ecology in the West and one of the last well-preserved ecosystems of its type in the United States.

Once you've taken in the wonder, continue straight along the trail, ignoring the dirt road to your right. Shortly after 3 miles, the trail passes beneath a set of power lines that seem to plunge straight down into the lake far below. Soon after, you'll be treated to views of the suspension bridge crossing the Crooked River arm and a set of lava rock walls—reminders of those who inhabited the area long ago.

A quarter-mile past the marked sign for 1.5 miles (of the top loop), round the corner and begin your return. Though not as spectacular in terms of cliffside views, the trail has you running through sagebrush and juniper directly toward Mount Jefferson and the Cascade peaks, offering great views of the mountainous horizon. Around 4.5 miles, be sure to take note of a particularly gnarly juniper tree by the trail that seems to epitomize (for me, at least) what the Oregon High Desert is all about. Around mile 5, reach the junction of the plateau's loop and begin your descent back toward your car.

DIRECTIONS

From Bend, take US 97 North toward Portland. About 15 miles north of Redmond, bear left on SW Culver Highway. After about 2.3 miles, turn left at SW Iris Lane in Culver. Drive 1 mile and turn right (north) on SW Feather Drive. Drive another 1.2 miles and turn left on SW Fisch Lane. After about 0.5 mile, Fisch Lane turns right and becomes SW Frazier Drive. Drive another 0.5 mile and turn left on SW Peck Road, which becomes SW Jordan Road as it enters The Cove Palisades State Park. Follow Jordan Road about 6 winding miles through the park. The Tam-a-láu Trailhead will be on the right, at the Upper Deschutes Day-Use Area.

21 Smith Rock State Park

TRAIL DETAILS AT A GLANCE

- **DISTANCE** 7.3- to 10-mile loop options
- **GPS TRAILHEAD COORDINATES** N44° 22.022' W121° 8.261'
- **DIFFICULTY** 5 • **SCENERY** 9 • **CROWDS** 7 • **SEASON** Year-round, sunrise–sunset
- **ELEVATION** +/–1,153' • **USERS** Hikers, runners, mountain bikers
- **CONTACT** Oregon State Parks, 541-548-7501, **tinyurl.com/smithrockstatepark**
- **PERMITS/FEES** $5 day-use fee • **RECOMMENDED MAP** *Sisters & Redmond High Desert Trail Map* by Adventure Maps, Inc. ($12, **adventuremaps.net**)
- **DOGS** Yes (leashed only)

THOUGH SMITH ROCK STATE PARK is one of the top rock-climbing destinations in the United States, it's also one of the best spots in Central Oregon for a trail run. Unique rock formations, meandering rivers, and stunning vistas combine for a perfect day out on the trail.

That beauty comes with a price, however: Many of the viewpoints require a good amount of climbing, and you can expect to be one of many people on the trails, particularly on weekends. But as with most running destinations, you'll have broken away from the crowds after a mile or two.

Several loop options are available and can be combined to fit your needs. The recommended starting point is at the main trailhead, near the visitor center.

From the visitor center, turn right on the Rim Rock Trail until it joins the Canyon Trail. After 0.1 mile, take a sharp right on The Chute toward the footbridge. There's a water fountain near the bridge where you can fill any bottles or reservoirs, along with a primitive restroom. Once over the footbridge, turn left on the River Trail, which you'll remain on for 1.6 miles.

Continue straight and you'll soon begin the long climb up the back of the park. If they haven't already, the crowds will begin to drop off at this point. A short section through private property connects you with the challenging Summit Trail, where you'll remain until the high point of the run. Numerous switchbacks take you up and up, providing views of Gray Butte to the northeast.

At the apex of the run, you'll reach the top of Burma Road. From here, outstanding views of the park abound below and to the south. Ignore the singletrack here—instead, run down the steep but manageable Burma Road as it winds down

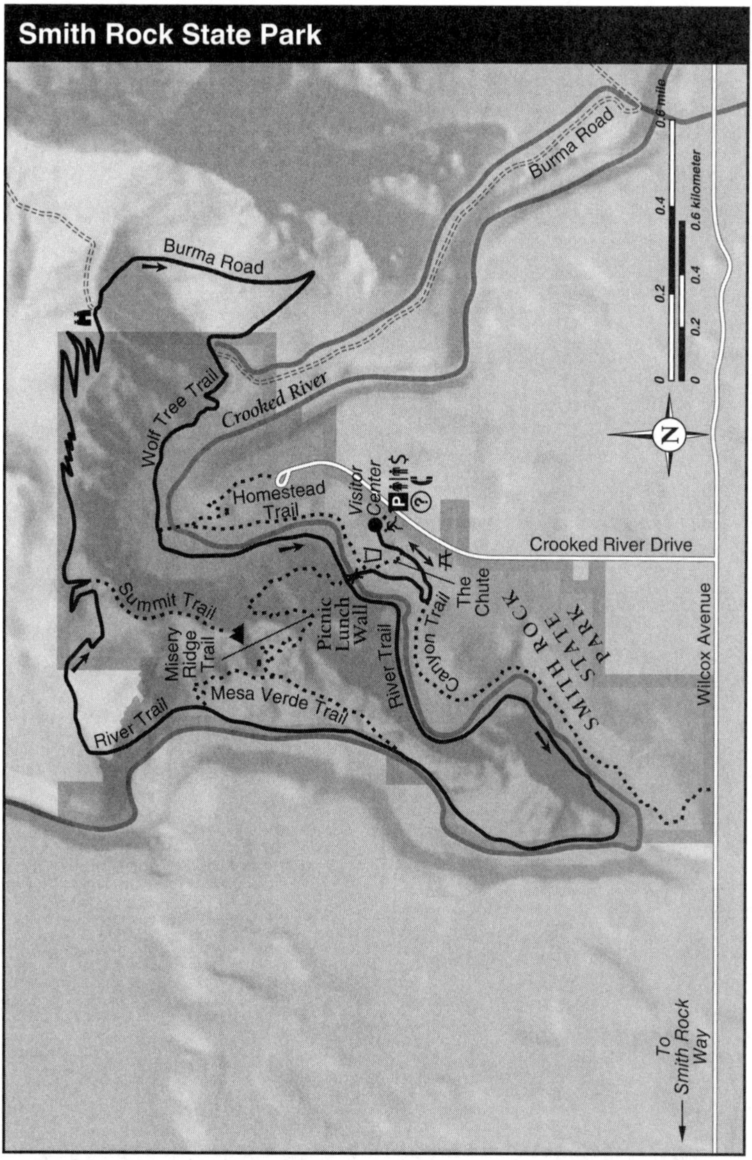

Smith Rock State Park

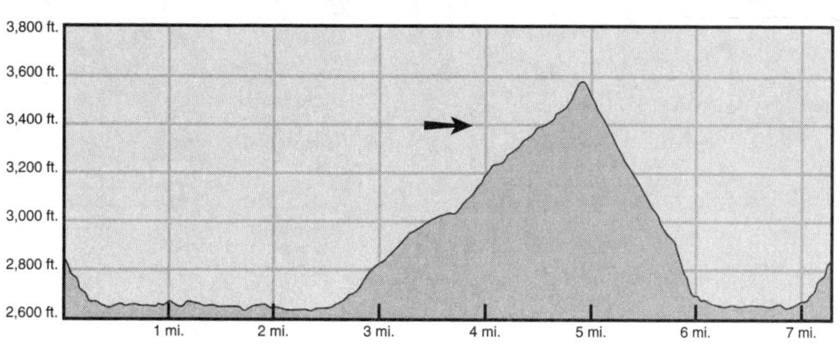

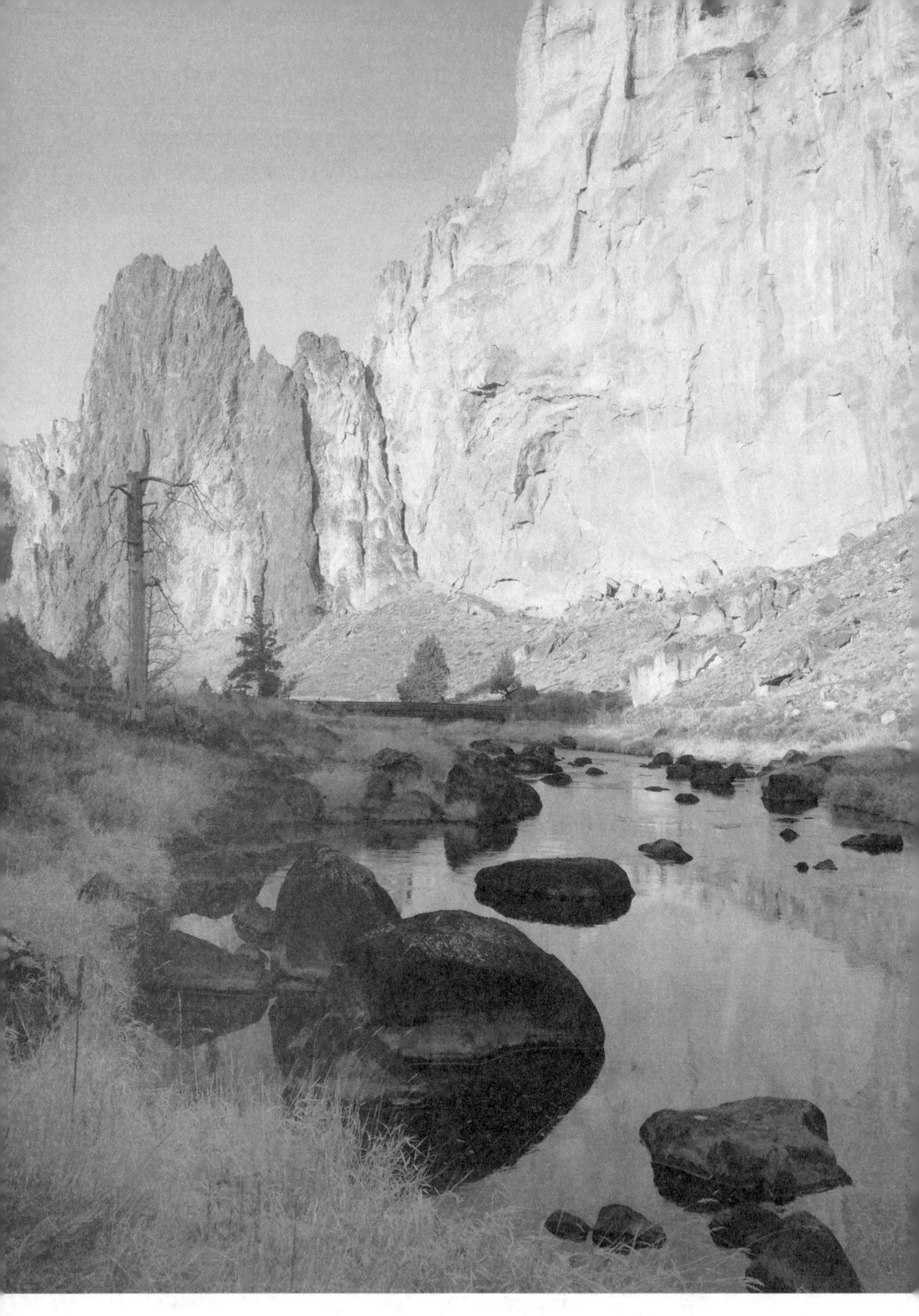

The Crooked River at Smith Rock

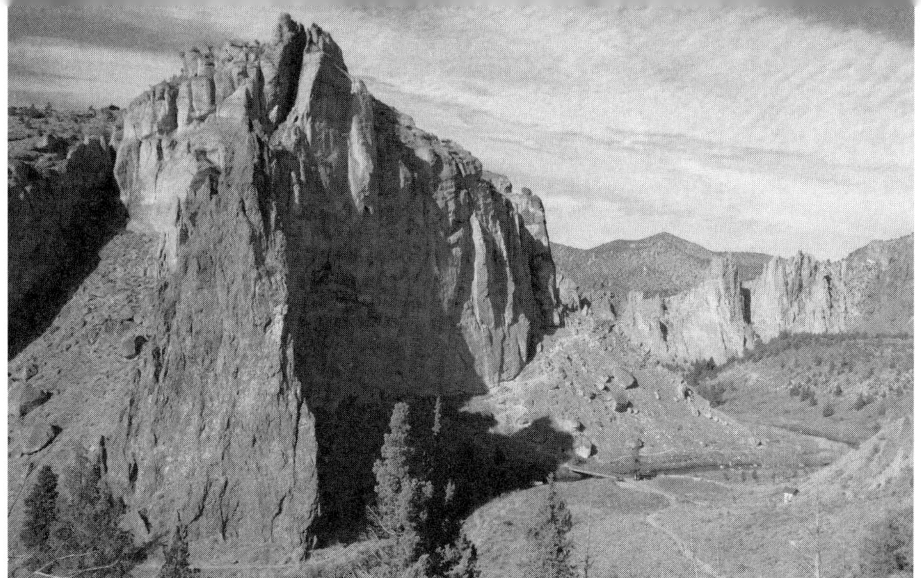

The east side of Smith Rock State Park

back toward the river. Just after the turn where the canal disappears under the rock, about 0.9 mile from the summit, look for the Wolf Tree Trail on your right. A quick, steep descent spits you out beside the Crooked River, where you'll continue on the north side back to the footbridge.

If you're feeling masochistic and want to add a few more miles, you can start up the Misery Ridge Trail from Picnic Lunch Wall by the footbridge, heading up and over the interior summit of Misery Ridge, then down the Mesa Verde Trail and back up the River Trail, where you started. This addition tacks on 700 feet of climbing in less than a mile, plus 3 miles back to the welcome center.

To take it a little easier, you can cross the footbridge and immediately turn left at the drinking fountain to connect to the Homestead Trail for an alternate route (and about 1.5 extra miles) back to the starting point. Or if you're just ready to be done, simply retrace your steps across the bridge and back up the quarter-mile to the parking lot.

DIRECTIONS

From Bend, take US 97 North about 18 miles. In Terrebonne, turn right on B Avenue/Smith Rock Way (look for the brown SMITH ROCK sign on the corner). After about 0.5 mile, turn left (north) on NE Lambert Road, keeping right on Lambert as it curves east. After 2 miles, turn left on NE Crooked River Drive, follow it 0.7 mile north, and park in one of the spots along the left side of the road.

22 Gray Butte

TRAIL DETAILS AT A GLANCE

- **DISTANCE** 9.1-mile loop • **GPS TRAILHEAD COORDINATES** N44° 23.882' W121° 3.870'
- **DIFFICULTY** 7 • **SCENERY** 6 • **SEASON** Year-round, sunrise–sunset
- **ELEVATION** +/–1,421' • **USERS** Hikers, runners, mountain bikers, horses
- **CONTACT** Crooked River National Grassland, Ochoco National Forest; 541-416-6640, **www.fs.usda.gov/ochoco** • **PERMITS/FEES** None
- **RECOMMENDED MAP** *Sisters & Redmond High Desert Trail Map* by Adventure Maps, Inc. ($12, **adventuremaps.net**) • **DOGS** Yes (leashed only)

THOUGH THE TALLEST LANDMARK IN THE AREA, Gray Butte is nearly always overshadowed by the beauty and popularity of nearby Smith Rock State Park (see previous profile). Overlooking Gray Butte, however, is a mistake. Not only does the area provide wonderful solitude on the trails, but parking is never an issue, nor are park fees. A combination of well-worn horse and mountain trails, combined with a bit of gavel road, makes for an excellent loop with an opportunity for 360-degree views around the butte. Plus, you get to see what many park goers never see at Smith Rock—the back side of it.

Start at the Skull Hollow Trailhead, just beyond the turnoff for Skull Hollow Campground. The trail begins at a flat grade as it parallels Forest Road 1395 a dozen yards to the west. In 0.3 mile, skirt the edge of a primitive campground and pass through a closed gate. Be sure to close this and all gates behind you, as portions of the land around Gray Butte are used for grazing cattle.

Once through, the trail begins to contour around the side of the hill before crossing another gated dirt road at 1 mile. Pick up the trail on the other side at the signed Cole Loop Trail 854. From here, climb your way gradually around the southwestern side of Gray Butte. Several rogue side trails appear in this area—keep right to stay on the intended loop.

At 2.4 miles, pass through another gate and an abandoned work site. A quarter-mile later, the trail crosses another jeep road and the Cole Loop Trail intersects the Gray Butte Trail 852 immediately after. Turn right and begin climbing up the steep, rocky trail as it zigzags its way to the west of the butte. Around 3 miles, the trail begins to flatten and views of Smith Rock State Park can be seen from the distance.

Gray Butte

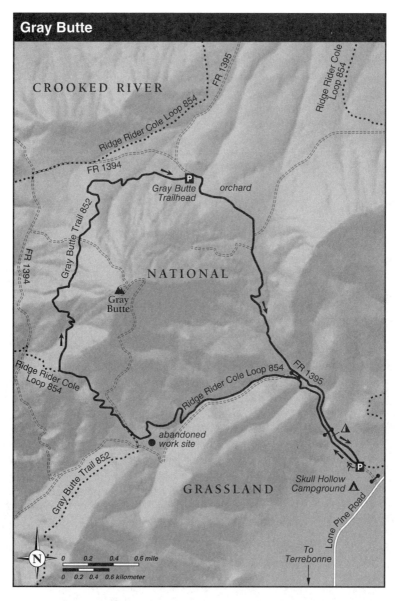

CROOKED RIVER
NATIONAL
GRASSLAND
FR 1395
Ridge Rider Cole Loop 854
FR 1394
Gray Butte Trailhead
orchard
Gray Butte Trail 852
Gray Butte
abandoned work site
Skull Hollow Campground
Lone Pine Road
To Terrebonne
0 0.2 0.4 0.6 mile
0 0.2 0.4 0.6 kilometer

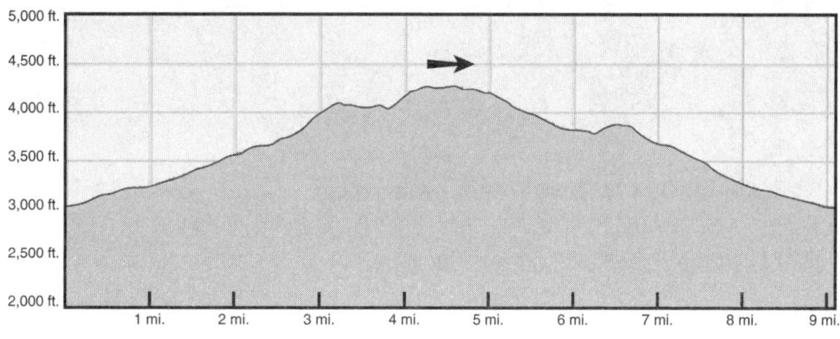

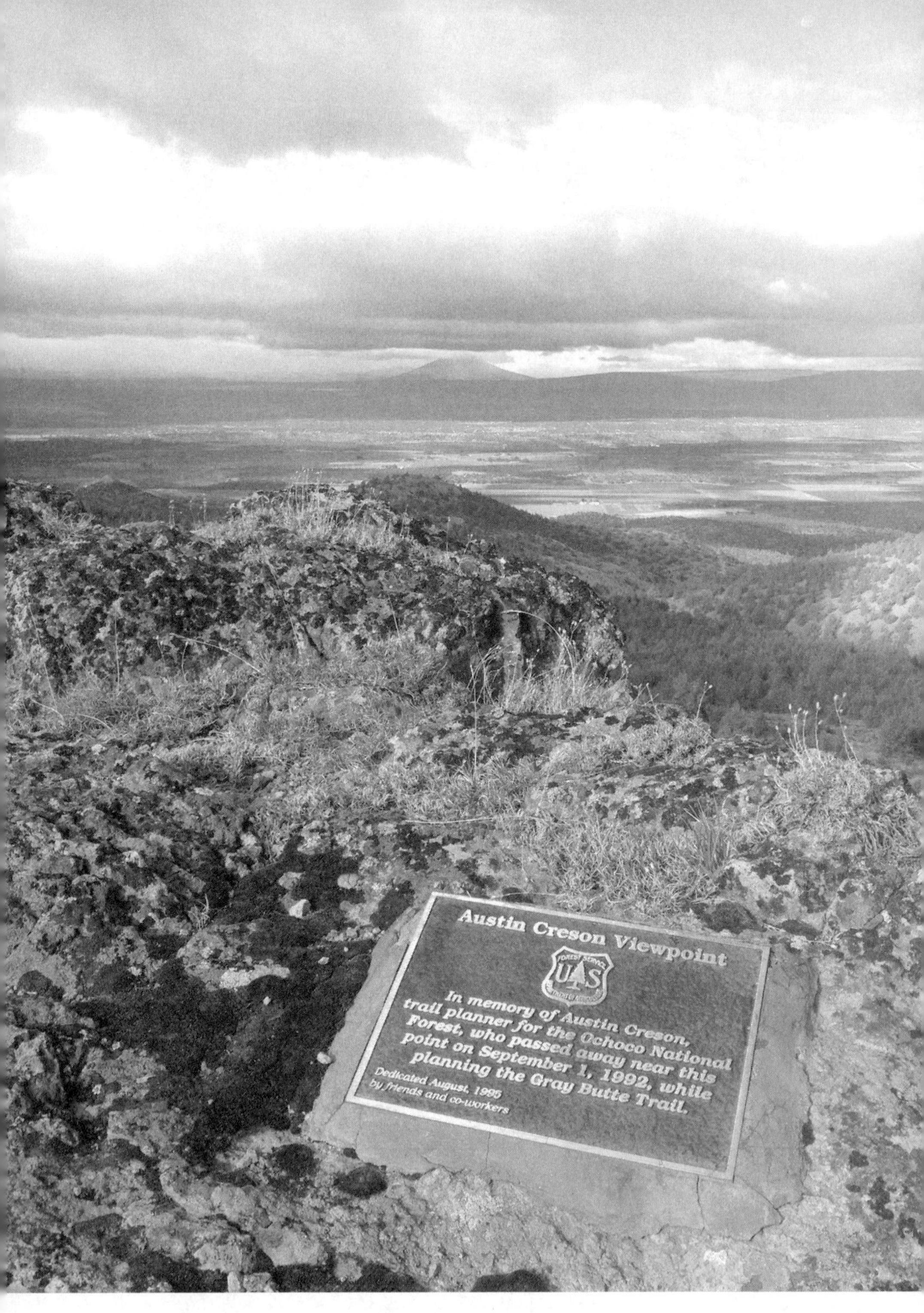

Looking west from the Austin Creson Viewpoint

Keep right at 3.5 miles after another gate and junction, and soon views of Black Butte and the Three Sisters, along with Mounts Jefferson and Hood, start to appear to the west. In 0.8 mile, an impressive overlook presents the Austin Creson Viewpoint and even more views to the west and the north. (Creson, a local trail planner for the Ochoco National Forest, participated in the planning of the Gray Butte Trail.)

From the viewpoint, the trail begins to flatten as you continue the loop. Keen eyes can pick out Haystack Reservoir to the north, glimmering in the distance. After crossing a jeep road at 4.8 miles, the trail begins to descend, with large, neatly piled rock cairns helping mark the way. Though the downhill is pleasant and gradual, watch your footing carefully as you descend through the loose rocks on the trail.

A mile and a half and a gate crossing later, the trail empties into the parking area for the Gray Butte Trailhead, near the old McCoin Orchard. The orchard was originally planted in 1886 by Julius and Sarah McCoin and privately run until the US Forest Service bought the land in the 1930s. From here, the remainder of your run will follow Forest Road 1395 back the nearly 3 miles to the Skull Hollow Trailhead parking and your car. With the exception of a Y-intersection at 6.9 miles (stay right), the forest road is easy to follow and makes for a very fast, very fun return and finish to the loop.

DIRECTIONS

Drive north from Bend on US 97 about 18 miles. In Terrebonne, turn right on B Avenue/Smith Rock Way (look for the brown SMITH ROCK sign on the corner). Follow Smith Rock Way east 4.8 miles until it Ts with Lone Pine Road at the cattle farm. Turn left on Lone Pine Road, following it east across the Crooked River and then north. After 4.2 miles, turn left at the sign for the Gray Butte Trailhead and Skull Hollow Campground. Cross the cattle guard and park at the sign for the Skull Hollow Trailhead, just beyond the turnoff for the campground.

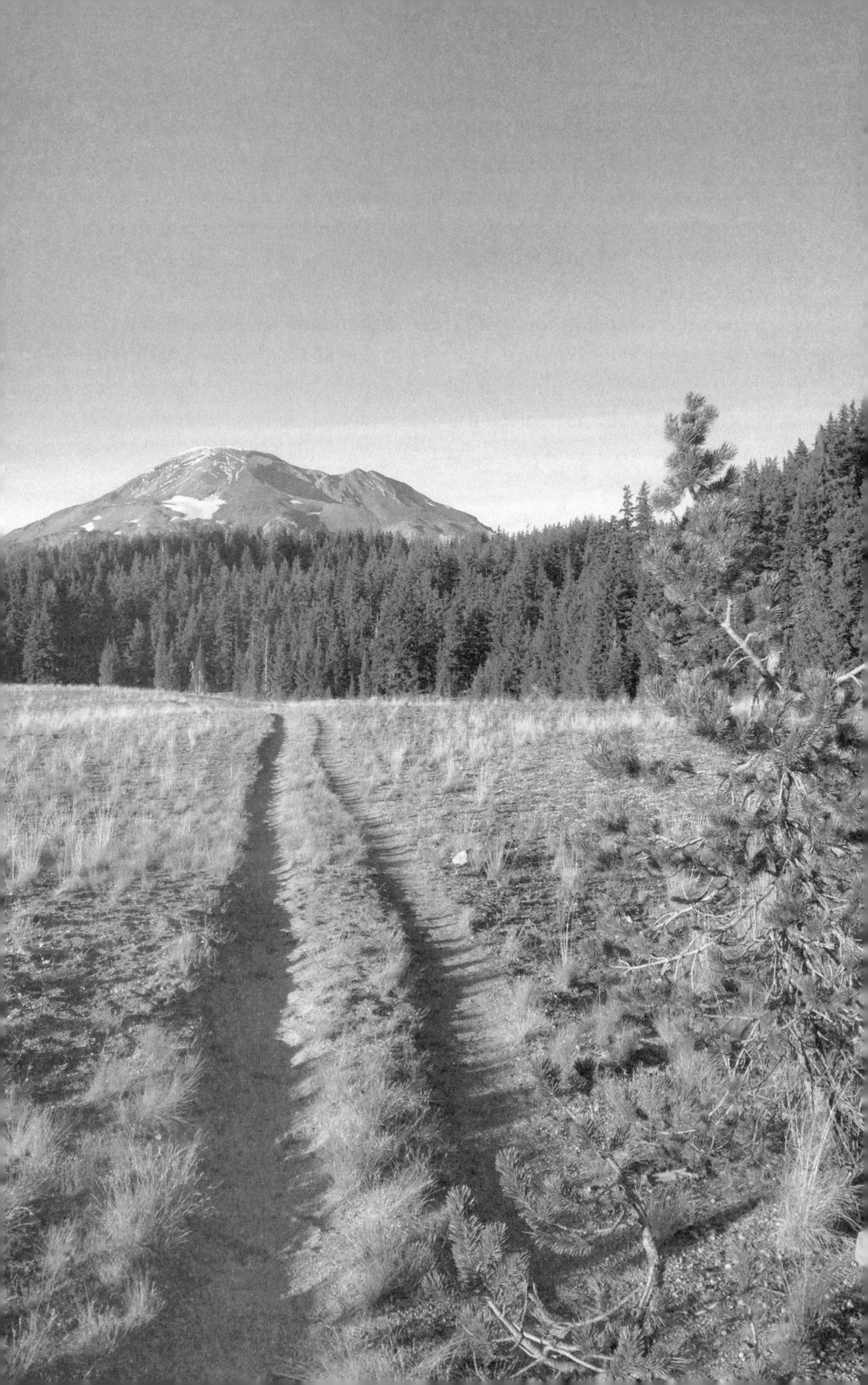

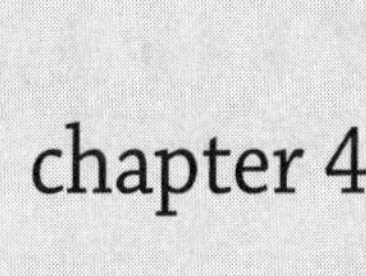

SUMMER RUNS

SUMMER TRAIL LIST

OPPOSITE: *Doubletrack across Wickiup Plains* (see Moraine Lake, page 164)

23 Tumalo Falls

TRAIL DETAILS AT A GLANCE

- **DISTANCE** 7.1-mile loop
- **GPS TRAILHEAD COORDINATES** N44° 1.919' W121° 33.984'
- **DIFFICULTY** 6
- **SCENERY** 7
- **CROWDS** 8
- **SEASON** Mid-June–October, sunrise–sunset
- **ELEVATION** +/–1,120'
- **USERS** Hikers, runners, mountain bikers
- **CONTACT** Bend–Fort Rock Ranger District, Deschutes National Forest; 541-383-4000, **www.fs.usda.gov/deschutes**
- **PERMITS/FEES** Northwest Forest Pass (see page 12)
- **RECOMMENDED MAP** *Bend, Oregon, Trail Map* by Adventure Maps, Inc. ($12, **adventuremaps.net**)
- **DOGS** Prohibited on the Bridge Creek Trail and inside the Bend Watershed

THE TUMALO FALLS–BRIDGE CREEK ROUTE is an attractive loop that's filled with plunging waterfalls, forested pine trails, and some good elevation for those seeking hill workouts. The area is popular among tourists, families, and countless hikers because of its accessibility and quick-payout-to-work ratio, but as with most wilderness trails, you'll find that the crowds quickly thin within the first 2 or 3 miles.

The main attraction for most is the namesake Tumalo Falls, which can be seen within a few steps from the parking lot. Though the falls is indeed impressive, the real gems are the countless other cascades farther up the trail, where you'll find more solitude and equally impressive scenery. And if the first half of the loop doesn't make you fall in love with the area, the picturesque return route down Bridge Creek and through the Bend Watershed most certainly will.

The recommended starting point is the North Fork Trail, which begins at the far end of the main parking lot by the restrooms. Follow the crowds as they head up toward the falls, and within 100 yards you'll notice the Bridge Creek Trail junction, which will serve as your return.

For now, continue uphill past Tumalo Falls (and the crowds), and in 0.9 mile you'll encounter Double Falls—a series of cascades churning over a set of 20-foot drops. A mile farther upstream is spectacular Upper Falls, which plunges 50 feet to the river below. From here, continue uphill, where you'll cross the middle fork of Tumalo Creek at 2.4 miles on a well-maintained footbridge and past numerous more unnamed falls, many of which can be seen from the trail.

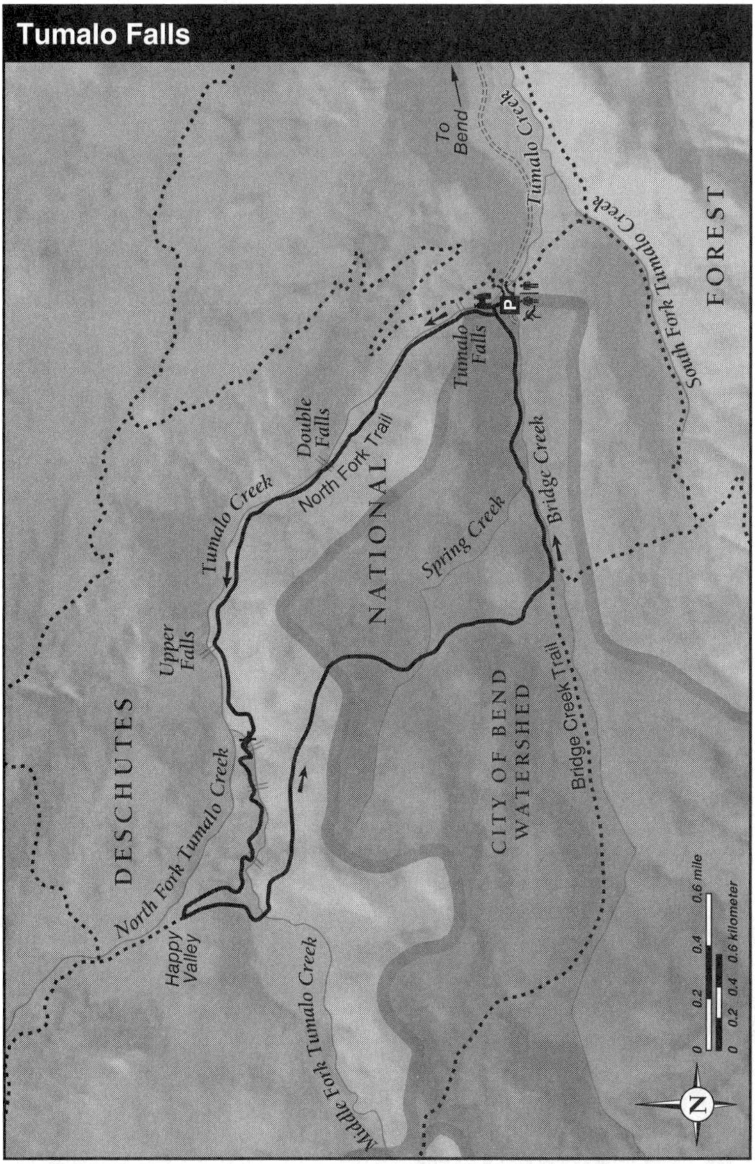

Tumalo Falls

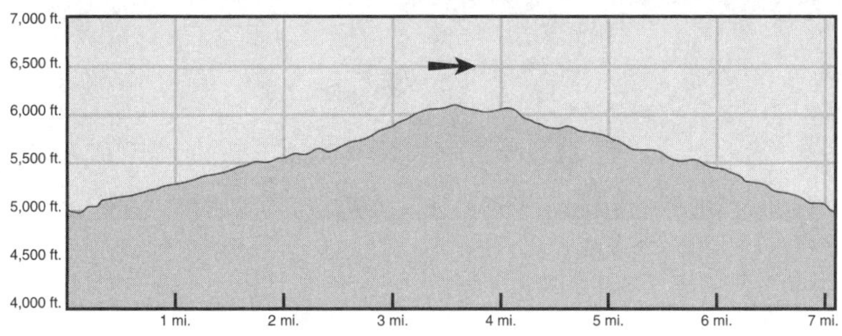

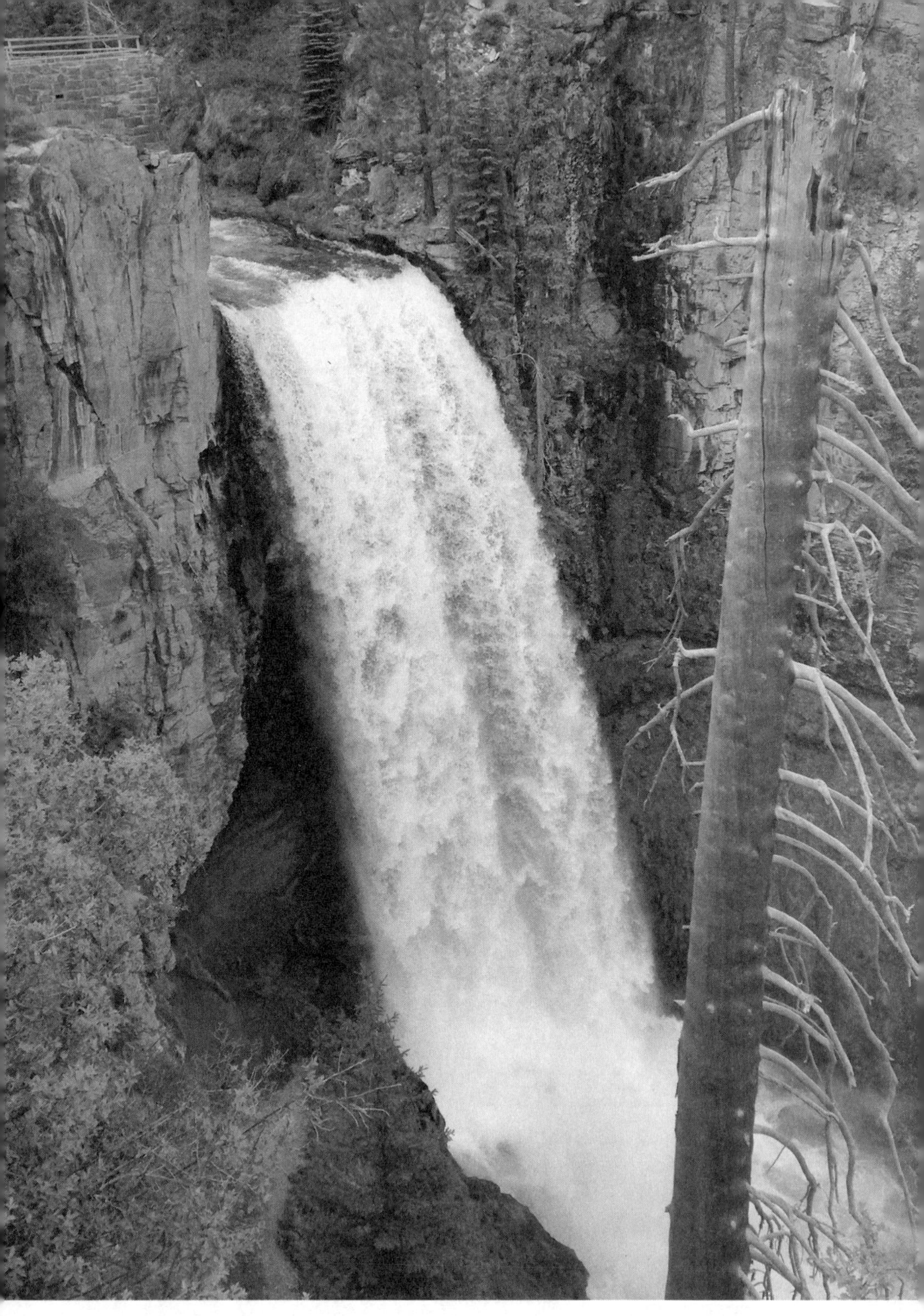

Tumalo Falls

At 3.4 miles, reach a T-junction noting Happy Valley and Bridge Creek—turn left for the Bridge Creek Trail, continuing slightly uphill before topping out at the high point of the loop just above 6,000 feet. Shortly after, you'll once again reach Tumalo Creek, where the trail seems to go straight into the wide creek. Rather than wade, follow the water 20 feet upstream via a faint path, and cross on a sturdy fallen log.

On the opposite side, the trail continues along the river for a short while before disappearing into the trees and coming out along a ridge overlooking the Tumalo Creek drainage. Enjoy the steady downhill grade as it takes you through ponderosa pines, spruce, and mountain hemlock while entering the Bend Watershed. Cross quaint Spring Creek and, in just under 6 miles, reach the junction and your final turn to complete the loop. Turning left here, follow the Bridge Creek Trail another 1.1 miles along the river, passing yet more waterfalls and scenic overlooks—this time without the crowds—before reaching the terminus of your loop at the Tumalo Falls Trailhead.

DIRECTIONS

In Bend, drive west on NW Galveston Avenue (Tumalo Avenue/Riverside Drive/Franklin Avenue east of the river), passing through the roundabout at NW 14th Avenue. At Flagline Drive (about 0.8 mile), Galveston turns into NW Skyliners Road. Continue through the roundabout at NW Mount Washington Drive, passing the Phil's Trail network, and continue out of town for about 10 miles, passing through a small residential area. When the pavement ends, bear right and continue 2.5 miles on Tumalo Falls Road/Forest Road 4603 to the Tumalo Falls Trailhead and parking lot.

24 Swampy Lakes

TRAIL DETAILS AT A GLANCE

- **DISTANCE** 7.5-mile loop
- **GPS TRAILHEAD COORDINATES** N43° 59.407' W121° 34.079'
- **DIFFICULTY** 6 • **SCENERY** 4 • **CROWDS** 3
- **SEASON** June–October, sunrise–sunset • **ELEVATION** +/–680'
- **USERS** Hikers, runners, mountain bikers
- **CONTACT** Bend–Fort Rock Ranger District, Deschutes National Forest; 541-383-4000, **www.fs.usda.gov/deschutes** • **PERMITS/FEES** Northwest Forest Pass (see page 12)
- **RECOMMENDED MAP** *Three Sisters Wilderness Trail Map* by Adventure Maps, Inc. ($12, **adventuremaps.net**) • **DOGS** Yes (leashed only)

THOUGH THE NAME ITSELF MAY NOT CONJURE UP inviting images of mountainous beauty, the Swampy Lakes area is nonetheless worth exploring. Popular with mountain bikers as a launching point to numerous trails in the area and beyond, Swampy Lakes also provides runners with multiple loop options offering just enough visual stimuli to keep things interesting. The Swampy Lakes Loop offers several routes of varying distances on rolling terrain and moderate elevation gain.

Start the loop to the left of the trailhead shelter and gently climb your way up through a forest of ponderosa pines, spruce, and mountain hemlock. Around 0.7 mile, you'll see your first cross-country-skiing sign, an indication of the area's popularity during the winter-recreation months. At just under 2 miles, take a left at your first junction to stay on the Ridge Loop Trail. For a short distance, the straight, flat trail pulls you in before it begins to climb along the side of Vista Butte.

At 2.6 miles, turn right at the marked junction toward the Flagline Tie Trail. Over the next mile, the trail remains fairly even and begins to offer glimpses of Mount Bachelor and Tumalo Mountain through the trees to your left. Gradually descending, run through a burn section before reentering thick forests of lodgepole pine as you get lower in elevation.

Turn right at 4 miles onto a T-junction and the Flagline Trail. Flagline, as it's simply known among locals, is one of the best mountain biking trails in the area. It's also a pretty darn good trail for running. *Note:* The trail is closed the first part of the summer until August 15 to protect elk-calving grounds.

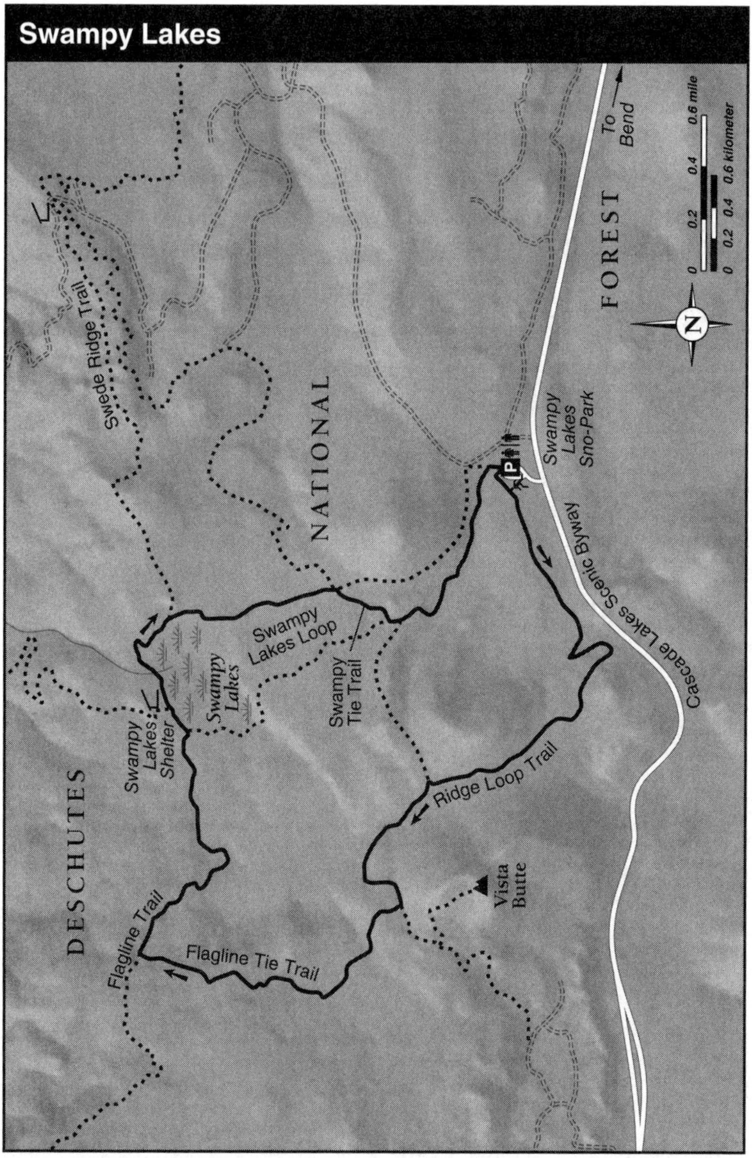

Swampy Lakes

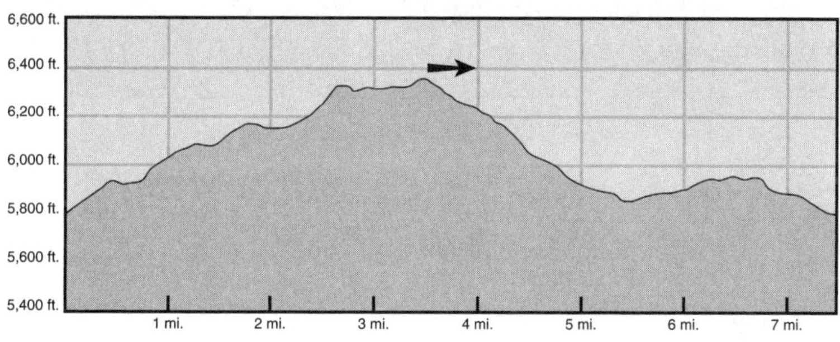

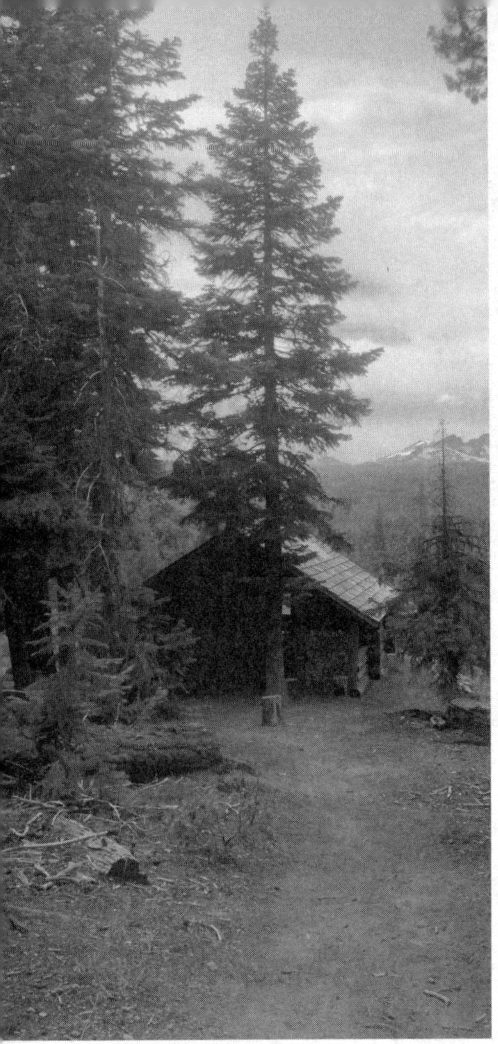

The Swede Ridge Shelter with Broken Top in the background

Run through this appealing section of Flagline, passing several log ramps for mountain bikers and small green meadows just off the trail. At 5.1 miles, intersect the Swampy Lakes Loop section, taking a left and running a quick 0.1 mile before reaching the old and rickety Swampy Lakes Shelter. Ignore the side trails here pointing toward South Fork and continue straight, crossing a small but scenic creek 0.25 mile down the trail.

Continue along the Swampy Lakes Loop, passing the marked side trail toward Swede Ridge (part of the Three Shelters Loop). A short time later, at 6.4 miles, reach another intersection pointing toward Swede Ridge (the return route of the Three Shelters Loop). For a more interesting return to the trailhead, turn right here onto the Swampy Tie Trail, a short 0.25-mile-long section that intersects back with the main Swampy Lakes Loop. Turn left here to complete the loop, keeping straight until the shelter and the Swampy Lakes Trailhead.

DIRECTIONS

From Bend, drive west on SW Century Drive, which becomes the Cascade Lakes National Scenic Byway toward Mount Bachelor. After 13.8 miles, turn right at the SWAMPY LAKES SNO-PARK sign, between Mile Markers 16 and 17, to reach the Swampy Lakes Trailhead.

25 Three Shelters Loop

TRAIL DETAILS AT A GLANCE

- **DISTANCE** 8.4-mile loop
- **GPS TRAILHEAD COORDINATES** N43° 59.407' W121° 34.079'
- **DIFFICULTY** 6 • **SCENERY** 5 • **CROWDS** 4
- **SEASON** June–October, sunrise–sunset • **ELEVATION** +/–708'
- **USERS** Hikers, runners, mountain bikers
- **CONTACT** Bend–Fort Rock Ranger District, Deschutes National Forest; 541-383-4000, **www.fs.usda.gov/deschutes** • **PERMITS/FEES** Northwest Forest Pass (see page 12)
- **RECOMMENDED MAP** *Three Sisters Wilderness Trail Map* by Adventure Maps, Inc. ($12, **adventuremaps.net**) • **DOGS** Yes (leashed only)

DESCHUTES NATIONAL FOREST is dotted with primitive log shelters throughout its high elevations. The Oregon National Guard built many of these huts as part of its training regimen for members during the 1980s. Called "forward bunkers" at the time, these small but stout structures have morphed over the years into key destination points and warming huts for Nordic skiing, snowshoeing, and snowmobiling outings in the winter. Local Nordic groups now maintain and repair the shelters as well as stock them with firewood during the winter-recreation season.

During the summer, these huts also make great destination points for warmer-weather activities such as trail running. The Three Shelters Loop offers runners a chance to visit three distinct and different shelters along its route and take in some scenery on the mostly rolling terrain in the process. The loop connects the (unnamed) trailhead shelter with the Swampy Lakes and Swede Ridge Shelters in a clockwise loop.

Start the loop on the wide singletrack trail 20 yards down from the trailhead shelter—*not* on the trail immediately to the left of the shelter). Follow the sandy path and signed XC (cross-country-skiing) markers slightly uphill, heading in a northwesterly direction. Just over a half-mile in, pass a signed ski junction for the Beginner Loop, continuing straight. A quarter-mile later, ignore signs pointing the way to the Ridge Loop Trail and, immediately after, signs for the Swampy Tie.

The next half-mile provides a gentle downhill grade, and around 1.5 miles in, the trees open up just enough to provide glimpses into the Swampy Lakes area

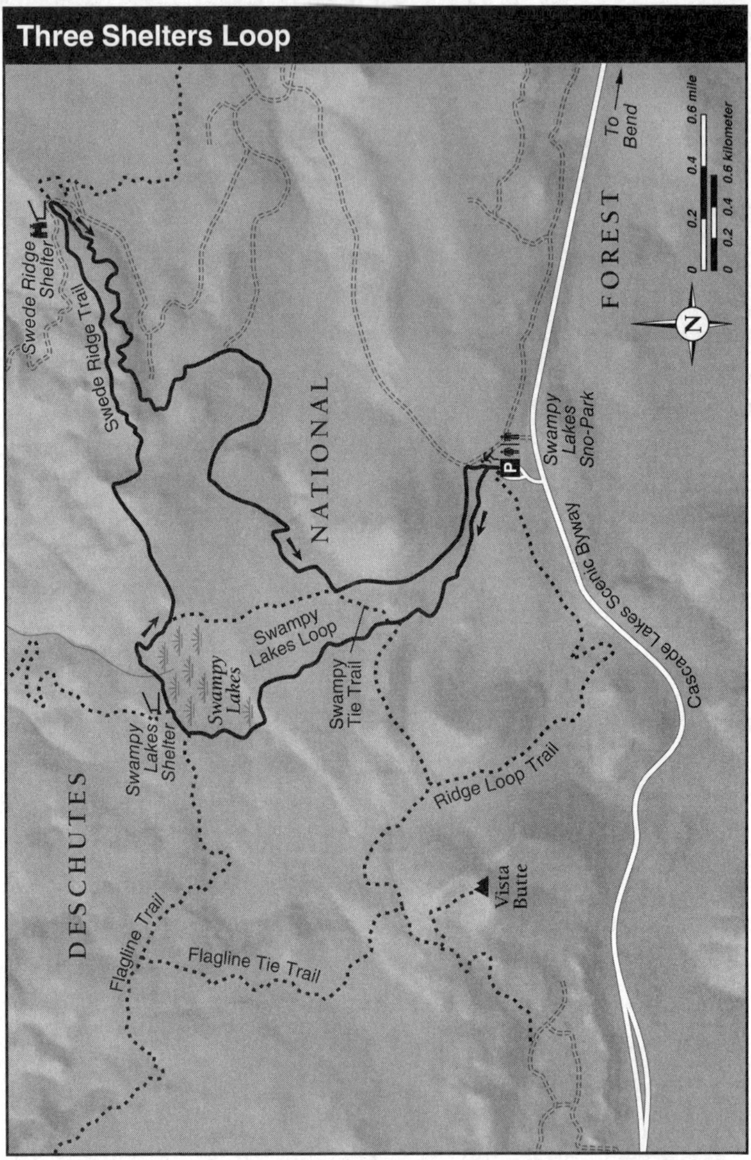

Three Shelters Loop

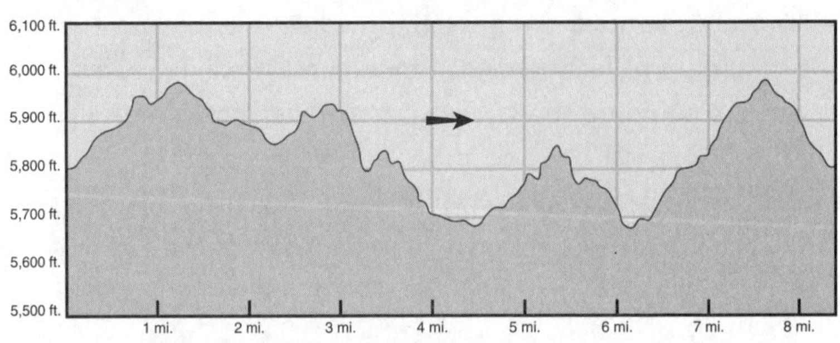

below and to your right. Though water is not always present, lush green grasses provide a pleasant respite from the dry, dusty trails and ponderosa pines. In early summer, be thankful you're running—any stops or breaks result in heavy mosquito swarms.

Near the bottom of the descent, cross several small streams to come upon signs for the Flagline Trail. Once again, ignore these and continue straight, meeting the Swampy Lakes shelter in 100 yards. Though not the most idyllic shelter, one can imagine the warmth a crackling fire would bring to cold fingers and toes in the winter months here.

From the shelter, continue straight on the Swampy Lakes Loop, keeping your eyes open for views of the meadows through the trees on your right. A short time later, cross a manageable stream and, at 2.5 miles, turn left at the signed junction for the Swede Ridge Trail. A series of short ups and downs gives way to a nice downhill at around 3 miles, through thick forests of pines and manzanita.

At 3.8 miles, emerge through the trees to wide open views of the Tumalo Valley and South Sister and Broken Top Mountains. Soon after, the Swede Ridge Shelter pops into view, and the singletrack spits you out onto a forest road bisecting the trail. Be sure to thoroughly check out the shelter here and, in particular, the views of the Cascades behind it. Once satisfied, make your way back up to the trail and look for an unmarked trail slightly up the road from whence you originally came.

The next stretch of trail features tight turns, quick ups and downs, and a fun bit of dodging and weaving through the trees. Keep straight (right) at an unmarked Y-junction around 5.8 miles, and soon after begin your steady, deceptive climb back toward the trailhead. At 7.5 miles, you encounter a four-way junction, where you'll turn left to return to the Swampy Lakes Loop. Fifty yards later, the singletrack empties onto an uneven, deeply rutted logging road, which takes you back to the final signed right turn back to the trailhead.

DIRECTIONS

From Bend, drive west on SW Century Drive, which becomes the Cascade Lakes National Scenic Byway toward Mount Bachelor. After 13.8 miles, turn right at the SWAMPY LAKES SNO-PARK sign, between Mile Markers 16 and 17, to reach the Swampy Lakes Trailhead.

26 Paulina Lake

TRAIL DETAILS AT A GLANCE

- **DISTANCE** 8.25-mile loop
- **GPS TRAILHEAD COORDINATES** N43° 42.727' W121° 16.542'
- **DIFFICULTY** 3 • **SCENERY** 7 • **CROWDS** 8
- **SEASON** May–October, sunrise–sunset • **ELEVATION** +/–680'
- **USERS** Hikers, runners • **CONTACT** Newberry National Volcanic Monument, 541-383-5700, **tinyurl.com/newberrynvm**
- **PERMITS/FEES** $5 day-use fee
- **RECOMMENDED MAP** *Bend, Oregon, Trail Map* by Adventure Maps, Inc. ($12, **adventuremaps.net**) • **DOGS** Yes (leashed only)

NEWBERRY NATIONAL VOLCANIC MONUMENT is a massive 500-square-mile volcano that features stunning scenery, beautiful alpine lakes, miles of basalt flows, and incredible rhyolite flows of obsidian. Designated a national monument in 1990, the area is a popular location for campers and recreationalists throughout the year and is about 45 minutes south of Bend.

The clear blue waters of picturesque Paulina Lake are the destination for this run. Sitting at an elevation of 6,340 feet on the western half of the 17-square-mile caldera, the lake is a must-see for the uninitiated and a quick favorite of those returning. The Paulina Lake Loop Trail circles the lake, hugging the shores in many areas while weaving in and out of ponderosa pines, open views, and rocky outcroppings.

The best place to begin the run is the day-use area, just after the turnoff for Paulina Lake Lodge as you enter the park. Start at the far end of the parking lot, near the edge of the campgrounds, running counterclockwise.

The well-maintained trail starts off meandering between the lakeshore and numerous campgrounds. After crossing a boat ramp, you'll notice signs of civilization begin to disappear as you enter the woods. Watch your feet during this section as the tempting blue waters beckon your glance while the numerous roots and rocky terrain beg to challenge your footwork.

At 1.4 miles, emerge from the solitude, passing a few campsites and a long, sandy beach. Shortly after, the trees disappear and the trail cuts through a swath of

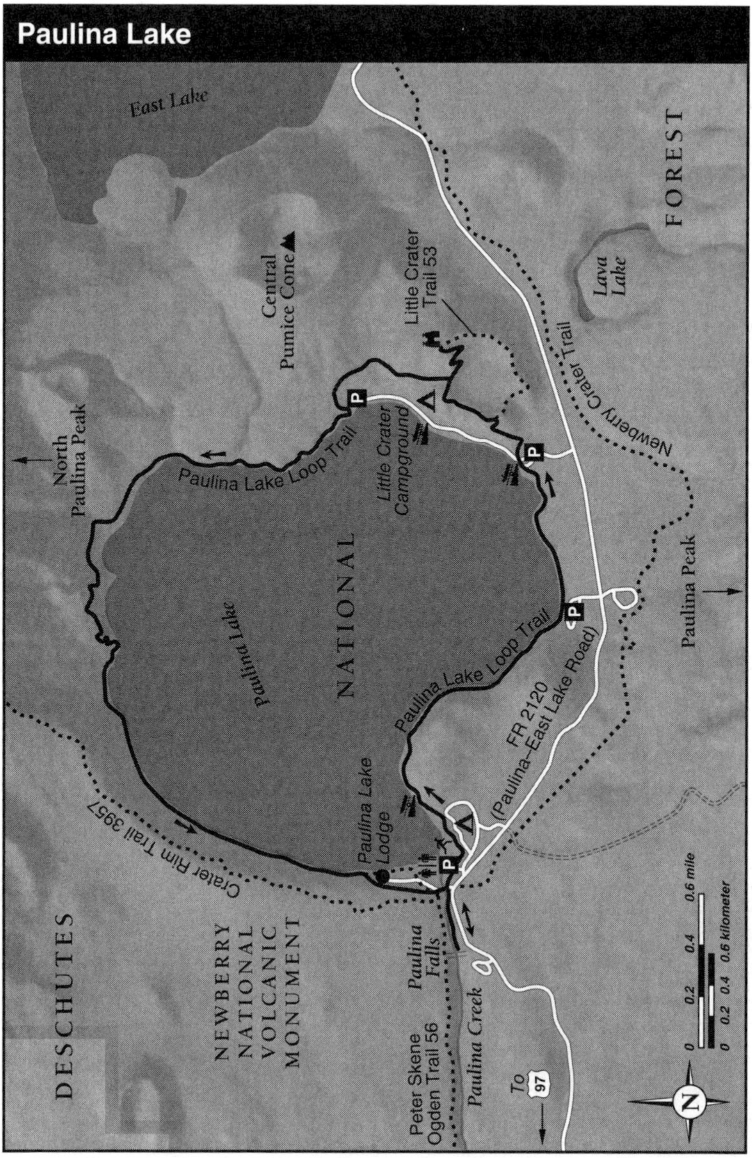

Paulina Lake

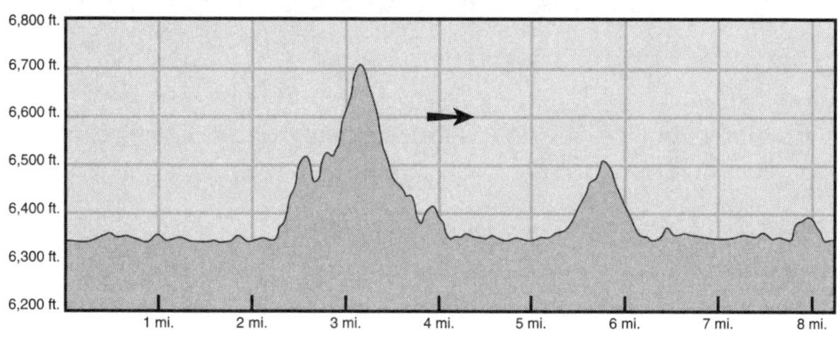

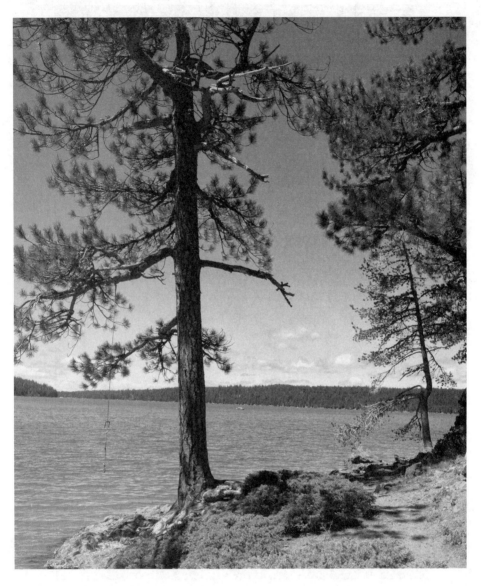

A rope swing dangling over the lake tempts runners to a take a dip on a hot day.

grasses with marshland to your right. A third of a mile later, watch for a faint trail to your right, which will allow you to bypass an inlet that cuts off the main trail.

Right at 2.0 miles, the trail dumps you onto a boat ramp. Here, the official Paulina Lake Loop Trail follows the road through Little Crater Campground to pick up on the far end. A more appealing diversion, however, is to turn right up the boat ramp, 25 yards to the trailhead for Little Crater Trail 53. This 1.5-mile loop trail allows you to bypass the campground and gain some outstanding views of the lake.

After you take the Little Crater Trail bypass, a steady climb brings you to the loop junction 0.3 mile from the trailhead. Though you can go in either direction, a left turn yields immediate views of Paulina Peak looming behind the lake. Continue in this direction until you reach a second junction in the loop 0.5 mile later. Turn right for a short, steep climb to a spectacular viewpoint of Paulina Lake and East Lake (the best views for the latter are slightly up the trail) and the Cascade mountains in the background. On clear days, views south reveal Mount Thielsen as well.

Once satisfied, return to the junction and take a right through a dense forest of pines back down to the opposite side of Little Crater Campground. A parking lot and large trailhead sign mark the continuation of the loop. The next mile of trail may be the best, with outstanding views of the lake and Paulina Peak while the trail hugs the rocky, pristine shore. At just under 4.5 miles, keep your eyes to the right, and soon you'll notice the glasslike, coal-colored obsidian rock underfoot. Be careful as you run through this area, as a fall onto the extremely sharp-edged obsidian can yield disastrous results.

At this point, the trail reenters the trees and begins to gain a bit of elevation as you continue around the lake. You'll notice boaters and anglers dotting the waterscape below. As you round the final corner, keep right at a fork in the trail at mile 7.25 to bypass the lodge and beaches. A short while later, the trail abruptly empties onto a logging road and trail junction to McKay Crossing—ignore the signs and turn left to find the bridge over Paulina Creek. If you're up for another side trip, just past the bridge on your right look for the trail to Paulina Falls, which is located a short half-mile down the creek. The falls are impressive and a worthwhile reason for extending your run. When finished, return the half-mile up the trail to the day-use area and your car.

DIRECTIONS

Travel south from Bend on US 97. After about 24 miles, look for signs for Newberry National Volcanic Monument and Paulina Lake. Turn left (east) on paved Paulina–East Lake Road (County Road 21/Forest Road 2120) and drive 13 miles until you reach Paulina Lake.

27 Patjens Lakes

TRAIL DETAILS AT A GLANCE

- **DISTANCE** 6.7-mile loop
- **GPS TRAILHEAD COORDINATES** N44° 22.647' W121° 52.843'
- **DIFFICULTY** 5 • **SCENERY** 7 • **CROWDS** 4
- **SEASON** June–October, sunrise–sunset • **ELEVATION** +/–619'
- **USERS** Hikers, runners, horses • **CONTACT** McKenzie River Ranger District, Willamette National Forest; 541-822-3381, **www.fs.usda.gov/willamette**
- **PERMITS/FEES** Northwest Forest Pass (see page 12) plus self-issued wilderness permit (free)
- **RECOMMENDED MAP** *Mount Jefferson and Mount Washington Trails Illustrated Topographic Map* by National Geographic ($11.95, **natgeomaps.com**) • **DOGS** Yes (leashed only)

DON'T LET THE FRENZY around the Patjens Lakes Trailhead fool you. Though the nearby campgrounds may be full, ATVs and dirtbikes within earshot, and water skiers visible off in the distance, all the clamor and noise stop and nature takes over within your first half-mile on this scenic and relatively easy loop.

The Patjens Lakes Loop hits three alpine lakes in addition to skirting several more ponds and the large and scenic Big Lake. Just south of 4,800-foot Santiam Pass, snow may linger into early summer and mosquitoes can be heavy in July, so be wary of any lakeside stops; better yet, visit in August or September.

After filling out your wilderness-use permit at the trailhead, begin your run through an open, burned forest area—a result of the 2003 B&B Complex fire. Scattered wildflowers dot the landscape in late July and throughout August. A quarter-mile from the trailhead, you'll hit the first junction and the start of the loop. The route described here runs clockwise.

Turn left at the junction and climb briefly before rounding a corner to see much of Big Lake laid out in front of you. The next half-mile provides stunning vistas while the trail parallels the lakeshore far below and Mount Washington looms over the water in the background. Ignore any side trails here—several pop up from the beaches below.

Past the lake, the trail weaves in and out of burned trees and wildflowers. Just after 2.5 miles, you'll begin to see the first lake through the trees to your right. It's well worth taking a break here and walking the sandy beach to the opposite side for a picture-perfect reflection of Mount Washington in the waters. Once satisfied,

Patjens Lakes

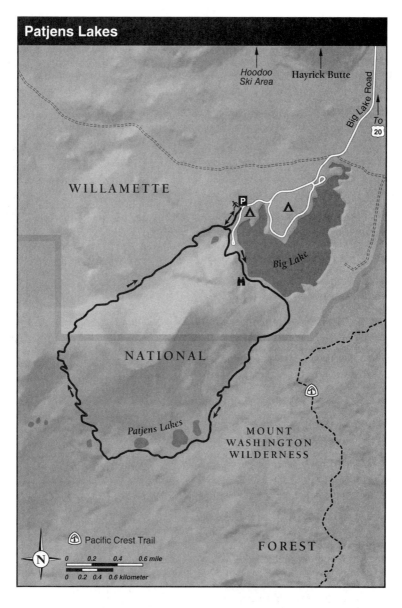

Hoodoo Ski Area
Hayrick Butte
Big Lake Road
To 20
WILLAMETTE
NATIONAL
FOREST
Big Lake
Patjens Lakes
MOUNT WASHINGTON WILDERNESS
Pacific Crest Trail
N
0 0.2 0.4 0.6 mile
0 0.2 0.4 0.6 kilometer

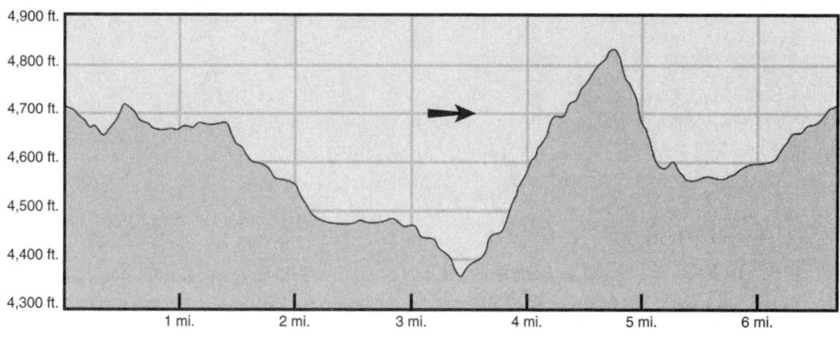

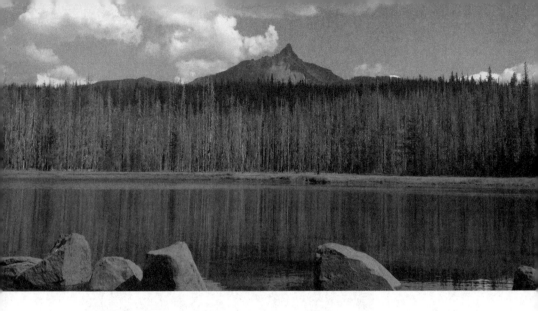

Mount Washington rises behind Patjens Lakes.

rejoin the trail, and within a quarter-mile you'll come to the second of the larger alpine lakes beside the trail. The path rounds the lake's contour briefly and passes several small meadows before ducking back into the pine-and-hemlock forest.

A short time later, a third lake begins to peek through the trees to your right. Several small trails provide an opportunity for further exploration and a brief reprieve in the shade. Back on the trail, duck in and out of the trees until the final Patjens Lake presents itself, this time on your left.

From here, begin a long, steady climb back out of the lakes area through a canopy of trees to eventually reenter the burn area and top out at 4,800 feet at mile 4.75. Be sure to glance behind you for nice views of Mount Washington and all three Sisters on the horizon. Meanwhile, Three Fingered Jack, Hoodoo Ski Area, and the very flat plateau of Hayrick Butte urge you forward.

A nice downhill over the next half-mile then flattens out for a relatively easy finish back to the loop junction at mile 6.5 and, a quarter-mile later, the Patjens Lake Trailhead and your starting point.

DIRECTIONS

From Bend, take US 20/OR 126 northwest to Santiam Pass. After about 38.5 miles, shortly after Mile Marker 80, turn left (south) toward Hoodoo Ski Area. Drive 4 miles on Big Lake Road to the trailhead, on the right about 0.5 mile after Big Lake Campground.

28 Canyon Creek Meadows

TRAIL DETAILS AT A GLANCE

- **DISTANCE** 6.6-mile loop
- **GPS TRAILHEAD COORDINATES** N44° 29.518' W121° 47.666'
- **DIFFICULTY** 6 • **SCENERY** 8 • **CROWDS** 7
- **SEASON** July–October, sunrise–sunset • **ELEVATION** +/–1,126'
- **USERS** Hikers, runners, horses • **CONTACT** McKenzie River Ranger District, Willamette National Forest; 541-822-3381, **www.fs.usda.gov/willamette**
- **PERMITS/FEES** Northwest Forest Pass (see page 12)
- **RECOMMENDED MAP** *Mount Jefferson and Mount Washington Trails Illustrated Topographic Map* by National Geographic ($11.95, **natgeomaps.com**) • **DOGS** Yes (leashed only)

FOR AN UP-CLOSE-AND-PERSONAL VIEW of Three Fingered Jack, Canyon Creek Meadows is your ticket. This popular route climbs to the base of the craggy mountain, through some of the state's most spectacular displays of wildflowers, and provides views of glaciers, meadows, and pristine mountain rivers in between. Few trails are able to get you up into the high alpine scenery quite as quickly as this one.

Due to the relatively short distance overall, Canyon Creek Meadows has become a popular area for many. So unless you're visiting during weekdays or in September, chances are you won't be alone. On the positive side, the Forest Service has helped to mitigate this somewhat by encouraging trail users to hike the route clockwise, reducing your chances of running into other users.

From the trailhead, veer right along Jack Lake, following signs distinguishing the main trail from side trails to the shore. As you make your way to the opposite end of the lake, you'll see Three Fingered Jack looming large over the water and the surrounding area. Make your way up the rocky trail through manzanita and pine snags caused from a fire in 2003. At 0.4 mile, you'll reach the beginning of the loop.

Keep left at the junction to stay clockwise and climb gradually uphill through the burn. As Three Fingered Jack urges you forward in front, Black Butte quietly bids you goodbye from a far-off ridge to your left. At 1.25 miles, run past a tarn and climb a short ways more before descending back through unburned pine and hemlock down to the top of the loop and your return point.

Canyon Creek Meadows

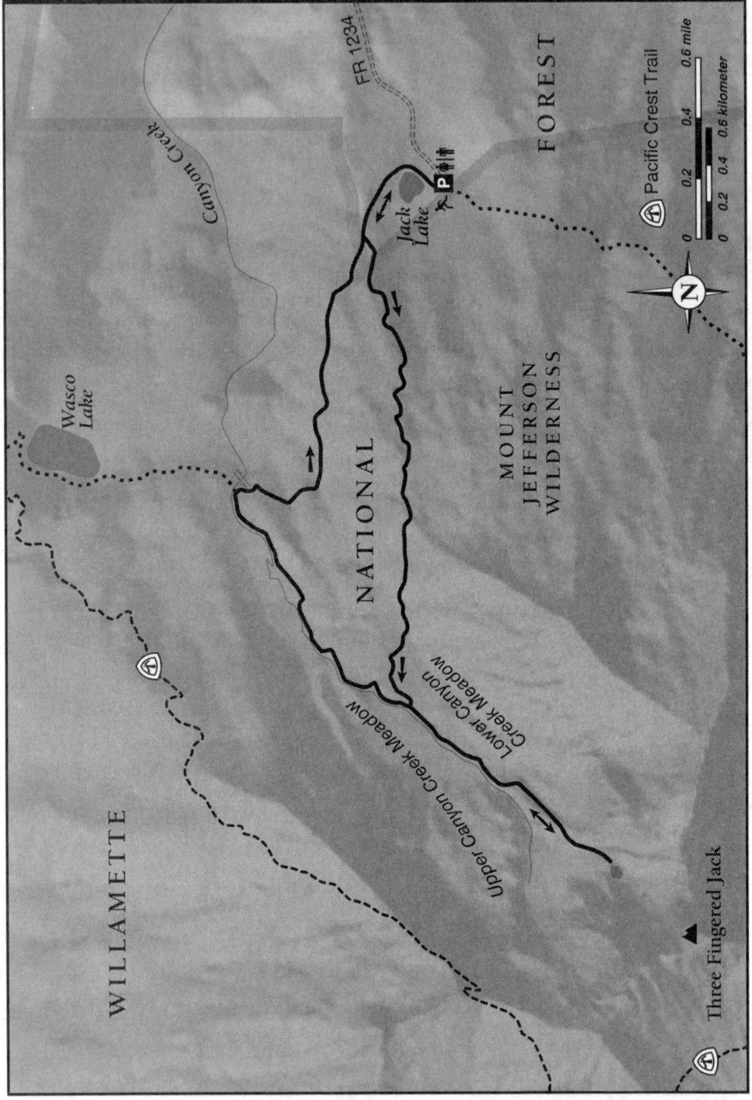

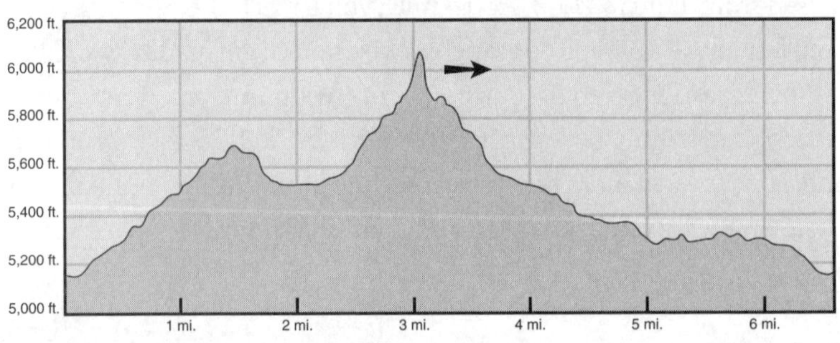

For now, continue left through a mostly flat area where you can hear the quiet murmur of Canyon Creek just beyond the grassy fields. Soon, your climb begins in earnest as the trail ducks in and out of the trees on its way up into Lower Canyon Creek Meadow. If you time your run in late July or early August, you'll soon be rewarded with gorgeous wildflowers spread through the meadow all around you. Lupine, subalpine daisies, and red paintbrush color the landscape and set the stage for your impending visit with Three Fingered Jack.

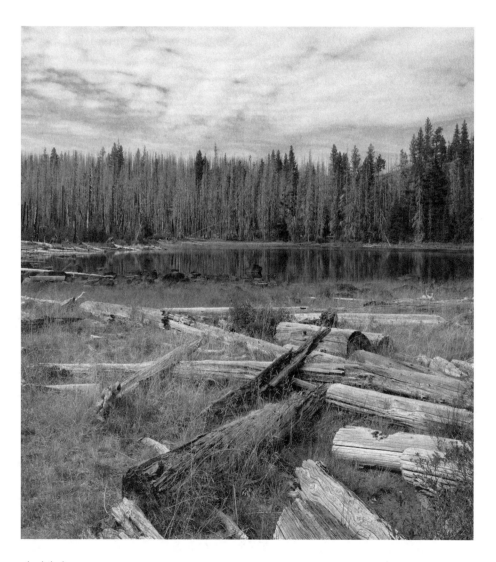

Jack Lake

Continue climbing and, after a brief jaunt back through the trees, Upper Canyon Creek Meadow appears below and to your right. Much larger than its sibling, the meadow spreads far and wide over a considerable distance. If you have the time, a number of side trails lead down the slopes, allowing further exploration. Remember to tread cautiously in alpine areas, and be mindful of where you're stepping.

As you emerge from the woods the final time, the trail splits off into a few directions. Most reconvene a short time later, so pick your route and make your way up to the saddle ahead of you. Once at the top, you'll be rewarded with impressive views of Three Fingered Jack immediately in front of you, along with an emerald-green cirque lake at the foot of a glacier on the mountain's flanks. A rough trail continues up along the ridgeline of the bowl for those who wish to take in even more. For those who do, impressive views to the north of Mount Jefferson and the Three Sisters await.

Once satisfied, carefully make your way down the rocky slopes and back onto firmer ground, returning to the last official junction. Here, at mile 3.9, make your return on the clockwise loop through both unspoiled and burned areas, following meandering Canyon Creek for the next mile. Around 4.5 miles, the trees open up to a marshy green meadow off to your left, and 0.4 mile later you reach the junction with Wasco Lake.

For those wishing to extend the run, Wasco Lake is a fairly flat 0.7 mile farther past the creek crossing. To finish the loop, keep right (straight) 1.1 miles back to the start of the loop and 0.4 mile back to your car. *Hint:* Just beyond the first curve on the return trail, you can see a lovely waterfall to your left.

DIRECTIONS

Drive 12 miles northwest of Sisters on US 20. Turn right just beyond Milepost 88, at the junction signed MT. JEFFERSON WILDERNESS TRAILHEADS, on Jack Lake Road/Forest Road 12. After about 1 mile, just past the four-way intersection with Suttle–Sherman Road/FR 1216, bear right at the Y-intersection, continue east on FR 12 another 3.4 miles, and follow signs indicating a left turn onto one-lane paved FR 1230 toward Jack Lake. After 1.6 miles, near Jack Creek Campground, veer left as the pavement ends onto gravel FR 1234—ignore the signs for Bear Valley and keep left. Stay on FR 1234 for 6 rough miles of tight turns and washboards to the Jack Lake parking lot.

29 Duffy Lake

TRAIL DETAILS AT A GLANCE

- **DISTANCE** 12.3-mile double loop
- **GPS TRAILHEAD COORDINATES** N44° 29.466' W121° 57.001'
- **DIFFICULTY** 7 • **SCENERY** 6 • **CROWDS** 6
- **SEASON** July–October, sunrise–sunset • **ELEVATION** +/–1,840'
- **USERS** Hikers, runners, horses • **CONTACT** McKenzie River Ranger District, Willamette National Forest; 541-822-3381, **www.fs.usda.gov/willamette**
- **PERMITS/FEES** Northwest Forest Pass (see page 12)
- **RECOMMENDED MAP** *Mount Jefferson and Mount Washington Trails Illustrated Topographic Map* by National Geographic ($11.95, **natgeomaps.com**) • **DOGS** Yes (leashed only)

THE CENTRAL OREGON CASCADES are filled with beautiful, clear lakes hidden deep within the forests. Most of these tranquil places rarely get visited because of location, but for those ardent souls who choose to venture beyond a few miles from the main roads and trailheads, rewards await aplenty.

The west side of Three Fingered Jack is one such place. Easily accessible from a short, paved road off of US 20, this run accesses the popular Duffy and Mowich Lakes, along with a few other less visited areas in two interconnected loops.

From the trailhead parking lot, run through a thick mixed-conifer forest to a junction with Big Meadows Horse Camp at less than 0.2 mile. If you'd like to do both loops, turn left here and descend a rough, rocky trail a half-mile before encountering a second junction. Following signs toward the Turpentine Trail, turn right and gradually gain back the elevation from the short downhill. Around the first mile marker, you'll encounter your first crossing of the North Santiam River. Though passable in late summer and bone dry in the fall, the river can be wide and difficult in early summer, so be prepared to rock-hop or get your feet wet.

Soon after the crossing, stay right at another junction to continue toward Turpentine. The trail here is in poor shape, with lots of large rocks, roots, and natural steps to make running difficult. The scenery in this area is nothing to write home about either, so as you're carefully watching your footing, know that you're not missing much around you.

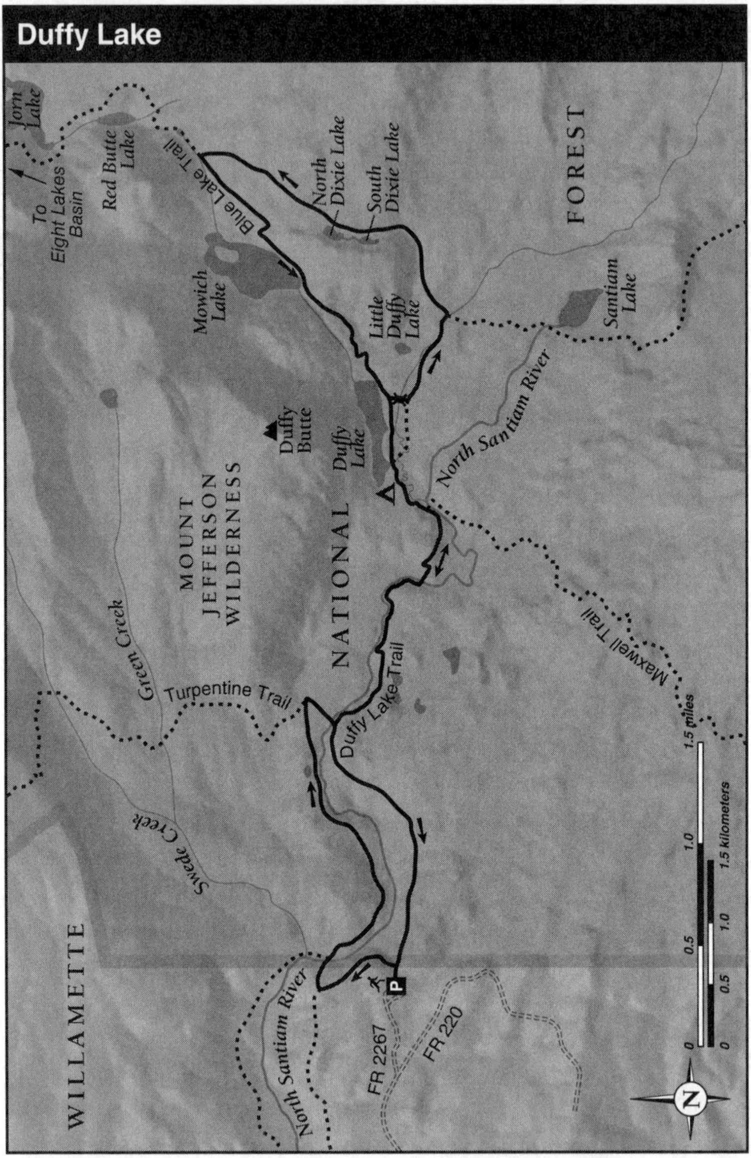

Duffy Lake
Jorn Lake
Red Butte Lake
To Eight Lakes Basin
Blue Lake Trail
North Dixie Lake
South Dixie Lake
FOREST
Mowich Lake
Little Duffy Lake
Santiam Lake
Duffy Butte
Duffy Lake
North Santiam River
MOUNT JEFFERSON WILDERNESS
NATIONAL
Green Creek
Turpentine Trail
Duffy Lake Trail
Maxwell Trail
Swede Creek
WILLAMETTE
North Santiam River
FR 2267
FR 220
P
0
0.5
1.0
1.5 miles
0
0.5
1.0
1.5 kilometers
N

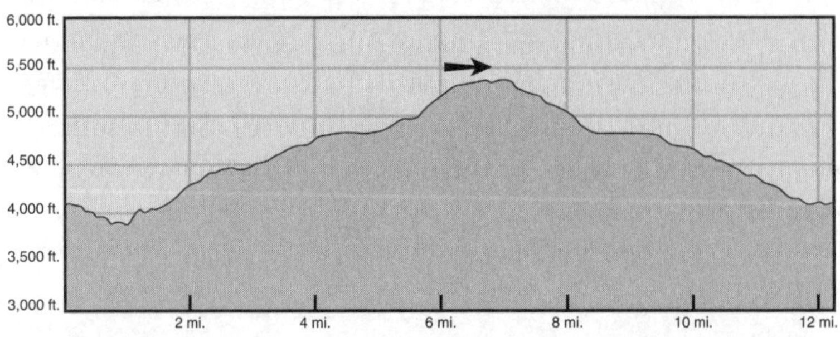

6,000 ft.
5,500 ft.
5,000 ft.
4,500 ft.
4,000 ft.
3,500 ft.
3,000 ft.
2 mi.
4 mi.
6 mi.
8 mi.
10 mi.
12 mi.

A brief respite comes at 2.2 miles, when you pass by a pretty pond before continuing uphill. At mile 2.6, turn right at the junction to complete the first loop. Be forewarned here, as the trail signs are old and rickety and are often barely hanging on to the tree in which they're tied. From here, it's a short jaunt—and one more river crossing—before the trail intersects the Duffy Lake Trail at mile 2.8.

At this point, the trail vastly improves, turning from narrow and overgrown with difficult footing to a wide, unmistakable footpath. Make your way up the nicer trail paralleling the river before crossing it at 3.9 miles. Continue past the Maxwell Trail junction at 4.3 miles and, 0.3 mile later, encounter a confusing intersection marking the presence of Duffy Lake. Choose the path ahead and to the right, toward the Santiam Lake pointer. Campsites and designated areas soon identify themselves when Duffy Lake emerges on your left. As you cross an attractive log bridge, you'll get a great view of the two-peaked Duffy Butte across the waters.

At the next junction, turn right toward Santiam Lake to begin the second loop. In 0.5 mile, follow the signed junction for Eight Lakes Basin before descending downhill and crossing a lovely, open meadow. Once back in the trees, begin a short but steep uphill over the next 0.5 mile before leveling out in the burned woods from the 2003 B&B Complex fire.

Around 6.3 miles, keep your eyes peeled for the lovely Dixie Lakes, both of which are worth checking out. North Dixie Lake in particular proves its scenic worth with Duffy Butte in the backdrop. At 7.1 miles, hit the final corner of the second loop at the intersection with the Blue Lake Trail. Begin your return route, and, in a quick mile, Mowich Lake presents itself around a corner. The largest lake in the vicinity, Mowich is well worth exploring and is also a great option for a midrun swim.

Once satisfied, run gradually downhill as you pass by the head of Duffy Lake and more familiar territory. Retrace your footsteps from here until the junction with the Turpentine Trail, which you'll ignore this time around, and continue straight to return to the trailhead via the Duffy Lake Trail.

DIRECTIONS

Drive northwest from Sisters on US 20/OR 126 for about 26 miles. At Santiam Junction, keep right at the large Y-intersection to continue on North Santiam Highway/OR 22. After 5.8 miles, immediately after Mile Marker 76, turn right onto paved Big Meadows Road. In 2.6 miles, turn left at the fork and drive a rough 0.3 mile on dirt to the Duffy Lake Trailhead.

30 Eight Lakes Basin

TRAIL DETAILS AT A GLANCE

- **DISTANCE** 15.3-mile loop
- **GPS TRAILHEAD COORDINATES** N44° 34.610' W121° 53.664'
- **DIFFICULTY** 9 • **SCENERY** 9 • **CROWDS** 4
- **SEASON** July–October, sunrise–sunset • **ELEVATION** +/–2,546'
- **USERS** Hikers, runners, horses • **CONTACT** McKenzie River Ranger District, Willamette National Forest; 541-822-3381, **www.fs.usda.gov/willamette**
- **PERMITS/FEES** Northwest Forest Pass (see page 12)
- **RECOMMENDED MAP** *Mount Jefferson and Mount Washington Trails Illustrated Topographic Map* by National Geographic ($11.95, **natgeomaps.com**) • **DOGS** Yes (leashed only)

MARION LAKE AND THE EIGHT LAKES BASIN are steeped in tradition. Ask many native Central Oregonians where they took their first backpacking trip or held their annual family campout, and more than likely many would name one of these places. Though much has changed over the years, including the removal of the beloved Forest Service cabin and rowboats on Marion Lake, the scenery remains as beautiful as ever.

For hardy trail-runners, the whole area makes for a spectacular loop. Difficult as it may be, the pristine alpine lakes, picturesque mountain streams, stunning vistas, and diversity from deep old-growth forests to flowering new growth in the burn help negate the distance and elevation.

Begin the loop at the Marion Lake Trailhead, about 4.5 miles down Forest Road 2255 (Marion Creek Road). The first 1.5 miles follow a well-trod path that climbs gradually through beautiful old-growth forests complete with a few tiny burbling streams that are easily stepped over. The trail then levels briefly before crossing the rocky outlet of Lake Ann. Though you can hear the water running beneath the rocks, it's completely hidden and out of sight. Run along the edge of the lake, following the trail another 0.25 mile to the junction with Marion Lake Outlet Trail 3495. Veer right on this trail and climb 0.1 mile to an unmarked side trail. For those adventurers, this meandering path takes you to Marion Falls, 0.3 mile away. It's a worthy side trip, but in order to catch a good view of the impressive falls, you have to do some scrambling.

Eight Lakes Basin

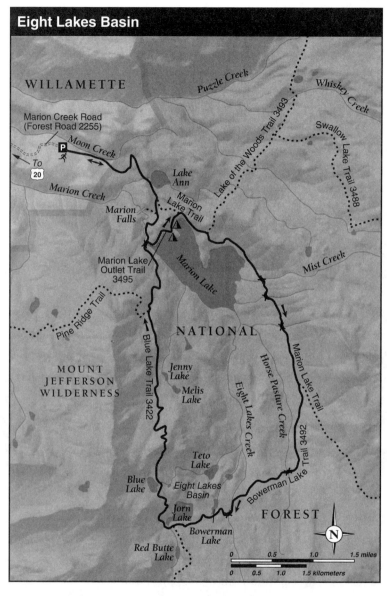

WILLAMETTE
NATIONAL
FOREST
MOUNT JEFFERSON WILDERNESS
Marion Creek Road (Forest Road 2255)
To 20
Moon Creek
Puzzle Creek
Whiskey Creek
Swallow Lake Trail 3488
Lake of the Woods Trail 3493
Lake Ann
Marion Creek
Marion Falls
Marion Lake Trail
Marion Lake Outlet Trail 3495
Marion Lake
Mist Creek
Pine Ridge Trail
Blue Lake Trail 3422
Jenny Lake
Melis Lake
Eight Lakes Creek
Horse Pasture Creek
Marion Lake Trail 3492
Teto Lake
Blue Lake
Eight Lakes Basin
Jorn Lake
Bowerman Lake Trail
Bowerman Lake
Red Butte Lake
N
0 0.5 1.0 1.5 miles
0 0.5 1.0 1.5 kilometers

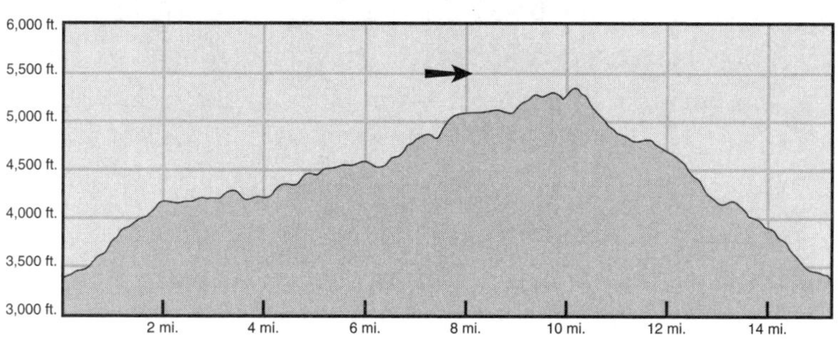

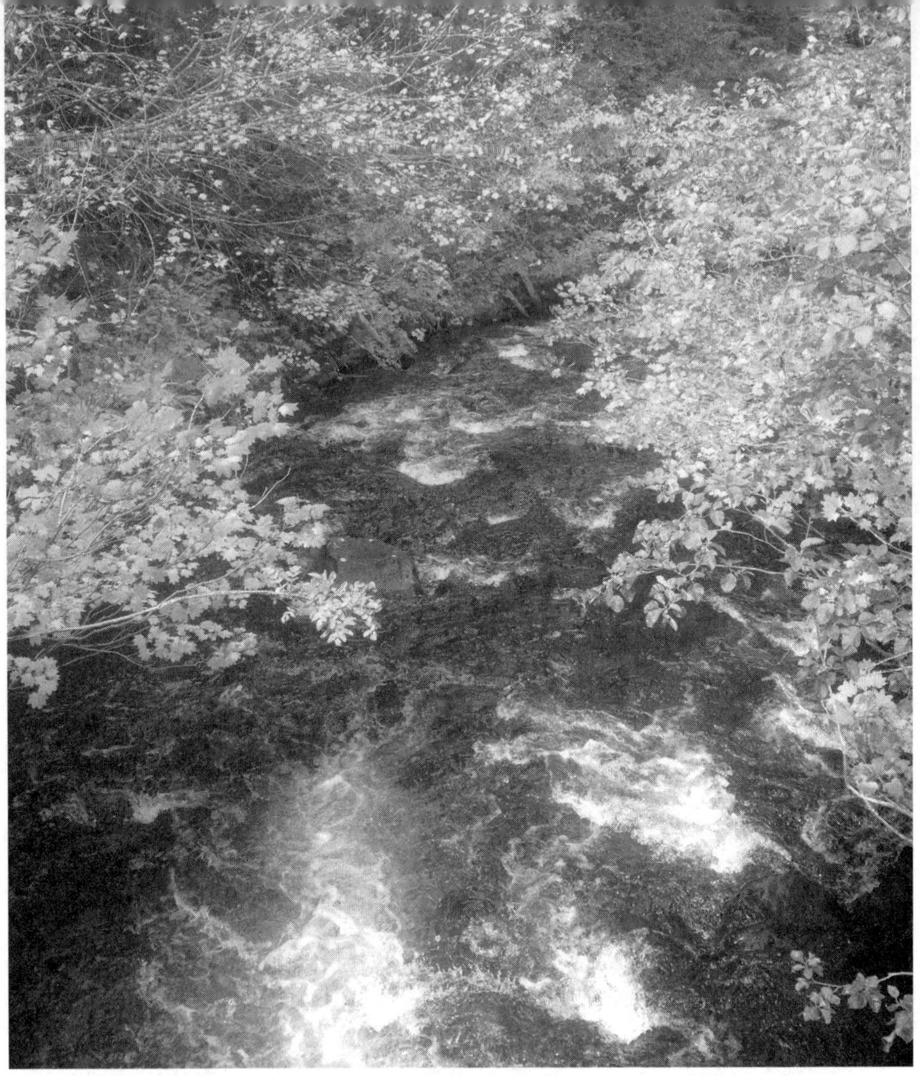

Marion Lake's outlet

Back on the trail, run toward the sound of the river, and soon you're ambling along the rushing waters. At 2.3 miles, the river's outlet and Marion Lake can be seen at the junction with the Blue Lake Trail 3422—this will be your return on the loop. For now, turn left to continue following the Marion Lake Outlet Trail as it hugs the contours of the lakeshore. Around 2.7 miles, a rocky outcropping on the lake's peninsula offers a great view of Three Fingered Jack on the opposite end.

Just under 3 miles and many campsites later, the trail Ts with the (unmarked) Marion Lake Trail. This is the former site of the Forest Service cabin, taken down many years ago but still standing proud in the minds of many Central Oregonians.

Turn right here to continue following the shore of the lake. Views of Three Fingered Jack continue to be outstanding as you run up the northeastern side.

At 3.4 miles, ignore the junction with the Lake of the Woods Trail 3493, keeping right. A short time later, cross a series of bridges and quaint wooden walkways over a creek and subsequent marshy patch. Marion Lake's many inlets begin to appear over the next mile as you rock-hop and log-jump many of these picturesque streams—some larger than others. At 4.4 miles, cross the largest creek on a log bridge, and soon the trail enters the burn area from the 2003 B&B Complex fire. Continue climbing gradually through the burn and turn right at the next junction to start on the Bowerman Lake Trail 3492.

The next 2.5 miles are difficult ones. Though pretty at points, with pearly everlasting lining much of the trail, running through the burn also means lots of sun exposure, overgrown paths, and fallen snags obscuring the trail. Make your way carefully up the long, steady climb until finally the trail begins to flatten around 8 miles. Reenter the woods, and soon the beauty of the Eight Lakes Basin is upon you.

At 8.25 miles, Bowerman Lake provides a stunning backdrop with Mount Jefferson sitting on the horizon behind it. Be sure to explore behind and on the other side of this lake as well, as many more bodies of water are hidden in the area (along with some well-coveted camping spots).

Once back on the trail, a quick half-mile later takes you to Jorn Lake, an even more impressive mountain lake with spectacular views of Mount Jefferson on one side and Three Fingered Jack on the other. Rogue paths descend from the main trail to camping areas and views along the shore. On the main trail, as you round the head of Jorn Lake, turn right at the junction to stay on the Blue Lake Trail (opposite the DUFFY LAKE TRAILHEAD pointer) at 8.8 miles.

From the junction, the scenery continues to impress as you make your way around Jorn Lake and climb the rocky trail on the west side. Soon, Three Fingered Jack and the long, burned valley you recently climbed begin to appear in view. At 9.5 miles, Blue Lake presents itself to the left of the trail, along with wildflowers such as buttercup and aster at your feet and Mount Jefferson pulling you forward in the distance. Round another corner to see Teto Lake down and to your right before zagging back the opposite way to see the continuation of Blue Lake. Multiple smaller, unnamed lakes can also be seen.

After a brief descent, the trail again climbs until you finally top out at 5,359 feet at 10.2 miles. From this rocky saddle, you can see Marion Lake and Mount

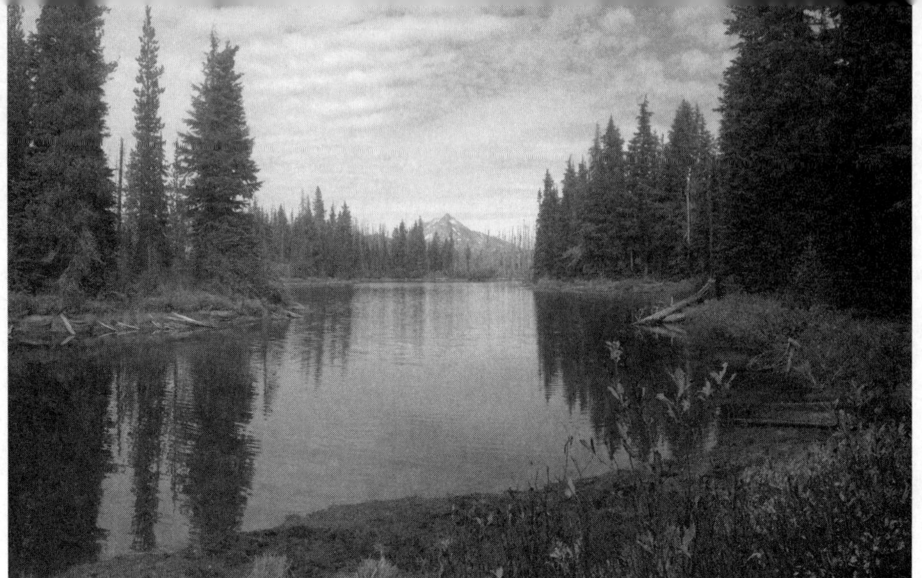

Mount Jefferson behind Bowerman Lake

Jefferson in front of you and Three Fingered Jack, along with many of the lakes you just passed, behind you. If you feel like you need a breather at this point, rest assured it's a wonderful place to soak in the views.

From here, the trail begins to work its way downhill through the burn—all the while with wonderful views of Mount Jefferson to the north. Eventually, the forest begins to reappear and, around 11.4 miles, Jenny Lake's blue waters can be seen from the trail. Continue downhill, passing the junction with the Pine Ridge Trail at 12.1 miles until Marion Lake once again makes itself known below the trail and to your right. Just before 13 miles, run carefully through a rocky section and cross the earlier bridge over Marion Creek to complete your loop. Keep left along the same Marion Outlet Trail and retrace your footsteps the 2.25 miles back to the trailhead and your car.

DIRECTIONS

From Bend, drive northwest on US 20 for 43.7 miles and keep straight at the Y-junction to merge on OR 22. After 1.9 miles, at Mile Marker 76 just beyond the fish hatchery, turn right on Marion Creek Road/Forest Road 2255 on the single-lane paved road. After 0.7 mile, pass through a gate and drive on the well-graded gravel road another 3.8 miles—keep right at mile 2.8 and then left at mile 3.4 to stay on FR 2255—to the trailhead parking lot, on the right.

31 Clear Lake

TRAIL DETAILS AT A GLANCE

- **DISTANCE** 4.8-mile loop
- **GPS TRAILHEAD COORDINATES** N44° 22.459' W121° 59.919'
- **DIFFICULTY** 2 • **SCENERY** 6 • **CROWDS** 8
- **SEASON** May–November, sunrise–sunset • **ELEVATION** +/–65'
- **USERS** Hikers, runners, mountain bikers • **CONTACT** McKenzie River Ranger District, Willamette National Forest; 541-822-3381, **www.fs.usda.gov/willamette**
- **PERMITS/FEES** Northwest Forest Pass (see page 12)
- **RECOMMENDED MAP** *Sisters & Redmond High Desert Trail Map* by Adventure Maps, Inc. ($12, **adventuremaps.net**) • **DOGS** Yes (leashed only)

CLEAR LAKE IS APTLY NAMED. Known for its deep, crystal-clear waters, the lake is the origin of the famed McKenzie River—arguably one of Oregon's most pristine and beautiful rivers. The lake itself is so clear that many of the ancient snags at the bottom are still visible more than 100 feet below the surface. Fed by numerous springs, the lake was originally created when the south end dammed up from the Sand Mountain lava flows more than 3,000 years ago.

The loop around Clear Lake is a gentle one with scenery ranging from old-growth forests to lava flows, deep blue springs, and even a quaint, rustic resort and campground. An additional 2.6-mile side loop around the nearby Sahalie and Koosah Falls makes extending the run into a 7.4-mile loop a very tempting one. Be cautious of other trail users during the summer months, because the lake is a popular camping and day-use spot.

To start the loop, park at the picnic area just before the resort. The trailhead is just in front of the log picnic shelter—a Civilian Conservation Corps project from the 1930s. From the trailhead, run counterclockwise on Clear Lake Trail 4341, starting out on a nice, even path shaded by old-growth ponderosa pines. In a quarter-mile, cross a small creek over a quaint log bridge before continuing on the wide dirt path. Just shy of the first mile, a sturdy bridge takes you over the beginnings of the McKenzie River—already a high-volume rushing river as it exits the lake.

Just beyond the bridge, reach the junction with the McKenzie River Trail. To add the 2.6-mile loop, keep right to follow the McKenzie downriver, but if you're

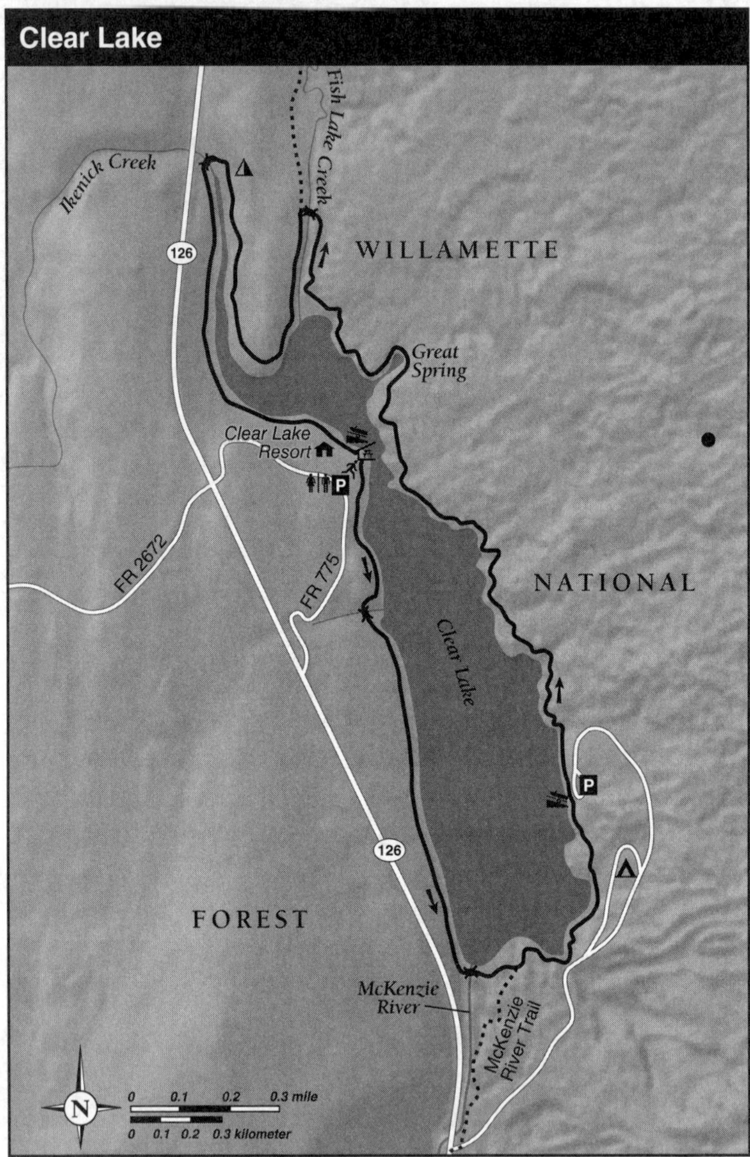

sticking to the main loop, turn left and proceed over the exposed tree roots that line the trail. Within 0.3 mile, the trail begins to enter the camping area and a short time later turns to pavement and then lava rock. After crossing a boat ramp, this pattern repeats itself once more before returning to dirt.

At 1.9 miles, cross a large lava rockslide and be cautious of your footing as the path begins to get more technical. For the next mile, the trail weaves around the

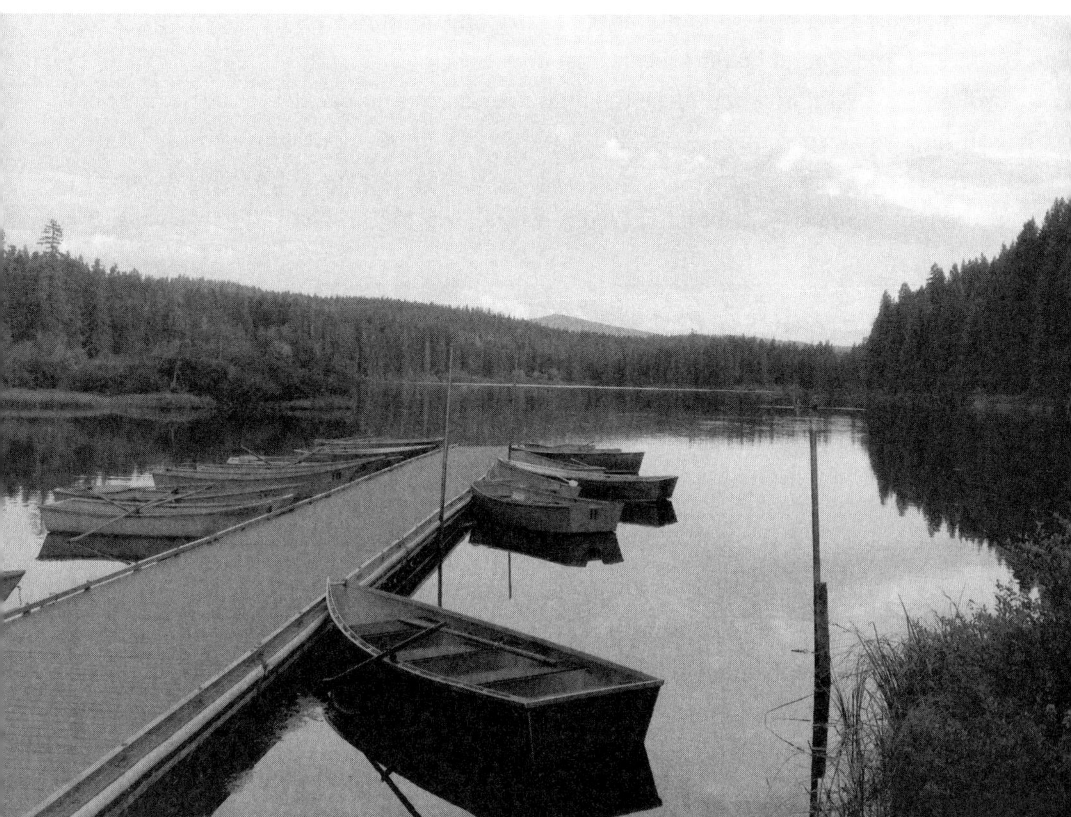

Boat dock at Clear Lake Resort

lake's contours, switching back and forth between shaded dirt trail and lava rock. As you run along the shores, it's easy to become mesmerized by the deep, blue waters of Clear Lake. The clarity of the lake also lends itself to being a popular dive spot, though the year-round frigid temperatures require divers to wear thickly lined suits. At 2.8 miles, a tight corner takes you around Great Spring—a brilliant-aquamarine spring and one of the feeder springs that forms the lake itself.

As you round the south end of Clear Lake, the trail once again meanders through dense old-growth forest. Cross the well-constructed Fish Creek bridge at 3.25 miles and immediately hit a T-junction on the other side. Turn left to again join Clear Lake Trail 4341 and follow Fish Creek (typically dry aside from a brief spring flow) back to the lake. Keep your eyes peeled to the horizon as you approach the lake for outstanding views of the Cascades directly opposite you.

From here, the trail follows the U-shaped contour of the lake before jutting back up and around Ikenick Creek. Just after the crossing, run through a rogue (but nicely kept) campsite and make the final turn as you run parallel to the nearby but unseen highway. A quick 0.6 mile later, the trail empties onto a paved road lined with rustic cabins. Follow this road past the cabins and the store (where you can also rent rowboats for a better view of the lake) back to the start and the picnic area.

DIRECTIONS

From Bend, drive northwest on US 20 for 43.7 miles. At Santiam Junction, bear left at the Y-junction to stay on US 20/OR 126 toward Eugene (straight turns into OR 22 toward Salem). About 3 miles later, US 20 and OR 126 split; turn left (south) to continue on OR 126/McKenzie Highway. Drive 3.8 miles and, just before Milepost 4, look for the signs for Willamette National Forest and Clear Lake Resort on your left. The parking area is 0.4 mile down the paved side road.

Footbridge across Fish Creek

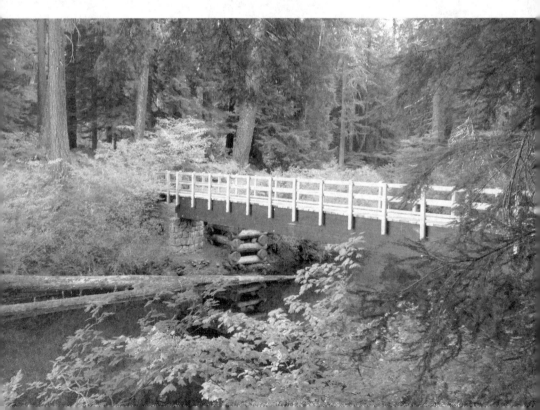

32 Iron Mountain

TRAIL DETAILS AT A GLANCE

- **DISTANCE** 6.5-mile loop
- **GPS TRAILHEAD COORDINATES** N44° 23.706' W122° 8.431'
- **DIFFICULTY** 8 • **SCENERY** 7 • **CROWDS** 6
- **SEASON** June–October, sunrise–sunset • **ELEVATION** +/–1,790'
- **USERS** Hikers, runners • **CONTACT** Sweet Home Ranger District, Willamette National Forest; 541-367-5168, **www.fs.usda.gov/willamette**
- **PERMITS/FEES** Northwest Forest Pass (see page 12)
- **RECOMMENDED MAP** *Mount Jefferson and Mount Washington Trails Illustrated Topographic Map* by National Geographic ($11.95, **natgeomaps.com**) • **DOGS** Yes (leashed only)

THE CASCADE RANGE IS KNOWN for its high volcanic peaks and open vistas. Mountains such as Hood, Jefferson, the Three Sisters, and Broken Top shine with their peaks adorned by glaciers and their profiles distinct against blue skies. These young mountains, technically part of the High Cascades, owe their stature to eons of hard work amassed by the Old Cascades. The foundation of the Cascade Range, the Old Cascades form the base from which the High Cascades rise, with most peaks in the lower-elevation ranges of 4,000–5,000 feet.

Iron Mountain is arguably the king of the Old Cascades in Oregon, and for good reason. Panoramic vistas and a spectacularly diverse ecosystem that includes more tree types than anywhere else in the state, along with nearly 60 plant species unique to the area, help this mountain stand above the rest. The icing on the cake, however, is the 300 different varieties of wildflowers that grow in the vicinity—from white bear grass and cat's-ear to red paintbrush and pink Washington lily and purple cliff penstemon.

The area's splendor makes it one of the most popular hiking destinations in the Old Cascades. For trail runners, this loop is spectacular, but you certainly work for the scenery, with nearly 2,000 feet of elevation gain in 6.5 miles.

To begin the run, park at the trailhead, 37 miles west of Sisters on US 20 just beyond the summit for Tombstone Pass between Mileposts 63 and 64. The trail begins by the message board at the far end of the parking lot, where it veers off from the old Santiam Wagon Road and into the old-growth forest below. After

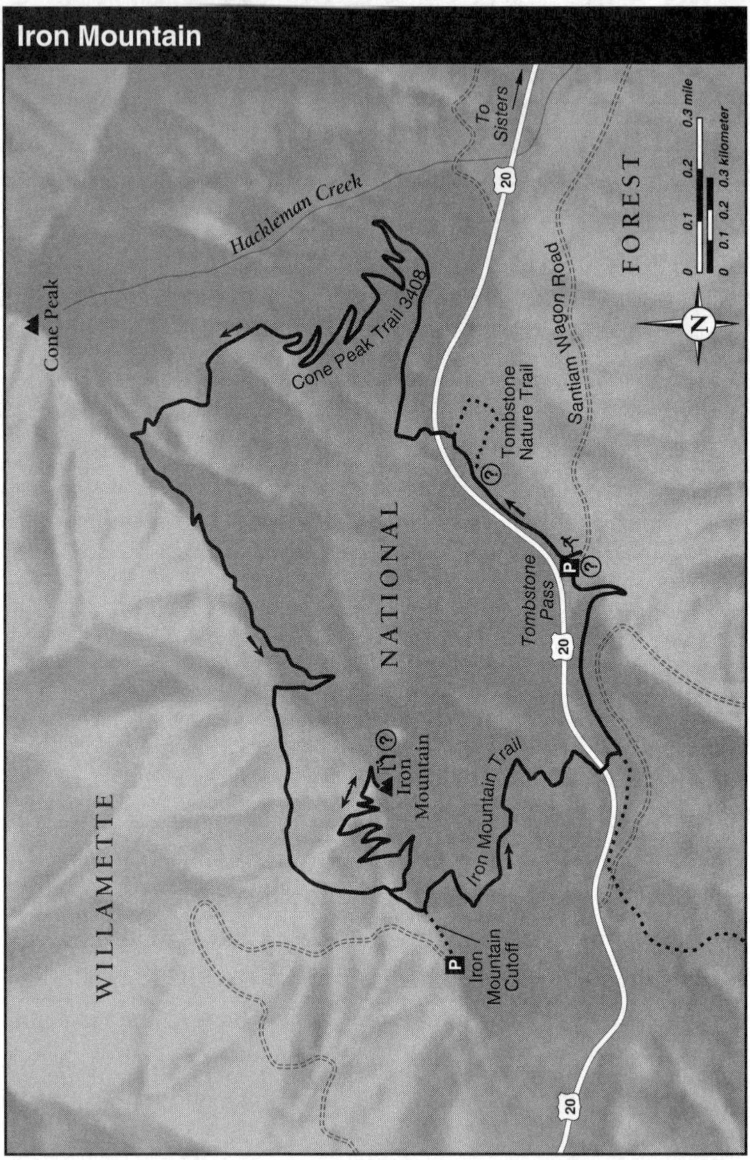

Iron Mountain

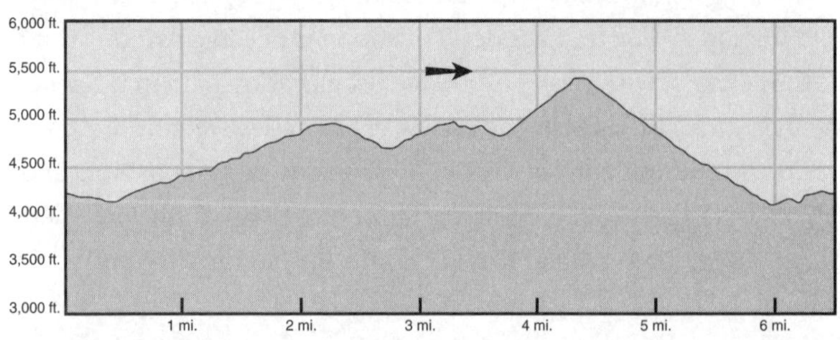

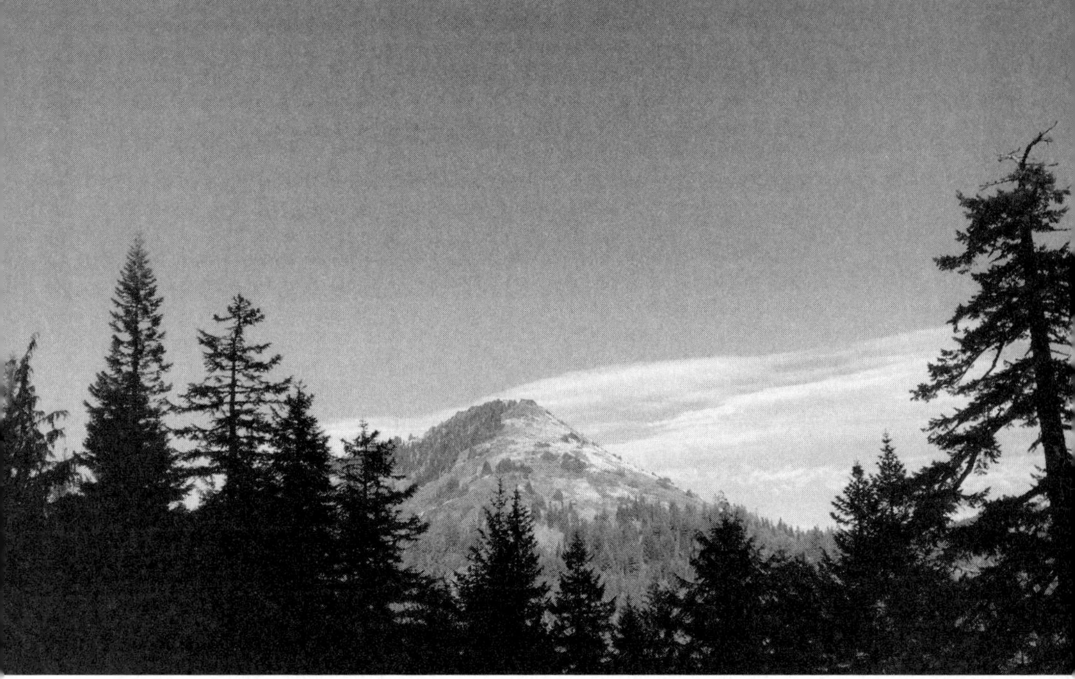

Cone Peak

0.3 mile, ignore the marker for the Tombstone Nature Trail and continue along Cone Peak Trail 3408. Soon after, carefully cross back over US 20 and look for the continuation of the trail up and across the highway 10 yards up.

From here, the trail begins a relentless uphill through the old growth via steep trails and several switchbacks. About 1.5 miles in, views of Echo Mountain, South Peak, and Cone Peak begin to open as you run through colorful fields of wildflowers. Iron Mountain soon becomes visible, and the trail levels out as you run back west across the saddle between Cone Peak and Iron Mountain. The next 1.5 miles are pleasant, with small, rolling hills as you make your way around the flanks of Iron Mountain.

At 3.67 miles, turn left at the signed junction for the Iron Mountain Trail and the summit. Run up the rocky, exposed switchbacks to the former fire lookout site where a sturdy deck and viewing platform now stand. Interpretive signs around the viewing deck describe the area's rich plant diversity, along with the geologic history of Iron Mountain. The present-day mountain was formed during the last two million years by the advancing and retreating of massive ice sheets, which removed much of the volcanic strata and exposed the magnesium and olivine, which give the area its reddish color.

More impressive than the area's history, however, are the 360-degree views. On clear days, the Cascades' major peaks can all be seen, from as far north as Mount Adams to Diamond Peak in the south. You'll be thankful for the many reasons to stop and catch your breath as well, as you've gained approximately 1,750 feet of elevation in less than 4.5 miles.

From the summit, carefully retrace your steps down the steep grade and turn left at the junction onto the Iron Mountain Trail. Ignore the side trail a short time later for the Iron Mountain Cutoff and Trailhead, and continue running down the steep but runnable downhill toward the Deer Creek Trailhead. At 5.9 miles, carefully cross US 20 once again and, shortly after, turn left at the signed junction toward Santiam Wagon Road and Tombstone Pass. Complete the loop and find the parking lot 0.5 mile later.

DIRECTIONS

From Sisters, take US 20 West to Santiam Pass, bearing left at the Y-junction to stay on US 20/OR 126 toward Sweet Home. About 37 miles from Sisters, look for the trailhead turnoff on your left, between Mileposts 63 and 64 near the summit of Tombstone Pass.

33 Scott Lake

TRAIL DETAILS AT A GLANCE

- **DISTANCE** 9.7-mile loop
- **GPS TRAILHEAD COORDINATES** N44° 12.846' W121° 53.585'
- **DIFFICULTY** 7 • **SCENERY** 7 • **CROWDS** 5
- **SEASON** July–October, sunrise–sunset • **ELEVATION** +/–1,514'
- **USERS** Hikers, runners • **CONTACT** McKenzie River Ranger District, Willamette National Forest; 541-822-3381, **www.fs.usda.gov/willamette**
- **PERMITS/FEES** Northwest Forest Pass (see page 12)
- **RECOMMENDED MAP** *Mount Jefferson and Mount Washington Trails Illustrated Topographic Map* by National Geographic ($11.95, **natgeomaps.com**) • **DOGS** Yes (leashed only)

SCOTT LAKE SITS AT AN ELEVATION of roughly 4,800 feet on the west side of McKenzie Pass. Reflected in its waters are spectacular views of North and Middle Sister. Popular with campers in August (and mosquitoes in July), the lake is the starting point for a running loop connecting a handful of subalpine lakes, along with a short detour to the open, wildflower-dotted summit of Scott Mountain overlooking the area in all directions. The lake itself is a worthy destination, too, so if you have the time, try camping the night before or after your run.

To begin the clockwise loop, start from the Scott Lake parking lot and take Benson Trail 3502. The trail begins with a wide, meandering path dotted with rocks and roots. A steady grade through a mature mixed-conifer forest of pine, fir, and hemlock brings you quickly to the first payout: beautiful blue Benson Lake. Lined with cliffs, the 26-acre lake hides a few rainbow and brook trout in its depths.

Continue running past Benson Lake, and within another mile, you'll reach the junction for Tenas Lakes. If you have time, spend a few hours exploring this area. In all, close to a dozen rock-rimmed lakes are grouped together in close proximity, beckoning visitors into their refreshing blue waters. Glacial features are in abundance on the rocks hugging the lakeshores, and unmarked (but obvious) paths in many directions offer hints to where the next water source lies. Tenas Lakes are a favorite for many swimmers; however, the sheer number of lakes and the few miles to get to them mean solitude is yours if you want it.

Once your exploration with the Tenas Lakes is complete, return to the main trail and turn left toward Scott Mountain. A half-mile later, ignore the side trail

Scott Lake

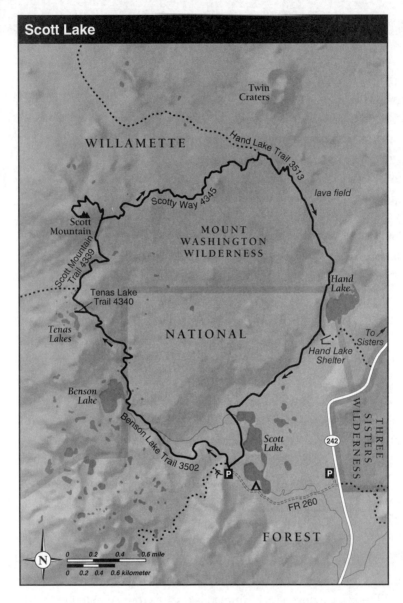

Twin Craters
Hand Lake Trail 3513
WILLAMETTE
lava field
Scotty Way 4345
Scott Mountain
MOUNT WASHINGTON WILDERNESS
Scott Mountain Trail 4339
Hand Lake
Tenas Lake Trail 4340
Tenas Lakes
NATIONAL
To Sisters
Hand Lake Shelter
Benson Lake
Scott Lake
THREE SISTERS WILDERNESS
242
Benson Lake Trail 3502
FR 260
FOREST
N
0 0.2 0.4 0.6 mile
0 0.2 0.4 0.6 kilometer

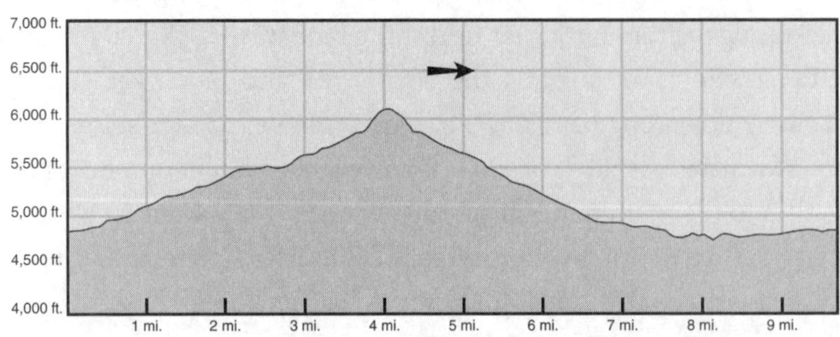

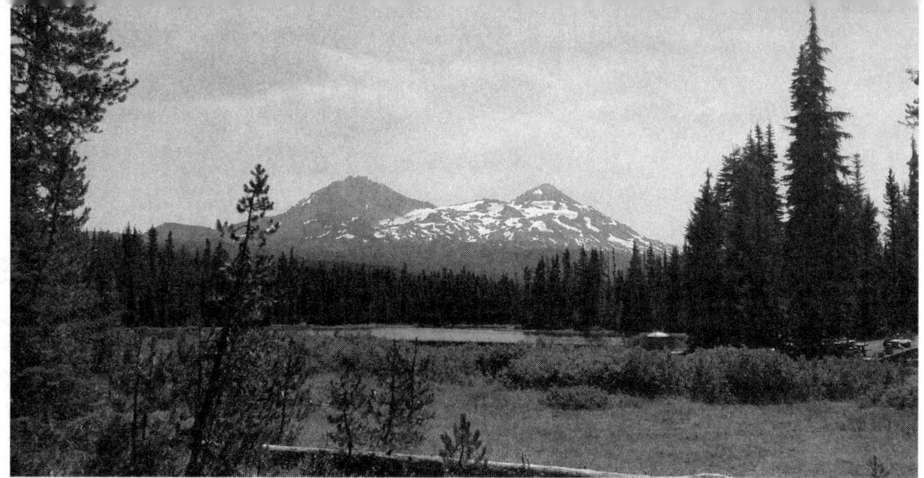

The Three Sisters from Scott Lake

pointing to the Knobs and keep straight. Around mile 3, after a sharp, short uphill corner, keep your eyes peeled to the right for a nice, moss-covered lake down below you through the trees. Shortly after, you earn your first views of Scott Mountain as you run down the trail.

At 3.4 miles, the junction for the Scott Mountain summit trail appears. Ultimately, you will want to turn right toward the obvious (but unmarked) trail to Hand Lake, but for now keep straight for the half-mile climb up Scott Mountain. The trail snakes its way up the backside of the mountain and offers a few glimpses on its way to the views ahead. In July and August, buttercups, lupine, and myriad other mountain wildflowers line the trail as you emerge through the trees to the open summit.

Once on top, you're rewarded with 360-degree views of the Sisters, Mount Jefferson, Mount Washington, Three Fingered Jack, Belknap Crater, and many more. You can also easily trace your running route from Scott Lake to Benson and Tenas Lakes and the return along the burn area to Hand Lake and back around. Those with keen eyes can also spot the McKenzie Scenic Highway working its way up the pass to the Dee Wright Observatory.

Once you've had your share of scenery, descend the same trail back to the junction and turn left toward Hand Lake. From here, the trail can be a bit overgrown and rough, as most hikers use Scott Mountain as a turnaround point back to Scott Lake. About 1.5 miles from the junction, the trail pops out from under the trees into an area burned from a long-ago fire. The exposed area means some overgrown trails, but you'll be rewarded with lupine-lined paths and strands of huckleberries dotting the landscape in August and September.

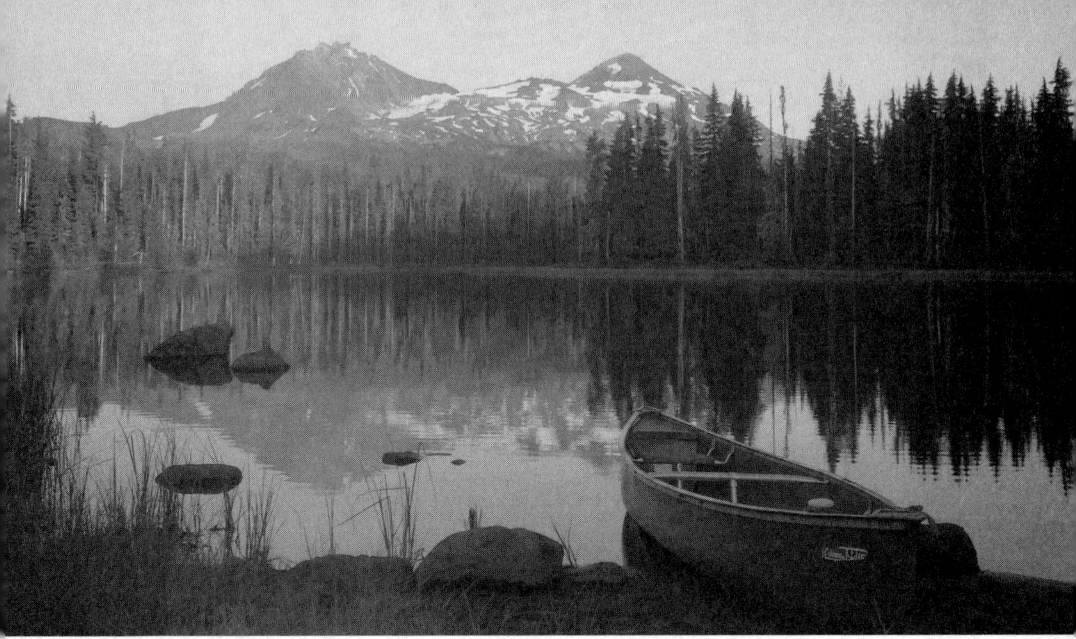

Another Three Sisters view from Scott Lake

At 6.4 miles, turn right at the signed junction toward Hand Lake. A half-mile later, the trail begins to run parallel with the massive lava field leading up to Belknap Crater. Soon after, impressive views of the Three Sisters begin to emerge. At 7.75 miles, the trail ducks back into the trees and veers right back toward Scott Lake. To get a closer look at Hand Lake, however, keep left along the lava rock down to the shore for views of the lake and the Sisters behind it.

Back on the trail, a signed junction for OR 242 leads runners to the Hand Lake Shelter just down the hill—a worthwhile detour. From the shelter, Mount Washington can be seen over the lava fields with Hand Lake in the foreground. Return to the main trail and continue 1.5 miles back to Scott Lake and the trailhead. Be sure to take in the views the last half-mile as the trail weaves in and out of the trees beside the lakeshore.

DIRECTIONS

Take OR 242 (the McKenzie Pass–Santiam Pass National Scenic Byway) about 15 miles west from Sisters toward McKenzie Pass and Dee Wright Observatory. About 6 miles from McKenzie Pass, look for signs for Scott Lake on the right.

34 Matthieu Lakes

TRAIL DETAILS AT A GLANCE

- **DISTANCE** 6.7-mile balloon loop
- **GPS TRAILHEAD COORDINATES** N44° 15.590' W121° 47.238'
- **DIFFICULTY** 6 • **SCENERY** 8 • **CROWDS** 5
- **SEASON** June–October, sunrise–sunset • **ELEVATION** +/–1,090'
- **USERS** Hikers, runners, horses • **CONTACT** Sisters Ranger District, Deschutes National Forest; 541-549-7700, **www.fs.usda.gov/deschutes**
- **PERMITS/FEES** Northwest Forest Pass (see page 12)
- **RECOMMENDED MAP** *Mount Jefferson and Mount Washington Trails Illustrated Topographic Map* by National Geographic ($11.95, **natgeomaps.com**) • **DOGS** Yes (leashed only)

THE MATTHIEU LAKES LOOP somehow flies under the radar of many hikers and runners. Encompassing all of the elements of what makes Central Oregon special, this balloon loop provides spectacular views of the Cascades, sweeping views of ancient lava fields, and pristine alpine lakes nestled among old-growth ponderosa pines. And if you time it just right, you might run into a smattering of northbound Pacific Crest Trail (PCT) hikers who are willing to share their trail stories from all the rugged miles leading to Oregon.

The loop starts just before Lava Camp Lake and its campground—a worthy place to pitch a tent if you prefer an overnight adventure. Be sure to watch for horses on this loop as well, as it's a popular area for riders. If you do encounter people on horseback, remember to be respectful and announce your presence before attempting to pass.

From the parking lot, begin on the wide, shaded trail through the pines. The dirt may be soft in some places due to horses and erosion. Within a quarter-mile, join the PCT and turn left at the signed junction. Here, the path saddles up beside a continuous bed of lava rock, which will accompany you a generous distance until the junction with Matthieu Lakes Trail 4602 and the start of the loop. Keep right, and within a few yards you'll pass your first of many tarns that add a nice bit of scenery along the forested path.

At just under 2 miles, the trail begins a series of long, gradual switchbacks leading up to signs for the North Matthieu Lake area. The northern lake, much

Matthieu Lakes

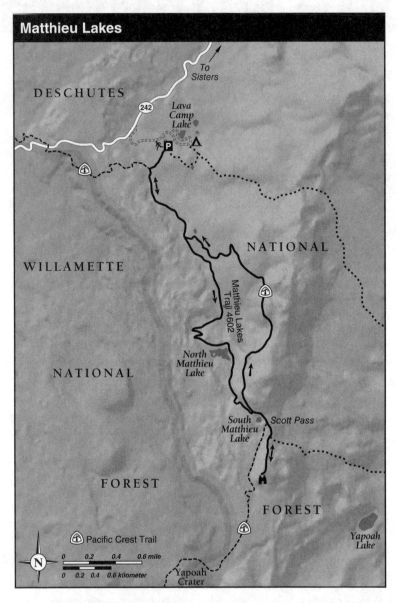

To Sisters
DESCHUTES
242
Lava Camp Lake
NATIONAL
WILLAMETTE
Matthieu Lakes Trail 4602
North Matthieu Lake
NATIONAL
South Matthieu Lake
Scott Pass
FOREST
FOREST
Pacific Crest Trail
0 0.2 0.4 0.6 mile
0 0.2 0.4 0.6 kilometer
N
Yapoah Lake
Yapoah Crater

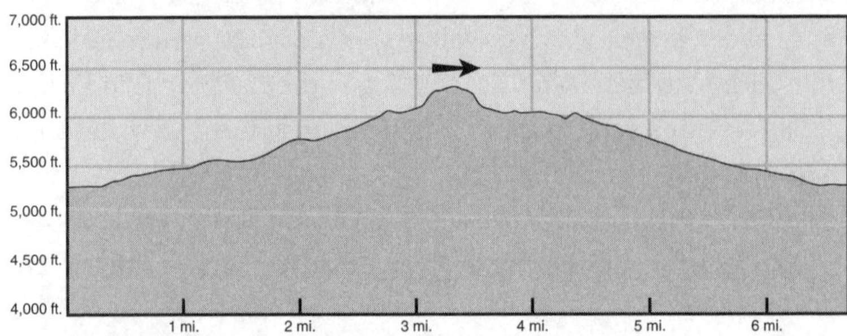

bigger than its southern sibling, contains a handful of nice campsites along the lakeshore, hidden among the trees. A rough, unmarked trail circles the lakeshore for those seeking a diversion and more views of the water.

From North Matthieu Lake, the trail continues to climb gradually until you reach the junction with the PCT and the route back. For now, however, continue a few more yards down the trail, now the southbound PCT, to come upon South Matthieu Lake. Though considerably smaller, the lake is arguably more scenic than North Matthieu Lake, providing a lovely alpine foreground with North Sister looming behind it.

South Matthieu Lake provides a good turnaround spot, but for those wishing to put in a bit more mileage for a scenic payout, continue around the lake to the junction with Scott Pass. Stay left here, leaving the PCT; at just under 3 miles, before the trail dips down into the woods, look for an unmarked but worn trail to the right, snaking its way steeply up the hill in front of you. Take this trail up and over the ridge, and soon you'll be rewarded with spectacular views of North and Middle Sister beyond a wildflower-lined pathway. The trail ends a quarter-mile later, and runners are amply rewarded with views in nearly all directions.

The Sisters stand proudly to the south, along with the deep reddish hues of Yapoah Crater. Those with a keen eye can spot the PCT wrapping its way around the base. For the truly adventurous souls, a steep scramble down the rock-strewn hill will pop you out on the PCT below. For those who prefer an easier (and safer) option, use this as your turnaround point. As you descend back toward South Matthieu Lake, the northern skyline is filled with spectacular views of Mount Jefferson, Three Fingered Jack, and Mount Washington in the distance.

Continue your run on the same route until you reach the junction with Matthieu Lakes Trail 4602. This time, stay right to continue on the PCT and complete the loop. The next half-mile offers breathtaking views of the mountains. (*Hint:* Be sure to turn around before rounding the corner at the apex of the small climb.) Soon, you'll spot North Matthieu Lake below and to your right and on hot summer days hear the cheerful elations of swimmers in its chilly waters.

From here, the trail starts as a fast, smooth downhill, hugging the side of the mountain, and gradually gives way to familiar terrain near the loop start. Around 5.75 miles, another tarn is visible through the trees to the right, and shortly after, you meet the loop terminus and the Matthieu Lakes Trail junction once again. Stay right and retrace your footsteps to the Lava Camp trailhead.

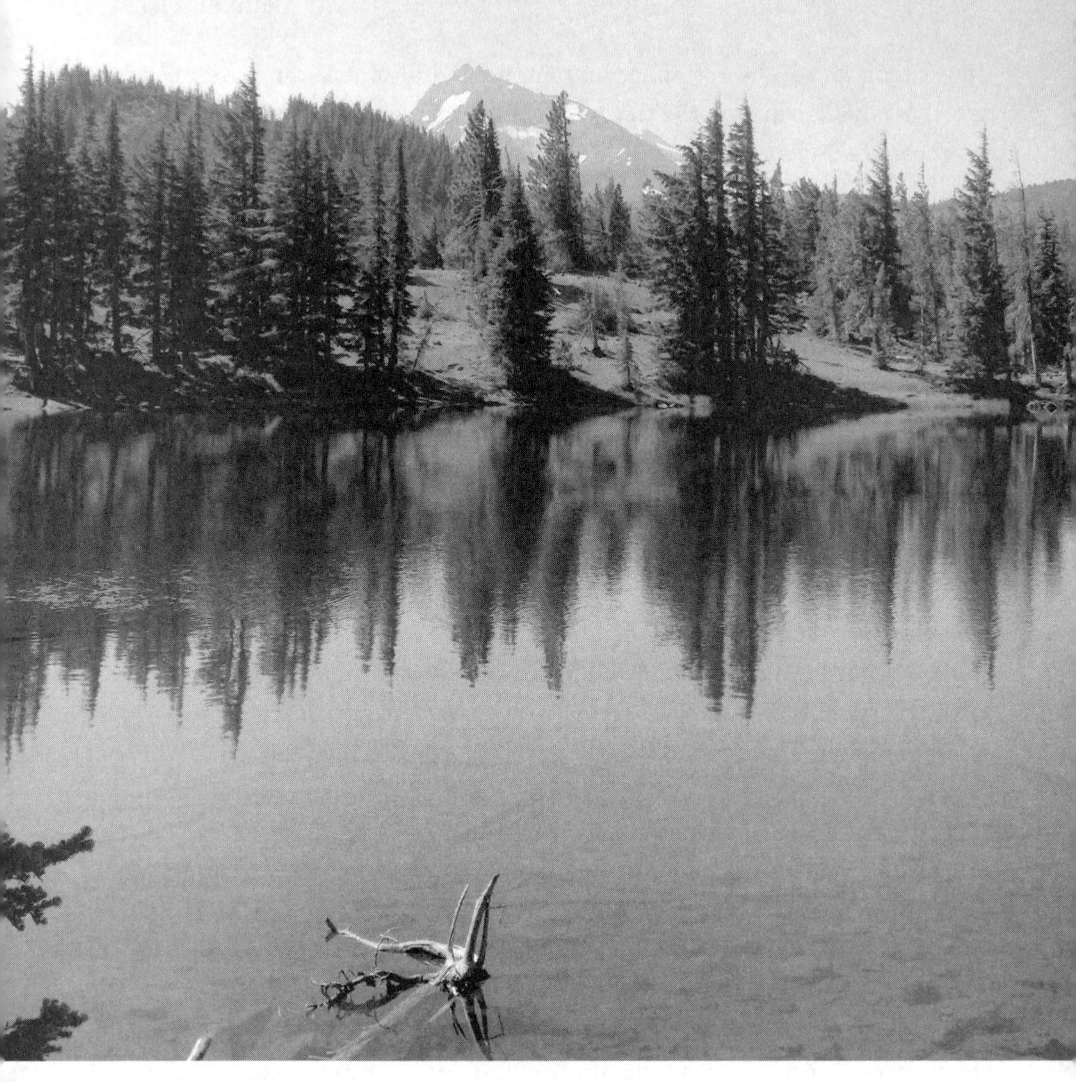

South Matthieu Lake with North Sister in the background

DIRECTIONS

From Sisters, pick up OR 242 (the McKenzie Pass–Santiam Pass National Scenic Byway) at the west end of town. After about 14 miles, just after Milepost 78, look for signs to Lava Camp Lake and the PCT, where you'll turn left. Turn right at the PCT and the Lava Camp Lake Trailhead parking lot, a quarter-mile up the road.

35 Obsidian Trail

TRAIL DETAILS AT A GLANCE

- **DISTANCE** 17.3-mile loop • **GPS TRAILHEAD COORDINATES** N44° 12.788' W121° 52.661' (Scott Trailhead), N44° 12.236' W121° 52.247' (Obsidian Trailhead)
- **DIFFICULTY** 10 • **SCENERY** 10 • **CROWDS** 4
- **SEASON** August–October, sunrise–sunset • **ELEVATION** +/–3,062'
- **USERS** Hikers, runners, horses (on some trails) • **CONTACT** Sisters Ranger District, Deschutes National Forest; 541-549-7700, **www.fs.usda.gov/deschutes**
- **PERMITS/FEES** Northwest Forest Pass (see page 12), Obsidian Limited Entry Area Permit (see page 13)
- **RECOMMENDED MAP** *Three Sisters Wilderness Trail Map* by Adventure Maps, Inc. ($12, **adventuremaps.net**) • **DOGS** Yes (leashed only)

THE OBSIDIAN TRAIL LOOP IS A SPECTACULAR FORAY into the heart of the Oregon Cascades volcanic landscape. The area is hugely popular with hikers and backpackers, and a permit is required to limit the number of people and minimize impact on the fragile alpine environment. For those who throw their names in the hat early, a landscape filled with mountain views, crystal-clear streams, wildflowers, and waterfalls awaits.

A long, arduous run with 3,000-plus feet of elevation gain, this loop is best tackled at a slow and steady pace. With the top-notch scenery here, however, you have many reasons to allow yourself to slow down and enjoy the surroundings. The loop can be started in multiple places, including the Scott Trailhead and the official Obsidian Trailhead—each just about a mile apart on OR 242. If you prefer to avoid the larger parking lot and crowds, choose the former option (described here).

From the Scott Trailhead, cross the McKenzie Pass–Santiam Pass National Scenic Byway and continue through forests of pines and hemlock to the first junction (your loop return). Stay left, following signs for the Pacific Crest Trail (PCT), and immediately begin climbing through the old-growth forest. After 1.25 miles, a switchback provides a brief glimpse back toward the valley before ducking back into heavy cover and into the trees.

At the 3-mile marker, the trail enters a large lava field and meanders its way up, through, and over the rough basalt flows before settling back down into a

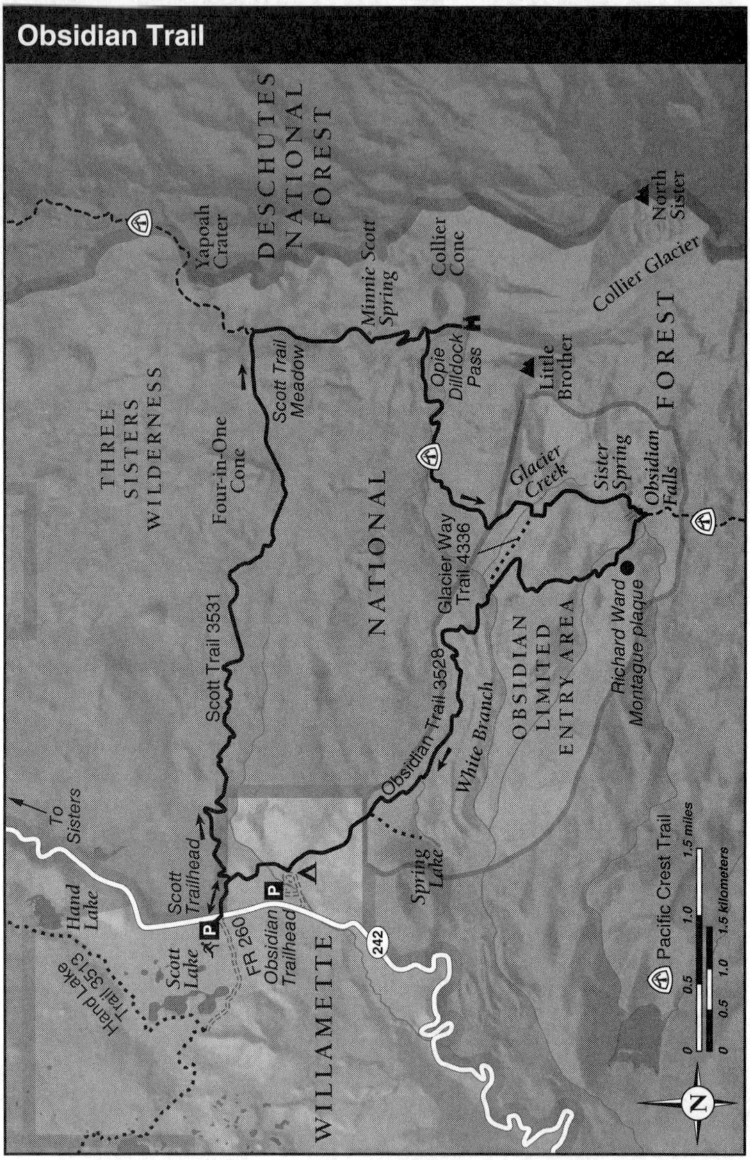

Obsidian Trail

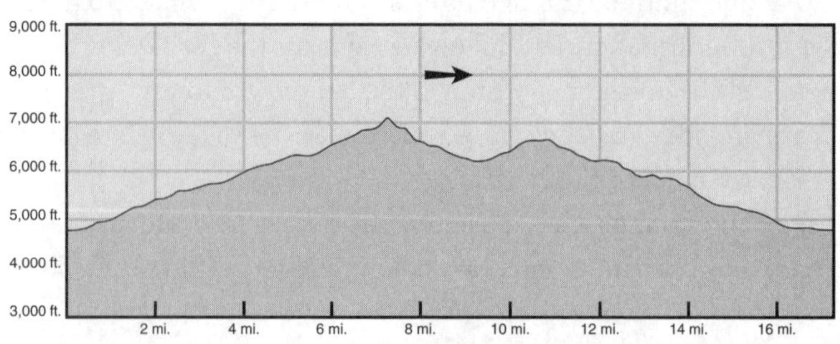

sandy trail. Over the next mile, this pattern repeats itself a few times until you emerge into a large, barren volcanic field carpeted with cinders at mile 4.4. North Sister greets you to the south, hovering above the horizon while the red mound of cinders that is Four-in-One Cone frames you in to the north. If you're looking to add another mile to the trip, veer left at the lava rock cairn, which snakes its way up over 0.5 mile to the top of each of the four cones. The short side trip is well worth it, with exceptional views of Mount Washington, Three Fingered Jack, and Mount Jefferson along the horizon.

Back at the main path, continue east on Scott Trail 3531 for another 0.8 mile until the trail drops down into Scott Trail Meadow and the junction with the PCT. In July and August, this area is a delight, with brilliant blue lupine coloring the landscape in all directions. Meanwhile, Yapoah Crater and its cinder red flanks add to the display.

From the meadows, climb steadily on the PCT, passing Minnie Scott Spring and cresting the windy, barren, 7,000-foot Opie Dilldock Pass at mile 6.8. After rounding the corner, you are immediately enveloped by Collier Cone and the spectacular surroundings. For an even better view, follow a rock cairn off the main trail to a saddle overlooking Collier Glacier, a spectacular green cirque lake at its base, and magnificent North Sister directly in front of you. On a clear day, this area is well worth spending some extra time for exploration.

Once satisfied, return to the PCT southbound and descend through a series of lava rock–strewn switchbacks before slightly leveling out and taking in the views of Little Brother in the foreground and North and Middle Sisters in the back. At this point, about halfway through the run, you're on cloud nine and congratulating yourself for making the decision.

Gradually descending into the trees, enter the Obsidian Limited Entry Area at 9.5 miles. Within a half-mile, cross Glacier Creek and ignore the side trail pointing up at North Sister—an unmaintained but popular route for those climbing the nontechnical but difficult route to the summit. Instead, keep south on the PCT and pass the junction with Glacier Way Trail 4336, which makes its way steeply down to your eventual path. (If you're looking to cut nearly 3 miles off your route, this is a great shortcut.)

Briefly climb your way back up through the trees until you emerge once again beside Glacier Creek and into obsidian country in earnest. From here to Sister Spring, shiny black obsidian in all sizes sparkles in the sunlight at every

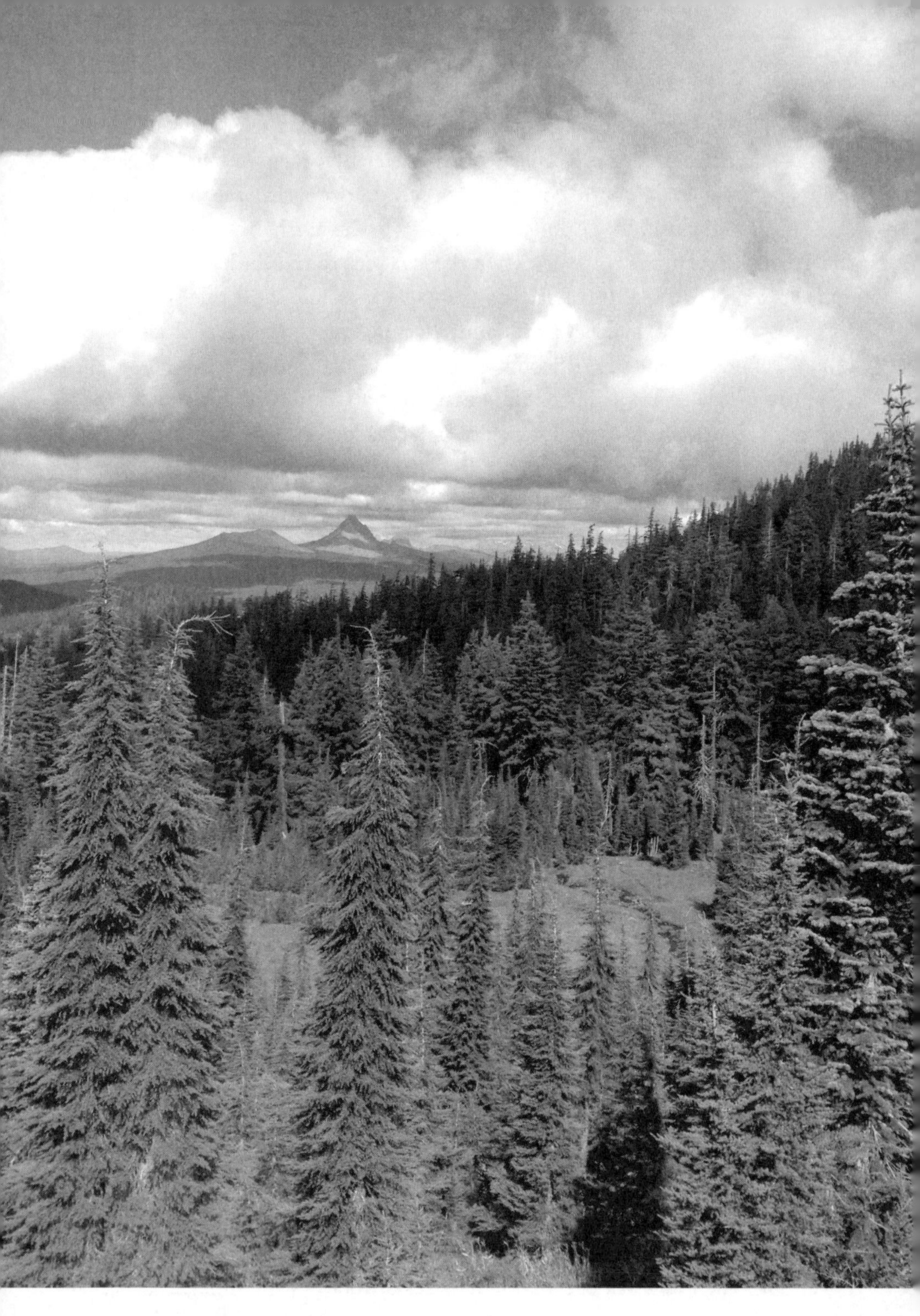

Scott Trail Meadow

turn, creating a magical feeling in the backcountry. The pristine spring waters and smooth, alpine landscape add to the feeling as you take in the mountainous beauty.

At mile 11, cross the creek and, shortly after descending, you'll hear the plunge of lovely Obsidian Falls to your right. Another quarter-mile takes you down to the junction with Obsidian Trail 3528, where you'll turn right, opposite a spectacular boulder split perfectly in two. After crossing the creek several more times, stop to investigate a seemingly out-of-place plaque just off the trail honoring Richard Ward Montague, a prominent and well-respected lawyer and politician in Portland from 1890 to 1913.

The trail soon makes its way back into the pine-and-hemlock forests, passing the terminus of the Glacier Way Trail at 13 miles, and back through a section of the Jerry Lava Flow. Over the next several miles, a steady, pleasant downhill through lush green forest takes you past a junction with Spring Lake (at mile 15.6) and eventually to the junction with the Scott Trail at mile 16.4. The Obsidian Trailhead parking lot is visible from the junction, roughly 100 feet ahead. Instead, turn right and run another half-mile before hitting the loop's end. Retrace your steps back the short distance on the Scott Trail, across the highway and back to your car.

DIRECTIONS

Drive west on OR 242 (the McKenzie Pass–Santiam Pass National Scenic Byway) from Sisters about 20 miles to the turnoff for Scott Lake. Turn immediately right on the gravel road, following the signs for the Scott Trailhead parking area. If you choose to begin at the Obsidian Trailhead, drive 1 mile farther on OR 242 and turn left at the signs, between Mileposts 70 and 71. Parking here can be cumbersome and difficult—look for the trail near the far end of the lot, by a message board and trailhead sign.

36 Broken Top

TRAIL DETAILS AT A GLANCE

- **DISTANCE** 12.3-mile loop
- **GPS TRAILHEAD COORDINATES** N44° 1.413' W121° 40.927'
- **DIFFICULTY** 7 • **SCENERY** 9 • **CROWDS** 4
- **SEASON** July–October, sunrise–sunset • **ELEVATION** +/–1,587'
- **USERS** Hikers, runners, horses • **CONTACT** Bend–Fort Rock Ranger District, Deschutes National Forest; 541-383-4000, **www.fs.usda.gov/deschutes**
- **PERMITS/FEES** Northwest Forest Pass (see page 12)
- **RECOMMENDED MAP** *Three Sisters Wilderness Trail Map* by Adventure Maps, Inc. ($12, **adventuremaps.net**) • **DOGS** Yes (leashed only)

THE CASCADES RANGE IS FILLED WITH ICONIC PEAKS, from Mount Hood to the north to Mount Thielsen to the south. In between, the Three Sisters, Mount Bachelor, and craggy Broken Top are the stars. It's Broken Top that many Central Oregonians call their favorite. And for good reason: Broken Top's ruggedly handsome peak, the accessible high alpine basins filled with streams and wildflowers, and the outstanding views of the surrounding area make it a must for outdoor lovers. A 12-mile loop provides a wondrous variety of scenery for trail runners who are willing to put in a few extra miles and feet of elevation.

From the parking area at Todd Lake, follow the well-beaten path to the start of Todd Lake Trail 34, just beyond the restroom. The trail climbs steeply for 1.25 miles through dense woods with glimpses of the lake as you zigzag up along the ridge. After entering into the Three Sisters Wilderness, the trees thin and the path begins to level out, with views of Broken Top appearing in front of you.

At 2.4 miles, keep straight at the Soda Creek Trail junction and, within a quarter-mile, cross the creek itself, which can be a bit tricky in July. Along the creek's shores is a great spot for wildflowers, with lupine, Indian paintbrush, monkeyflower, and senecio all making appearances in late July and early August. The trail then gently climbs its way toward Broken Top, with views of Mount Bachelor and Sparks Lake along the way to your left.

Turn right onto Broken Top Trail 10 at 3.25 miles and take in the spectacular views as the trail winds in front of Broken Top's crater. The trees slowly fade

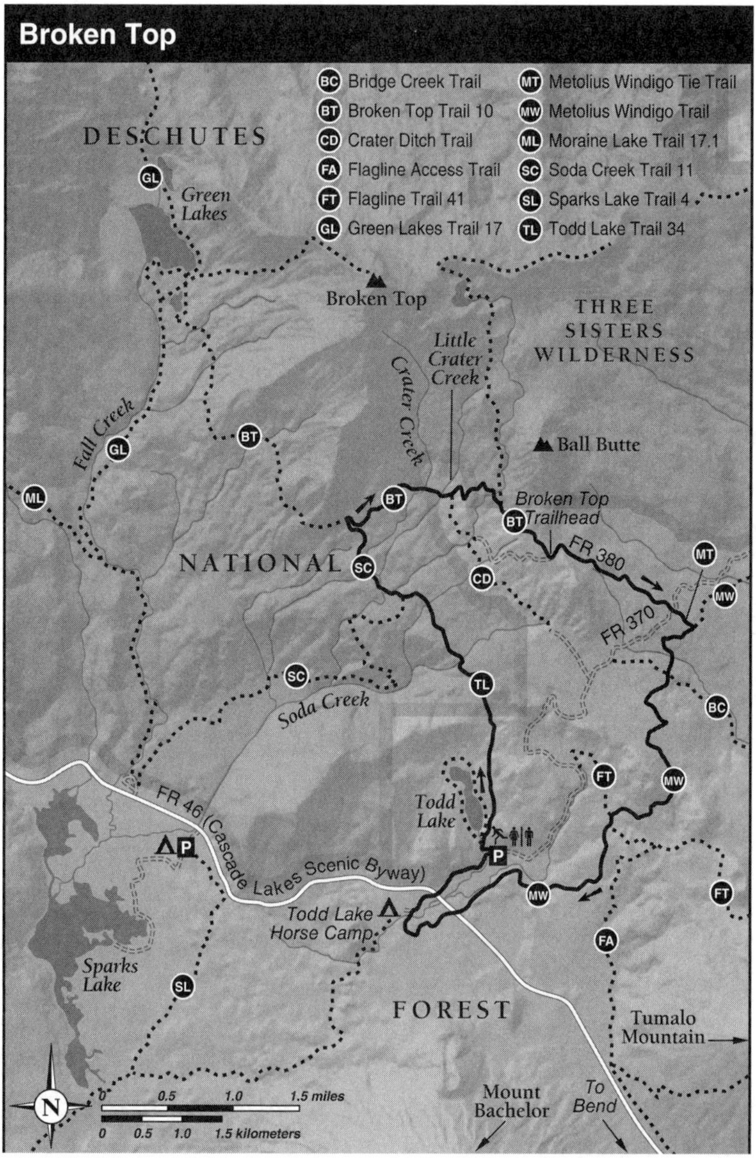

Broken Top
BC Bridge Creek Trail
BT Broken Top Trail 10
CD Crater Ditch Trail
FA Flagline Access Trail
FT Flagline Trail 41
GL Green Lakes Trail 17
MT Metolius Windigo Tie Trail
MW Metolius Windigo Trail
ML Moraine Lake Trail 17.1
SC Soda Creek Trail 11
SL Sparks Lake Trail 4
TL Todd Lake Trail 34
DESCHUTES
Green Lakes
Broken Top
THREE SISTERS WILDERNESS
Little Crater Creek
Crater Creek
Fall Creek
Ball Butte
Broken Top Trailhead
FR 380
FR 370
NATIONAL
Soda Creek
Todd Lake
FR 46 (Cascade Lakes Scenic Byway)
Todd Lake Horse Camp
Sparks Lake
FOREST
Tumalo Mountain
Mount Bachelor
To Bend
N
0 0.5 1.0 1.5 miles
0 0.5 1.0 1.5 kilometers

7,200 ft.
7,000 ft.
6,800 ft.
6,600 ft.
6,400 ft.
6,200 ft.
6,000 ft.
2 mi.
4 mi.
6 mi.
8 mi.
10 mi.
12 mi.

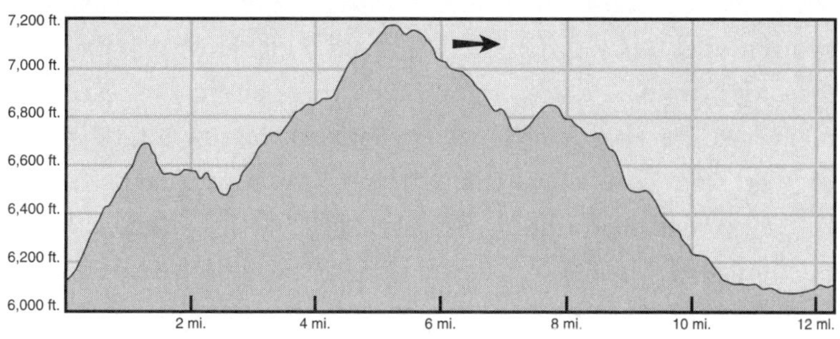

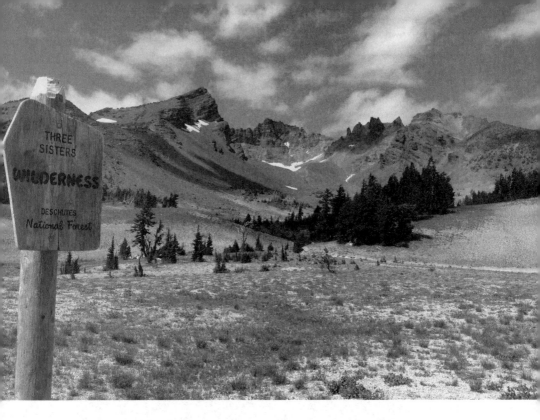

Broken Top

as you run across expansive pumice fields with far-reaching views toward Sparks Lake, Mount Bachelor, and beyond.

At the 4.2-mile mark, cross a small creek and exit (for the moment) the Three Sisters Wilderness. Shortly after, you'll reach Crater Creek and the junction with the Crater Ditch Trail. If you have some time and want to extend your run, turn left and follow the creek up toward the crater for some spectacular views. Back at the junction, cross the creek and continue on toward Broken Top Trailhead, meandering your way up and through a small section of forest before popping back out on the pumice fields.

After another crossing, this time of Little Crater Creek, follow the trail as it heads toward Ball Butte. Ignore the well-trod (but unmarked) junction for No Name Lake at 4.8 miles and keep right for another half-mile to reach the Broken Top Trailhead. At this point, you'll need to connect the singletrack with a stretch of Forest Road 380. Keep left at the bottom of the hill from the trailhead, and follow the very rough road until it Ts out at FR 370 at 6.5 miles. Look for the Metolius Windigo Tie Trail and trailhead sign on the opposite side of the road.

A quarter-mile after entering the singletrack, turn right at the junction with the Metolius Windigo Trail, a popular horse and mountain bike trail that is also a national recreation trail. Wind your way downhill through lovely old-growth forests of pine and hemlock, keeping straight through the watershed at 7.3 miles. At 9.1 miles, ignore the side trail to FR 370 and, a short time later, keep right at an incorrectly marked junction for Swampy Lakes.

Continue running downhill and cross a couple of jeep trails at miles 10.2 and 10.7 before eventually meeting up with the Cascade Lakes National Scenic Byway at 10.9 miles. Look for the continuation of the Metolius Windigo on the opposite side, and follow this sandy section of trail up and around a field of lava rocks before emptying into the Todd Lake Horse Camp area.

To find your way back to your car, follow the short dirt road back to the highway and continue up the road you drove in on to make the loop complete at Todd Lake.

DIRECTIONS

From Bend, drive west on SW Century Drive, which becomes the Cascade Lakes National Scenic Byway, about 19 miles. Two miles beyond the turnoff for Mount Bachelor ski resort, turn right at the signs for Todd Lake. The parking area is up the road about 0.5 mile.

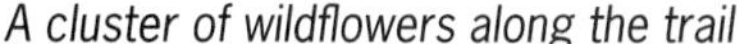

A cluster of wildflowers along the trail

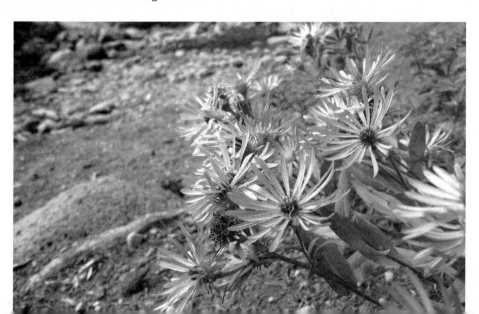

37 Green Lakes

TRAIL DETAILS AT A GLANCE

- **DISTANCE** 12.3-mile loop
- **GPS TRAILHEAD COORDINATES** N44° 1.867' W121° 44.186'
- **DIFFICULTY** 7 • **SCENERY** 10 • **CROWDS** 5
- **SEASON** July–October, sunrise–sunset • **ELEVATION** +/–1,499'
- **USERS** Hikers, runners, horses • **CONTACT** Bend–Fort Rock Ranger District, Deschutes National Forest; 541-383-4000, **www.fs.usda.gov/deschutes**
- **PERMITS/FEES** Northwest Forest Pass (see page 12)
- **RECOMMENDED MAP** *Three Sisters Wilderness Trail Map* by Adventure Maps, Inc. ($12, **adventuremaps.net**) • **DOGS** Yes (leashed only)

THE GREEN LAKES/SODA CREEK LOOP is the pinnacle of Central Oregon trail running—it just doesn't get much better than this. It's a spectacular loop run that visits high alpine scenery, mountain lakes, an abundance of wildflowers, crystal-clear running streams, cascading waterfalls, and well-maintained trails. If it sounds tempting, it is. As you'd expect from the description, it's also pretty popular, especially among hikers. Crowds or not, though, this loop is a must if you love trail running.

The loop starts at the Green Lakes Trailhead, on the Cascade Lakes National Scenic Byway just after Sparks Lake on your left. (There is no sign for the short trailhead-access road, so keep your eyes peeled for the turnoff.) About 20 yards from the trailhead, you'll immediately cross a footbridge over Fall Creek before the trail gradually climbs alongside the snowmelt-fed creek. A number of small waterfalls dot the length of the creek as you climb up past a junction for Moraine Lake and through an idyllic small meadow split by Fall Creek.

After another short log bridge crossing, the trail takes you up a steeper section through ponderosa pines before you emerge with the South Sister summit peaking over the ridgeline. Within a half-mile, you'll reach a sign noting entry into the Green Lakes area. (This area is day-use only—camping is not permitted on the lakeshores.) Continue to your left, where you'll crest a hill before descending into the largest of the lakes with spectacular views across the water of South Sister and Broken Top mountains.

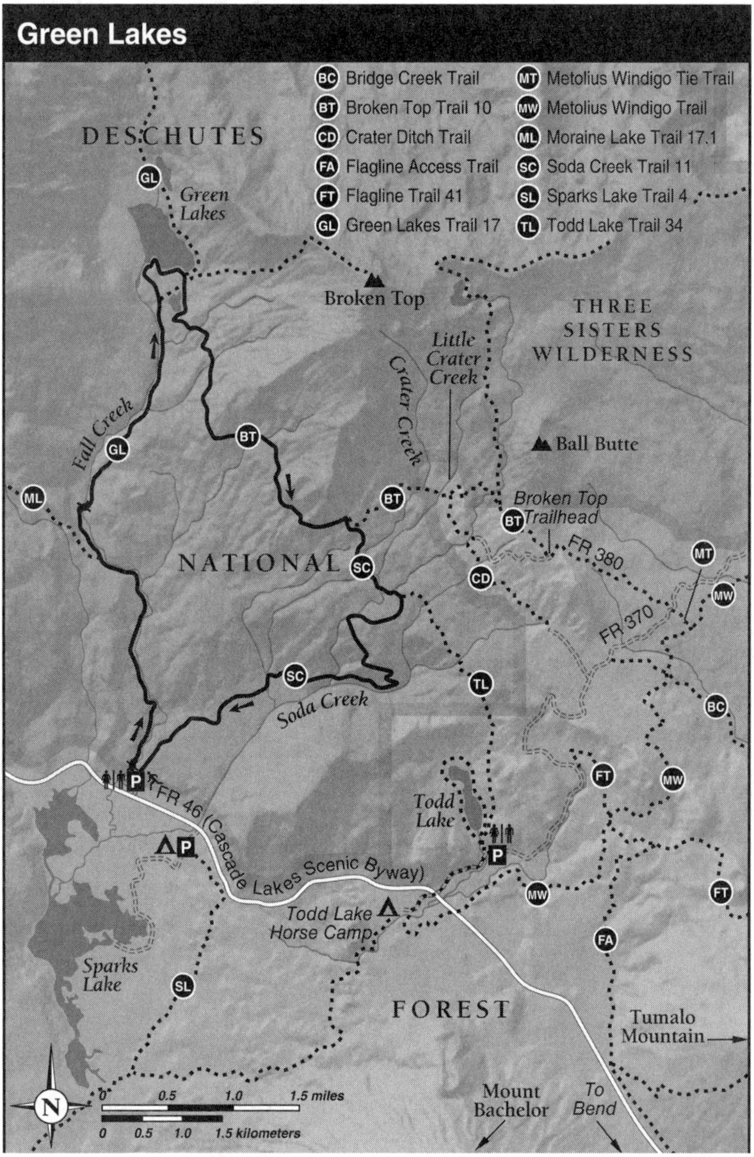

Green Lakes

- BC Bridge Creek Trail
- BT Broken Top Trail 10
- CD Crater Ditch Trail
- FA Flagline Access Trail
- FT Flagline Trail 41
- GL Green Lakes Trail 17
- MT Metolius Windigo Tie Trail
- MW Metolius Windigo Trail
- ML Moraine Lake Trail 17.1
- SC Soda Creek Trail 11
- SL Sparks Lake Trail 4
- TL Todd Lake Trail 34

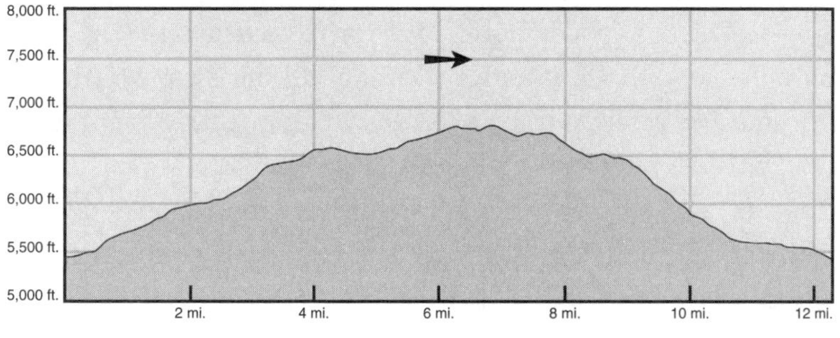

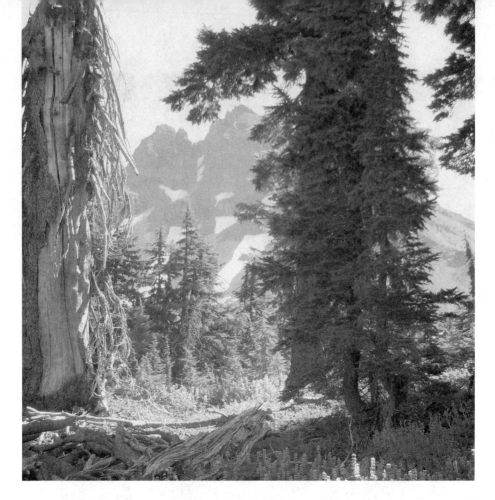

Broken Top is framed by a field of lupine in the foreground.

Once you've taken in the glory of the area, continue along the shoreline toward the east, where you'll wrap slightly around the lake before noticing a number of side trails. Pick the more established trail, which will take you behind the smaller of the two Green Lakes and to a junction. Turning right will take you back to the Green Lakes entry, so instead turn left to continue the loop. In a few yards, you'll see a posting for a campsite, one of 28 posted signs marking the designated camping areas. This is a good indicator that you're headed in the right direction.

Continue along the Broken Top Trail for 2.8 miles as you wind past several more campsites before turning a corner and disappearing back into the trees. Soon enough, you'll see wonderful views of Broken Top, Mount Bachelor, and Sparks Lake as you run past the bright-red cinder cone dubbed Cayuse Crater. Around 7.8 miles, turn right at the marked junction for the Broken Top Trailhead onto the Soda Creek Trail.

As popular as the Green Lakes area is, once you hit the Soda Creek Trail the crowds seemingly disappear, as most people make the journey into an out-and-back to Green Lakes only. This is a mistake—or fortunate for the loop fan—because Soda Creek holds its own wonders, with beautiful clear streams and lovely trails in its own right. As you take in the beauty of the quieter side of this loop, you can't help but count yourself lucky about being able to trail run in such beautiful terrain. Thinking positive thoughts, enjoy the tranquility as you descend the remaining 4.5 miles of the Soda Creek Trail and eventually back to the Green Lakes Trailhead parking lot.

DIRECTIONS

From Bend, drive west on SW Century Drive, which becomes the Cascade Lakes National Scenic Byway, about 19 miles. About 0.6 mile past the Sparks Lake turnoff, turn right on the next paved, unmarked road, which will take you into the Green Lakes Trailhead parking lot.

A runner cruises past Green Lakes with South Sister in the background.

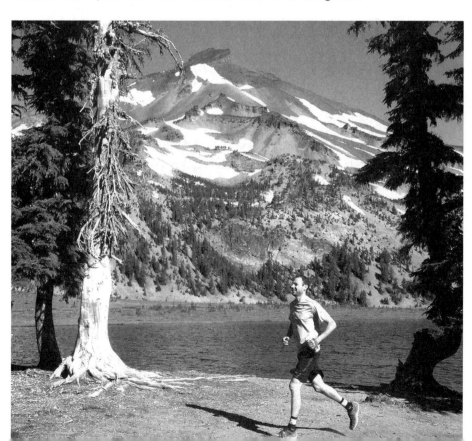

38 Moraine Lake

TRAIL DETAILS AT A GLANCE

- **DISTANCE** 7.5-mile loop • **GPS TRAILHEAD COORDINATES** N44° 2.237' W121° 45.857'
- **DIFFICULTY** 8 • **SCENERY** 9 • **CROWDS** 6
- **SEASON** August–October, sunrise–sunset • **ELEVATION** +/–1,557'
- **USERS** Hikers, runners, horses (on some trails) • **CONTACT** Bend–Fort Rock Ranger District, Deschutes National Forest; 541-383-4000, **www.fs.usda.gov/deschutes**
- **PERMITS/FEES** Northwest Forest Pass (see page 12), self-issued wilderness permit (free)
- **RECOMMENDED MAP** *Three Sisters Wilderness Trail Map* by Adventure Maps, Inc. ($12, **adventuremaps.net**) • **DOGS** Yes (leashed only)

THE SCENERY AROUND MORAINE LAKE doesn't get much better: classic high alpine views with a pristine mountain lake sparkling in the sunshine, volcanic peaks that feel so close you can touch, and plenty of spots to admire them all in between. The beauty comes at a price, however: Nearly all of the 1,500 feet of elevation occurs within the first 2 miles. Luckily, the return portion of the loop is much gentler and friendlier to runners.

To start out, park at the Devils Lake Trailhead or just to the side of the road by the culvert if the parking area is full—since Devils Lake is a popular trail, chances are your car will be one of many. The official trail begins on the opposite side of the highway through the small, scraggly pine trees.

After filling out your self-issued wilderness permit, follow a burbling stream up through the forest. Soon you veer from the water but continue up and up and up the rocky, root-strewn path. After the first mile, you'll get a very brief reprieve for 100 yards before the trail shoots back up. At 1.7 miles, you finally crest the ridgeline and are rewarded with views of South Sister looming directly in front of you.

At the four-way junction, turn right to go to Moraine Lake. This portion of the run is an absolute delight, with vast, sweeping views of Mount Bachelor to the southeast, Broken Top to the northeast, and South Sister straight north. As you descend into the mountain basin, you can't help but forget the steep, burley trail that brought you here.

Another junction at mile 2.3 marks your return route, but for now continue straight, following signs to Moraine Lake. After cresting the hill, descend to the

Moraine Lake

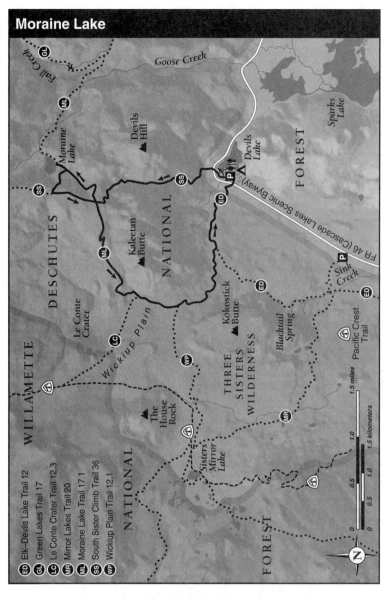

ED Elk–Devils Lake Trail 12
GL Green Lakes Trail 17
LC Le Conte Crater Trail 12.3
MR Mirror Lakes Trail 20
ML Moraine Lake Trail 17.1
SS South Sister Climb Trail 36
WP Wickiup Plain Trail 12.1

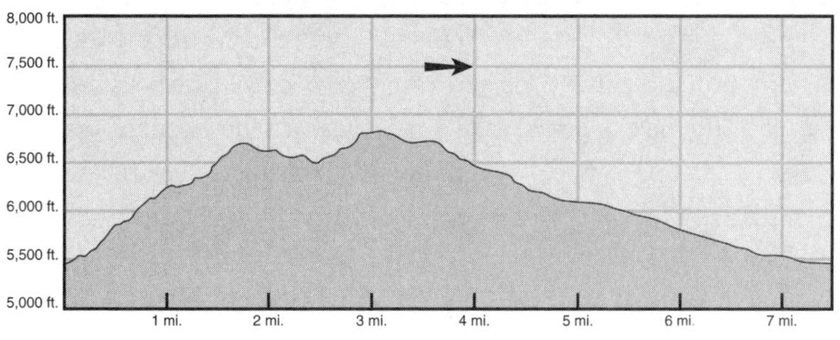

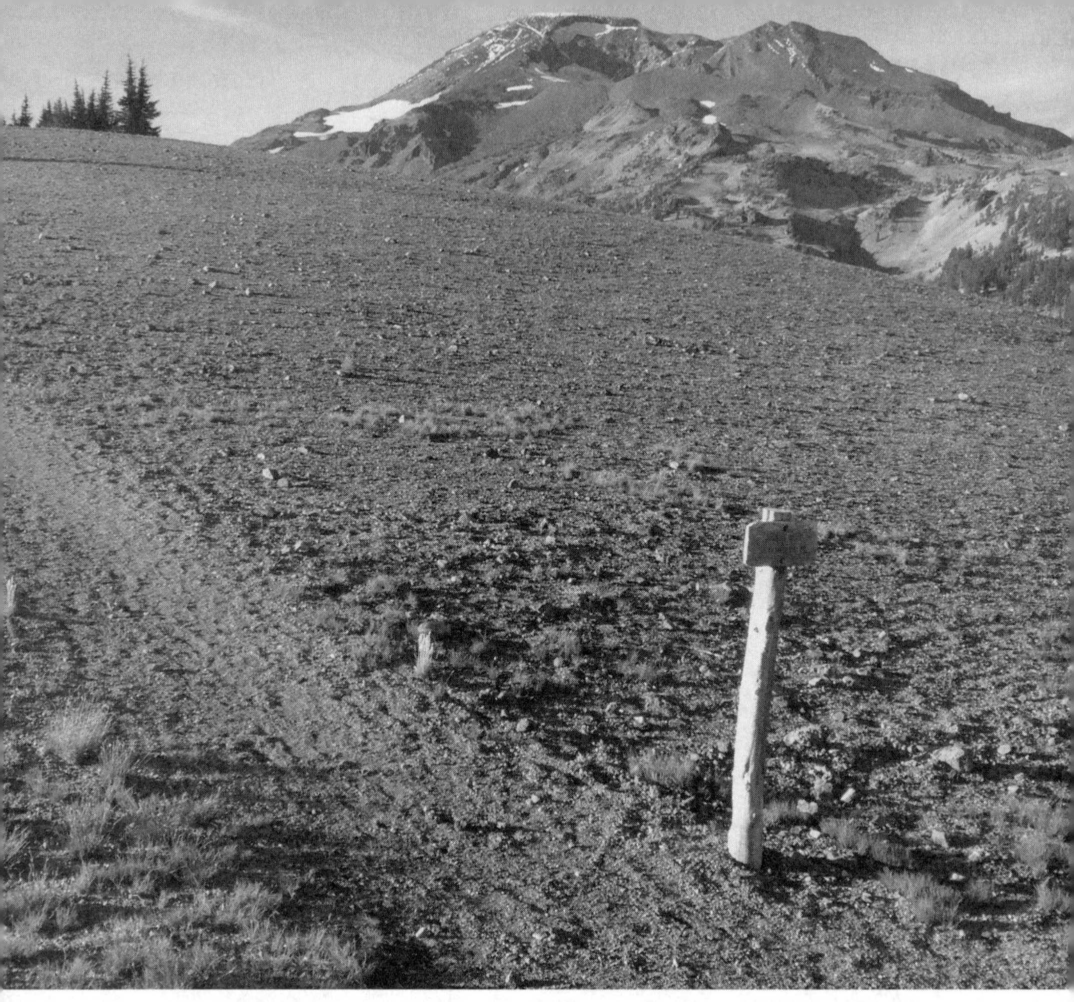

The trail up from Moraine Lake

lake, where you'll enjoy gorgeous views of South Sister reflected in its waters. When satisfied, return your way back to the junction and turn right up the ridgeline (and actual moraine). As you zigzag up, each turn presents a new glorious view with Moraine Lake, Broken Top, and South Sister.

When reaching the climbers' trail, turn left for 0.5 mile to meet back up with your first junction. This time, turn right toward Wickiup Plains to complete the larger loop. The next quarter-mile offers pleasant views of the open tableland and alpine scenery. Soon after, the trail begins to descend back through the trees, popping out briefly for views a few times before gradually descending at a very pleasant, runnable grade.

At 4.8 miles, you encounter a junction. Turn left toward Devils Lake Trailhead, following fast, flat doubletrack through the open landscape. In a quick mile, ignore the junction for the Sisters Mirror Lake trail to the right and continue straight, following signs for Devils Lake. At this point, you quickly lose the outstanding views as the trail winds its way down gradually through the pines.

Turn left at one last junction at mile 6.25 before passing under the Cascade Lakes National Scenic Byway less than a mile later and emerging into the Devils Lake Trailhead parking lot a quarter-mile later. Depending on where you parked, the trail resumes directly across the parking lot just to the right of the bathrooms. From there, a short jaunt through the trees and across the inlet to Devils Lake brings you back to the highway and your starting point.

DIRECTIONS

From Bend, drive west on SW Century Drive, which becomes the Cascade Lakes National Scenic Byway, 25.5 miles until you reach the turnoff for Devils Lake, on your left. There is a large parking lot for campers and day users. The trail begins just to the right of the bathrooms at the far end of the lot.

Broken Top behind Moraine Lake

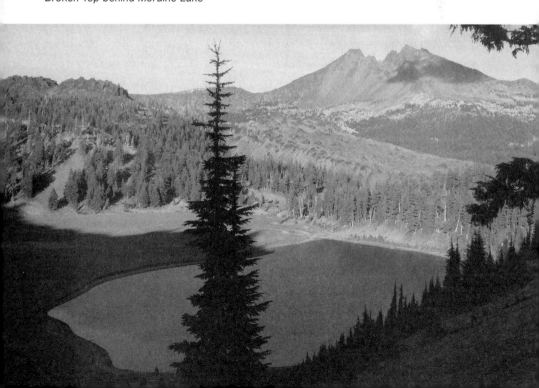

39 Sisters Mirror Lake

TRAIL DETAILS AT A GLANCE

- **DISTANCE** 9.3-mile loop
- **GPS TRAILHEAD COORDINATES** N44° 1.006' W121° 46.936'
- **DIFFICULTY** 5
- **SCENERY** 7
- **CROWDS** 5
- **SEASON** July–October, sunrise–sunset
- **ELEVATION** +/–732'
- **USERS** Hikers, runners, horses
- **CONTACT** Bend–Fort Rock Ranger District, Deschutes National Forest; 541-383-4000, **www.fs.usda.gov/deschutes**
- **PERMITS/FEES** Northwest Forest Pass (see page 12)
- **RECOMMENDED MAP** *Three Sisters Wilderness Trail Map* by Adventure Maps, Inc. ($12, **adventuremaps.net**)
- **DOGS** Yes (leashed only)

SISTERS MIRROR LAKE IS A BIT DECEPTIVE. When you reach the namesake lake for this run, you find that there really isn't much of the Sisters mountains to reflect in the lake—in fact, only the uppermost portion of South Sister peeks over the ridgeline. The alpine lake setting of the area more than makes up for it, however, as the inviting blue waters and the picturesque shoreline stand out here. Even more of a highlight, though, may be the countless "hidden" lakes around Sisters Mirror Lake. Just beyond the lake to the west and southwest lie lake after lake after lake, including many comparable in size to Sisters Mirror Lake. So for those who like a little exploration and adventure off the beaten path, this run is for you.

The run starts from the trailhead parking lot, just off the Cascade Lakes National Scenic Byway. A quick half-mile through ponderosa pines brings you to your first junction and the point at which the loop begins. For now, continue straight on the Mirror Lakes Trail, crossing the small but lovely Sink Creek just past the junction. For the next few miles, the trail takes a very gradual uphill as it heads west toward the lakes. At 1.2 miles, take a moment to stop at the first small pond to your right. Note the carefully made stone path at the outlet by the trail and the looming volcanic peak hovering over the lake on the opposite side.

In another 1.4 miles (around the 2.5-mile mark), the trail begins to bend northwest, and soon you'll catch your first views of South Sister in the distance. A brief mile later brings you to the junction with the Pacific Crest Trail (PCT). For now, take a left on the PCT, then stay left at another junction marking the PCT once more. The unmarked fork here at this junction will be your return route as you run around the lake.

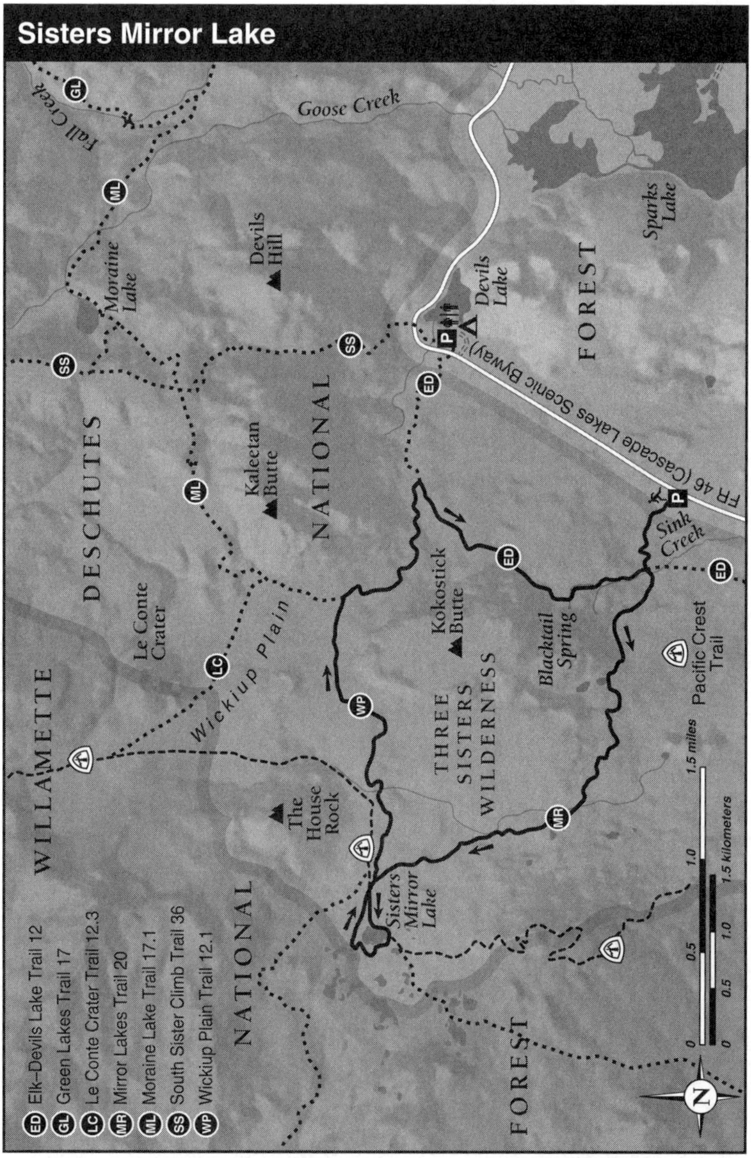

Sisters Mirror Lake

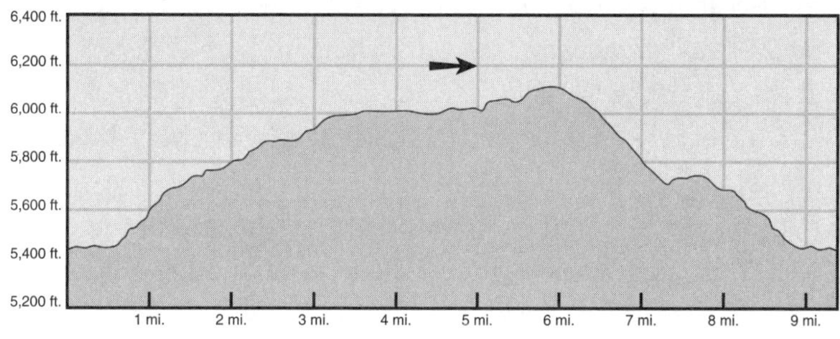

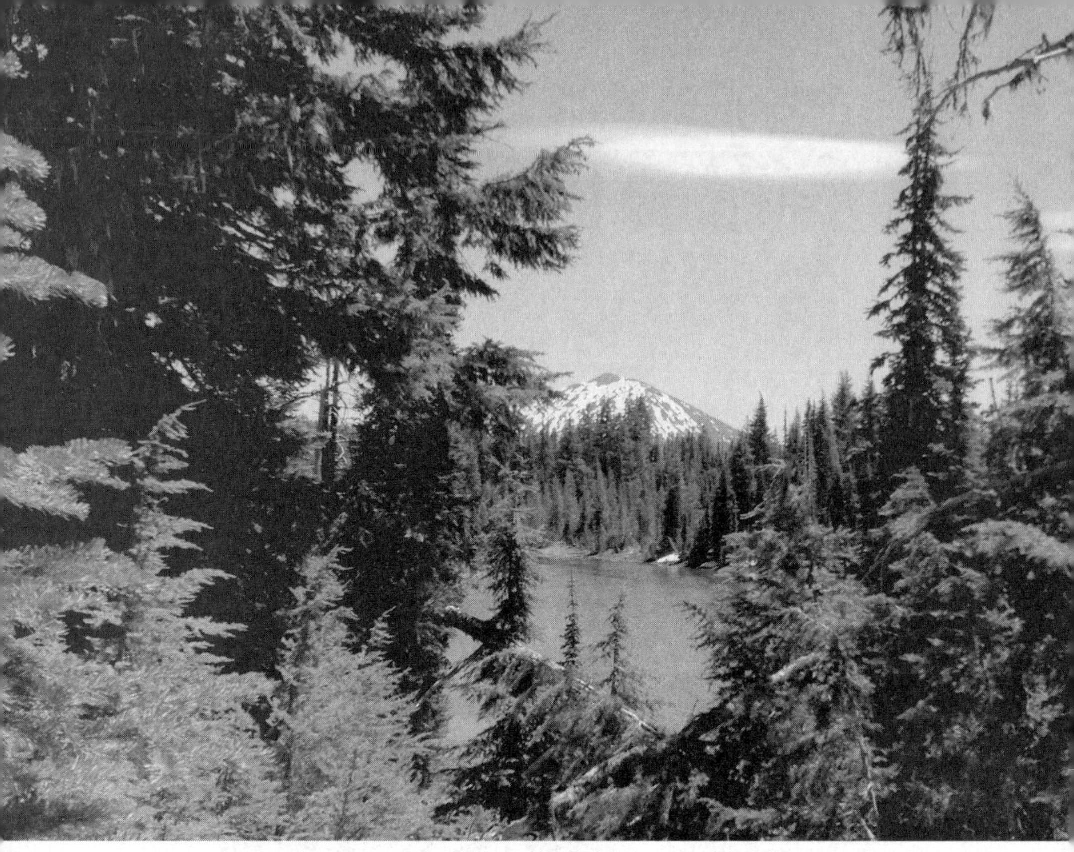

Mount Bachelor looms over Sisters Mirror Lake.

Within moments, the lake will pop into view to your right, and soon you're faced with another option of unmarked trails. This time, take a right on the trail that follows the shoreline around the south end of the lake. Remember here that your ultimate goal is to simply loop around the lake and back to the junction on the northeast side. However, the real fun begins at this point, as you can use this area as a launching point for exploration. Most lakes lie in a north–south line just to the west of Sisters Mirror Lake. Be sure to take a compass and a good map if you decide to venture off-trail. For those who want to play it a bit safer, there are plenty of well-beaten paths to a few of the closest lakes.

Eventually, make your way back to the shoreline path of Sisters Mirror Lake and round the top end of the lake, catching views of Mount Bachelor in the process. As a frame of reference, without the extra exploring, you should reach the same junction to the PCT around 4.4 miles.

At this point, run back the way you came but, instead of returning on the Mirror Lakes Trail, continue straight on the PCT for another quarter-mile until you reach a T-junction. Ignore the signs for Moraine Lake on the PCT and instead turn right through the rolling, heavily forested path. The trail remains well shaded but interesting as it winds through forest and lava flow islands.

Just shy of 6 miles, views begin to open up and South Sister looms in front of you. Another 0.3 mile brings you to a signed junction for the PCT (north)/ Moraine Lake and Elk Lake/Devils Lake Trailhead. Take a right toward the latter and begin your gradual descent back toward the highway. In a mile, arrive at your penultimate junction, taking a right and following signs for Elk Lake. Here, the trail is wide and smooth, as most likely the path was once a logging road.

At 8.25 miles, cross a small stream and a small, lush meadow at Blacktail Spring. Crisscross the stream a few more times as you head back south on the trail and back to your initial junction at 8.85 miles. At this point, a left puts you back on the now-familiar path, and then it's a short half-mile back to the Mirror Lakes Trailhead and parking lot.

DIRECTIONS

From Bend, drive west on SW Century Drive, which becomes the Cascade Lakes National Scenic Byway, for 26.9 miles and look for the turnoff for the Mirror Lakes Trailhead to your right (it's signed on the left side of the road). If you pass the Quinn Meadow Horse Camp turnoff, you've gone too far.

South Sister peeks above the ridge behind the lake.

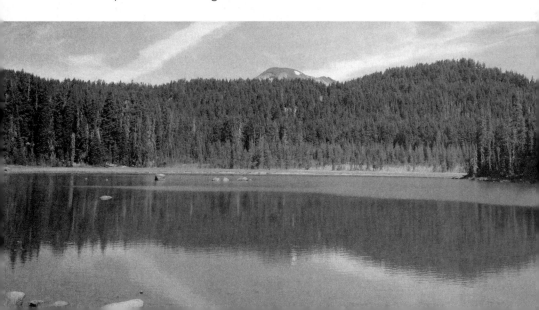

40 Horse Lake

TRAIL DETAILS AT A GLANCE

- **DISTANCE** 7.6-mile loop
- **GPS TRAILHEAD COORDINATES** N43° 59.014' W121° 48.708'
- **DIFFICULTY** 5 • **SCENERY** 5 • **CROWDS** 4
- **SEASON** July–October, sunrise–sunset • **ELEVATION** +/–631'
- **USERS** Hikers, runners, horses • **CONTACT** Bend–Fort Rock Ranger District, Deschutes National Forest; 541-383-4000, **www.fs.usda.gov/deschutes**
- **PERMITS/FEES** Northwest Forest Pass (see page 12)
- **RECOMMENDED MAP** *Three Sisters Wilderness Trail Map* by Adventure Maps, Inc. ($12, **adventuremaps.net**) • **DOGS** Yes (leashed only)

THOUGH LITERALLY RIGHT ACROSS THE STREET from the main entrance to Elk Lake, the Horse Lake Trailhead sees very little traffic by comparison. This is primarily due to the small bit of extra effort required for the payout on this run. There is no perfect trail leading to the shores of Horse Lake, nor does any distinct trail lead to the number of smaller lakes just off the main loop trail. Finding the gems requires a little bit of off-trail navigation and gusto. For those up for an adventure, though, it's well worth the small effort.

Begin at the main Horse Lake Trailhead, directly across the Cascade Lakes National Scenic Byway from the entrance to Elk Lake Resort. The trail begins with a wide, sandy path owing in part to the horse traffic seen on the trail. Unfortunately, this loose dirt will be a trend throughout the run in certain places. Within a quick 0.3 mile, pass a side junction pointing the way to Quinn Meadow Horse Camp to your right. Continue straight and begin a gradual climb on a wooded path through old-growth ponderosa forest.

At 1.4 miles, continue straight through the junction with the Pacific Crest Trail (PCT) and begin the downward side of the first of two small climbs on the run. It's important to note that the trail from here down to Horse Lake can be a bit rough, so be mindful of logs, rocks, roots, and other obstacles that are perfect for catching toes. A downhill tumble can lead to more than just injured pride, as the author well knows firsthand.

Horse Lake
Sink Creek
Quinn Creek
Hosmer Lake
Quinn Meadow Horse Camp
NATIONAL
FOREST
Elk Lake Resort
Elk Lake
Elk–Devils Lake Trail 12
DESCHUTES
FR 46 (Cascade Lakes Scenic Byway)
NATIONAL
THREE SISTERS WILDERNESS
Pacific Crest Trail
WILLAMETTE
Colt Lake
Sunset Lake
FOREST
Horse Lake
Horse Creek
Mile Lake
0 0.5 1.0 1.5 miles
0 0.5 1.0 1.5 kilometers
N

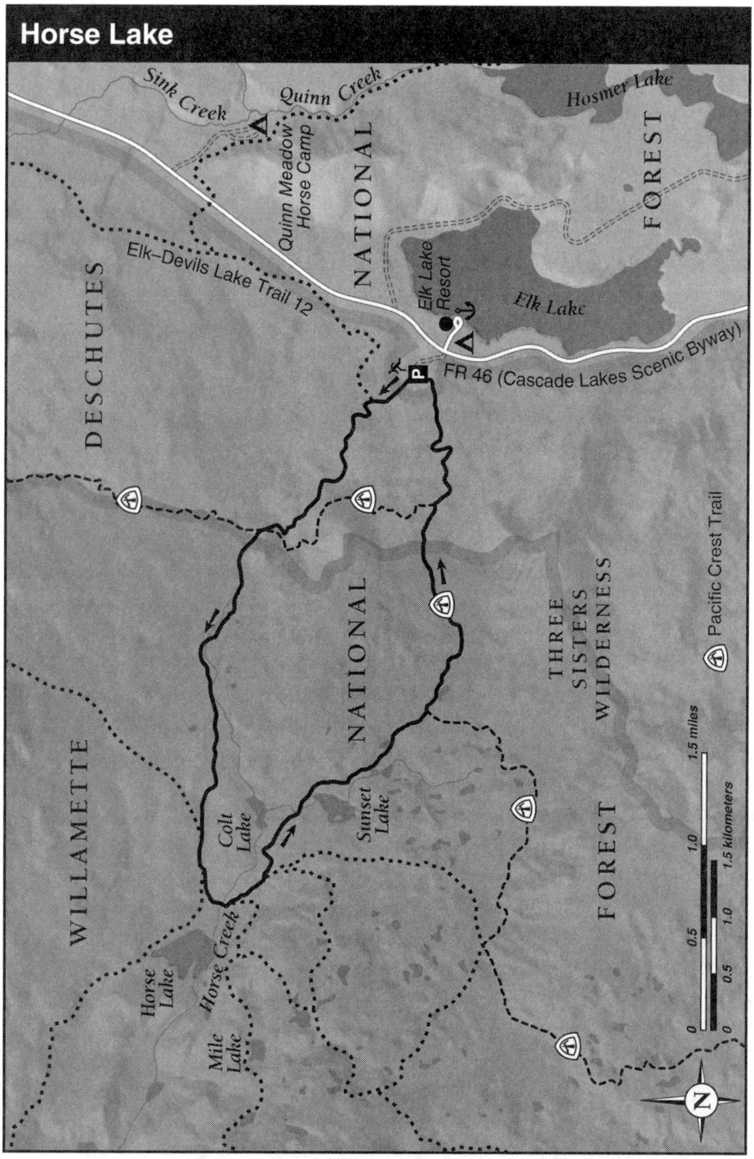

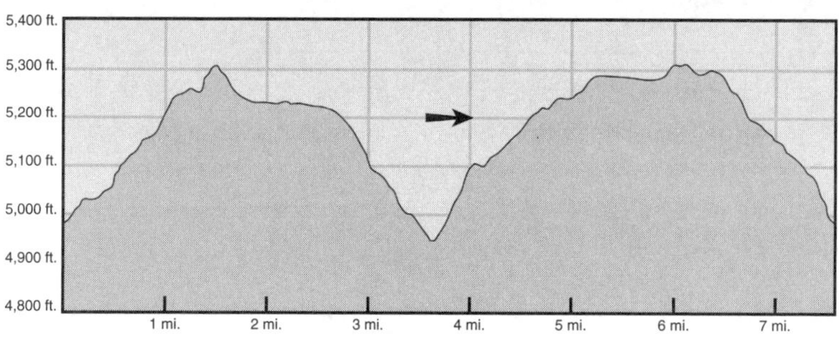

5,400 ft.
5,300 ft.
5,200 ft.
5,100 ft.
5,000 ft.
4,900 ft.
4,800 ft.
1 mi.
2 mi.
3 mi.
4 mi.
5 mi.
6 mi.
7 mi.

Around 3.25 miles, ignore a side trail toward Sisters Mirror Lakes and continue straight. Shortly after, you'll reach a junction signed HORSE CREEK TRAILHEAD. For those wishing to explore Horse Lake, it's here that you'll want to take a detour. The trail does not go directly to the lake, however, so after a quarter-mile on the trail, keep your eyes peeled for signs of water through the trees to your left. A few smaller footpaths will emerge in spots to take you closer toward the shores for further exploration.

Once satisfied, return to the previous junction and follow the signs pointing to Dumbbell Lake. Within a few dozen yards, cross picturesque Horse Creek and immediately take a left up the hill at an unsigned intersection. For those wishing for a little more exploration, continue straight for a dozen yards, where you'll see a vast, open meadow through the trees to your right. The meadow is perfect for a bit of midrun meandering.

Back on the trail, turn right (if coming from the meadow) and come to signs for Mile Lake—ignore these and continue straight up the hill toward Dumbbell. At 4 miles, the trail comes to a Y-junction, where you'll veer left toward Sunset Lake. Around 4.25 miles, look for a faint side trail on your left that sneaks its way through to the smaller Colt Lake. A quarter-mile later, this time on your right, keep your eyes peeled for the slightly larger Sunset Lake 20 yards down the hill through the trees. If you have a map and compass, these will help guide you to the spots.

Over the next mile, several other small ponds lie just off the trail and provide some nice opportunities for further exploration. At 5.3 miles, the trail enters a large, open meadow where it joins the PCT northbound. Stay left here to continue on the loop run, and another mile later, at around 6.6 miles, look for a signed marker for Elk Lake Trailhead 3. Here, views open up from Elk Lake in front of you to South Sister to the north. Continue on this trail for a quick downhill mile through the recovering forest and back to your starting point.

DIRECTIONS

From Bend, drive west on SW Century Drive, which becomes the Cascade Lakes National Scenic Byway, for 29.7 miles until you see a brown TRAILHEAD sign on the right, just before the sign for Elk Lake Resort. Turn right here to get to the trailhead.

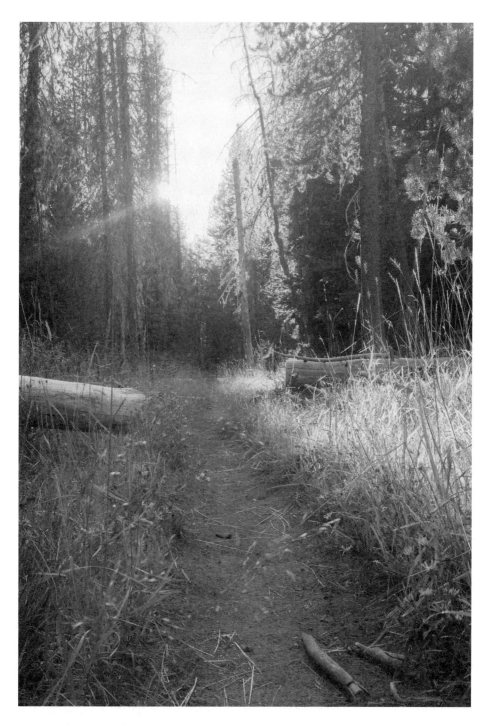

Wildflower-lined singletrack

41 Lemish Lake

TRAIL DETAILS AT A GLANCE

- **DISTANCE** 9.2-mile loop
- **GPS TRAILHEAD COORDINATES** N43° 47.637' W121° 54.171'
- **DIFFICULTY** 6 • **SCENERY** 4 • **CROWDS** 2
- **SEASON** June–November, sunrise–sunset • **ELEVATION** +/–767'
- **USERS** Hikers, runners, mountain bikers • **CONTACT** Bend–Fort Rock Ranger District, Deschutes National Forest; 541-383-4000, **www.fs.usda.gov/deschutes**
- **PERMITS/FEES** Northwest Forest Pass (see page 12)
- **RECOMMENDED MAP** *Bend, Oregon, Trail Map* by Adventure Maps, Inc. ($12, **adventuremaps.net**) • **DOGS** Yes (leashed only)

SOMETIMES YOU JUST WANT TO GET AWAY FROM PEOPLE and have a solitary outing in the woods. If this is what you're feeling, then Lemish Lake is a perfect run for you. Though not the most scenic on the list, it's pleasant enough, and you're guaranteed to be able to count the number of other trail users seen on one hand.

From the trailhead, run up the well-worn singletrack through forests of ponderosa pine and hemlock. At 0.5 mile, you'll encounter your first junction and the beginnings of Lemish Lake. Several campsites dot the shores just to the left of the junction. Turn right toward Charlton Lake, following the mountain bike pointers. Cross the outlet creek for Lemish Lake and keep left at the second junction, staying on the Charlton Lake Trail 19. From here, the trail parallels the lakeshore with nice views until it veers back up into the thicker forests.

Over the next 3 miles, the trail gradually steepens as it meanders through thick, moss-covered trees. Be wary of this area early in the season, as there tends to be much blowdown across the trail. The trails between Lemish Lake and Charlton Lake are some of the last cleared by crews.

At 3.4 miles, you'll reach the signed junction for Lily Lake and the Pacific Crest Trail. If you're looking for an extension on your run, take this side trail to check out appealing Lily Lake, a circular lake roughly equivalent in size to Lemish Lake. If you're content with the loop as is, keep left toward Clover Meadow/Charlton Lake, gently climbing your way up for a quarter-mile until another junction. Ignore this one and continue along the main path toward Clover Meadow. The next 1.5 miles are quick and fast as the path descends gradually through the forest.

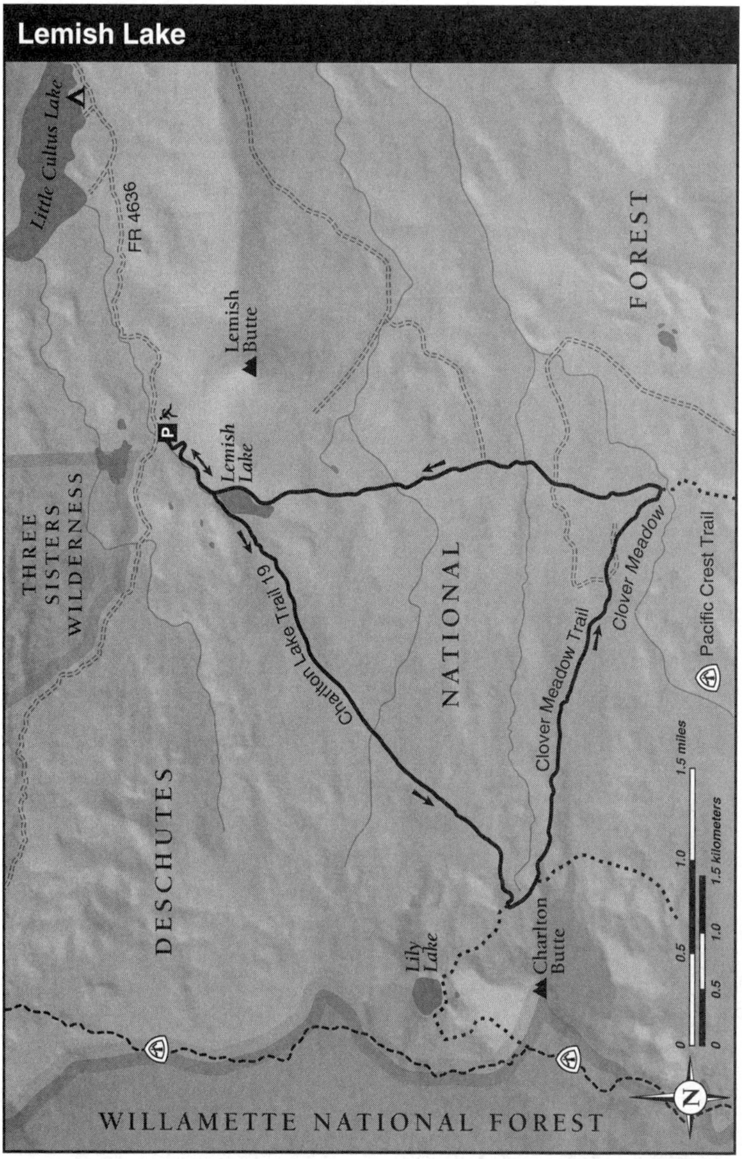

Lemish Lake

Little Cultus Lake
FR 4636
Lemish Butte
Lemish Lake
THREE SISTERS WILDERNESS
DESCHUTES
NATIONAL
FOREST
Charlton Lake Trail 19
Clover Meadow Trail
Clover Meadow
Pacific Crest Trail
Lily Lake
Charlton Butte
WILLAMETTE NATIONAL FOREST
0 0.5 1.0 1.5 miles
0 0.5 1.0 1.5 kilometers
N

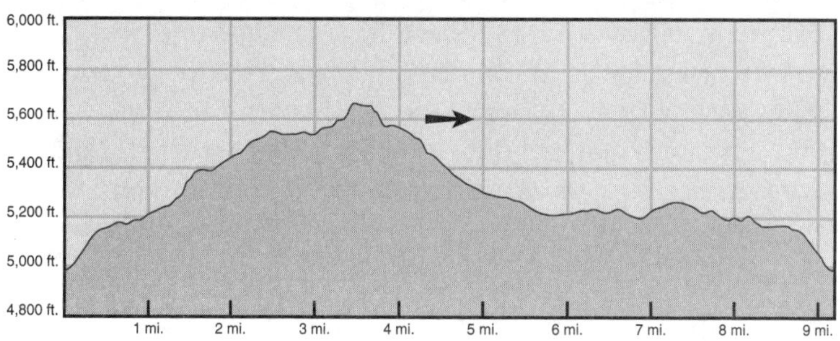
6,000 ft.
5,800 ft.
5,600 ft.
5,400 ft.
5,200 ft.
5,000 ft.
4,800 ft.
1 mi.
2 mi.
3 mi.
4 mi.
5 mi.
6 mi.
7 mi.
8 mi.
9 mi.

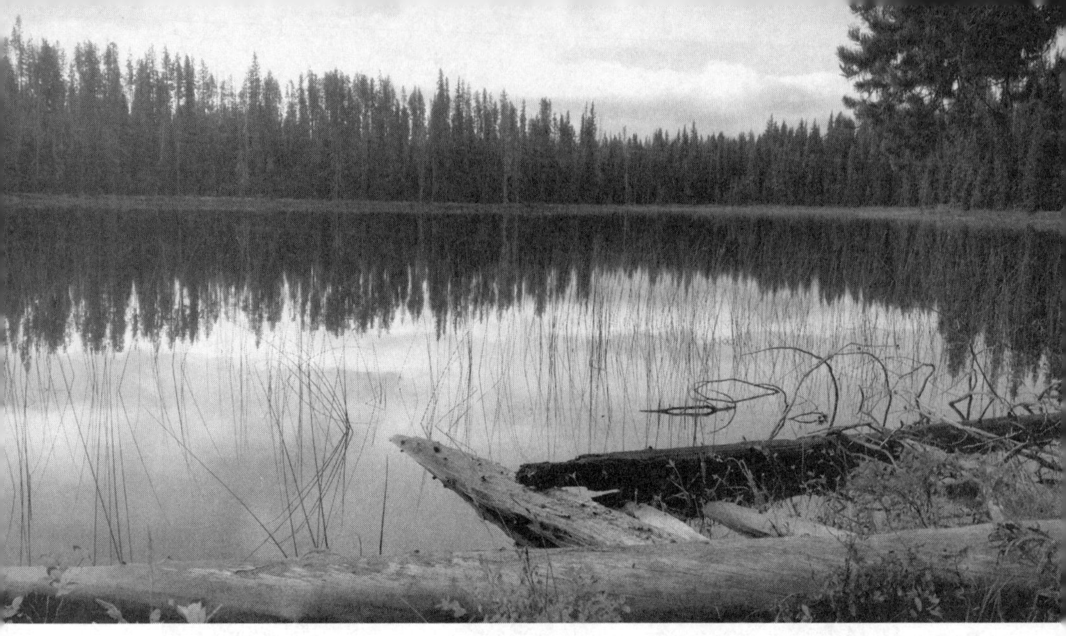

Lemish Lake

Around 5.4 miles, you begin to transition into an older burn and new-growth area as the path levels out. A brief quarter-mile later, the singletrack dumps you out onto an old jeep road, which you'll follow for 10 yards before ducking back into the trees on singletrack to your right. It's here that the path begins to turn sandy for the next few miles.

Take a sharp left turn at the junction toward Lemish Lake at 6.0 miles, crossing several rough roads and a burbling creek as you begin to exit the burn. Pass a horse camp at 7.1 miles and run through the forest until Lemish Lake starts to emerge once again around 8.4 miles. The trail soon begins to parallel the eastern shore until you complete the loop at the junction near the outlet. Retrace your original steps down the half-mile of trail through the forest and to your car.

DIRECTIONS

From Bend, follow the Cascade Lakes Scenic Byway for 41.1 miles until the right turn for Cultus Lake, on Forest Road 40. A short 0.7 mile after the turnoff, take a left on FR 4630, which becomes FR 4636 toward Little Cultus Lake. After 3.1 miles, turn left on FR 640, then immediately right back onto FR 4636 toward Irish and Taylor Lakes. Continue 2.4 miles (rough but passable in a passenger car) on FR 4636 and look for the trailhead on the left.

42 Lookout Mountain

TRAIL DETAILS AT A GLANCE

- **DISTANCE** 7-mile loop • **GPS TRAILHEAD COORDINATES** N44° 20.959' W120° 20.884' (Round Mountain Trailhead), N44° 20.391' W120° 21.548' (Independent Mine Trailhead)
- **DIFFICULTY** 6 • **SCENERY** 7 • **CROWDS** 4
- **SEASON** June–November, sunrise–sunset • **ELEVATION** +/–1,150'
- **USERS** Hikers, runners, mountain bikers, horses
- **CONTACT** Lookout Mountain Ranger District, Ochoco National Forest; 541-416-6500, **www.fs.usda.gov/ochoco**
- **PERMITS/FEES** Northwest Forest Pass (see page 12)
- **RECOMMENDED MAP** *Sisters & Redmond High Desert Trail Map* by Adventure Maps, Inc. ($12, **adventuremaps.net**) • **DOGS** Yes (leashed only)

THE OCHOCOS ARE A RELATIVELY SMALL MOUNTAIN RANGE in Central Oregon that often get overshadowed by the more grand Cascades range to the west. Not to be overlooked, the area is filled with highlights, including an array of gorgeous wildflowers during summer and some interesting man-made history—including a former lookout, an abandoned mine shaft, and a rustic ski shelter to warm winter-sports enthusiasts during the colder months.

Lookout Mountain is the tallest of the Ochoco peaks and on clear days offers views of nearly all the Cascades to the west, the Strawberry Mountains to the east, and 360-degree views of the Ochocos from the summit plateau. The well-maintained trails and gentle grades make it a popular spot for hikers, mountain bikers, and horseback riders, but the terrain is also perfect for trail running.

From the Independent Mine Trailhead, runners are presented with three different starting options. The recommended route is at the far end of the parking area on Lookout Mountain Trail 808 (not to be confused with the shorter, steeper 808a). Begin here by winding your way through thick groves of ponderosa pine and climbing gradually until the trail begins to level out after a mile. The trees thin as you crest the vast summit plateau and views of the surrounding mountains begin to open up.

Starting in June, bright wildflowers light up the sagebrush canvas plateau. Balsamroot, lupine, shooting star, mountain bluebell, Indian paintbrush, lark-spur, and columbine can all be found throughout the area. Shortly after crossing

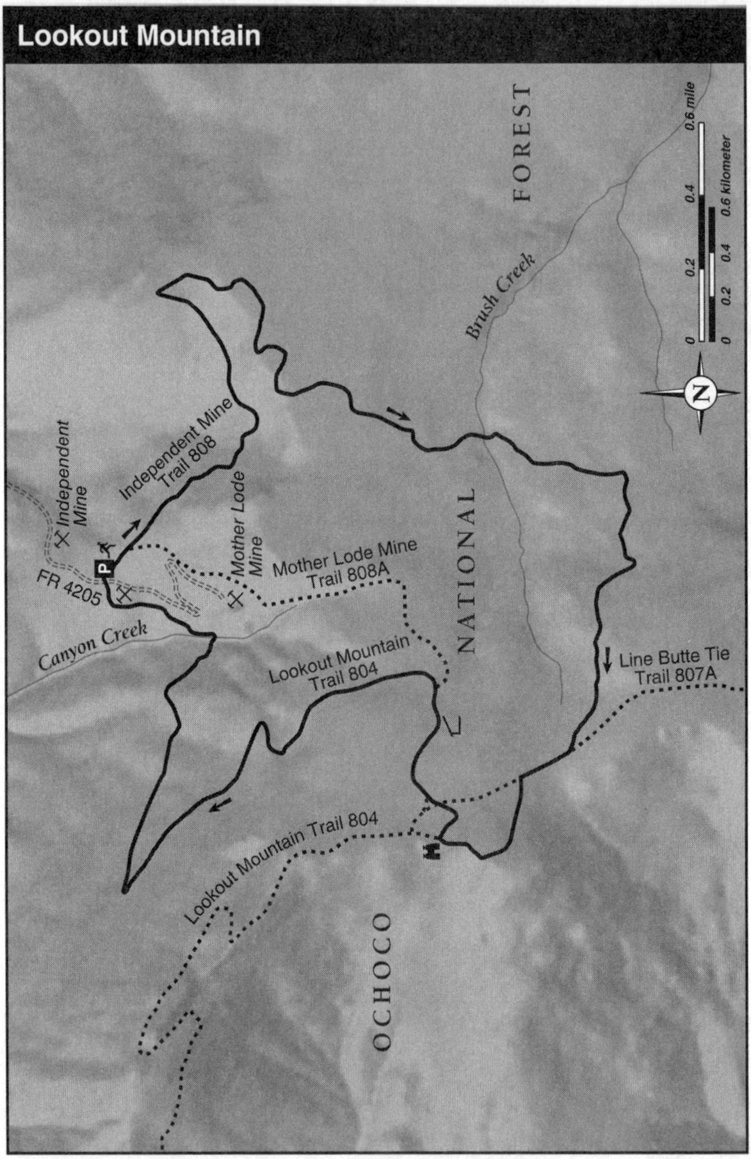

Lookout Mountain
FOREST
NATIONAL
OCHOCO
0.6 mile
0.4
0.2
0
0.6 kilometer
0.4
0.2
0
N
Brush Creek
Independent Mine Trail 808
Independent Mine
Mother Lode Mine
Mother Lode Mine Trail 808A
FR 4205
Canyon Creek
Lookout Mountain Trail 804
Line Butte Tie Trail 807A
Lookout Mountain Trail 804
P

7,000 ft.
6,800 ft.
6,600 ft.
6,400 ft.
6,200 ft.
6,000 ft.
5,800 ft.
1 mi.
2 mi.
3 mi.
4 mi.
5 mi.
6 mi.
7 mi.

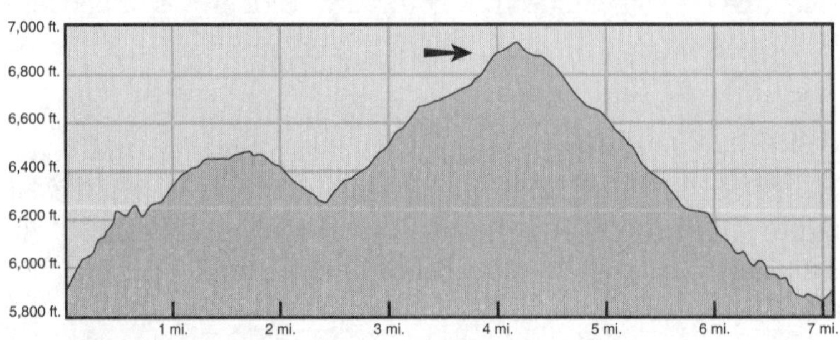

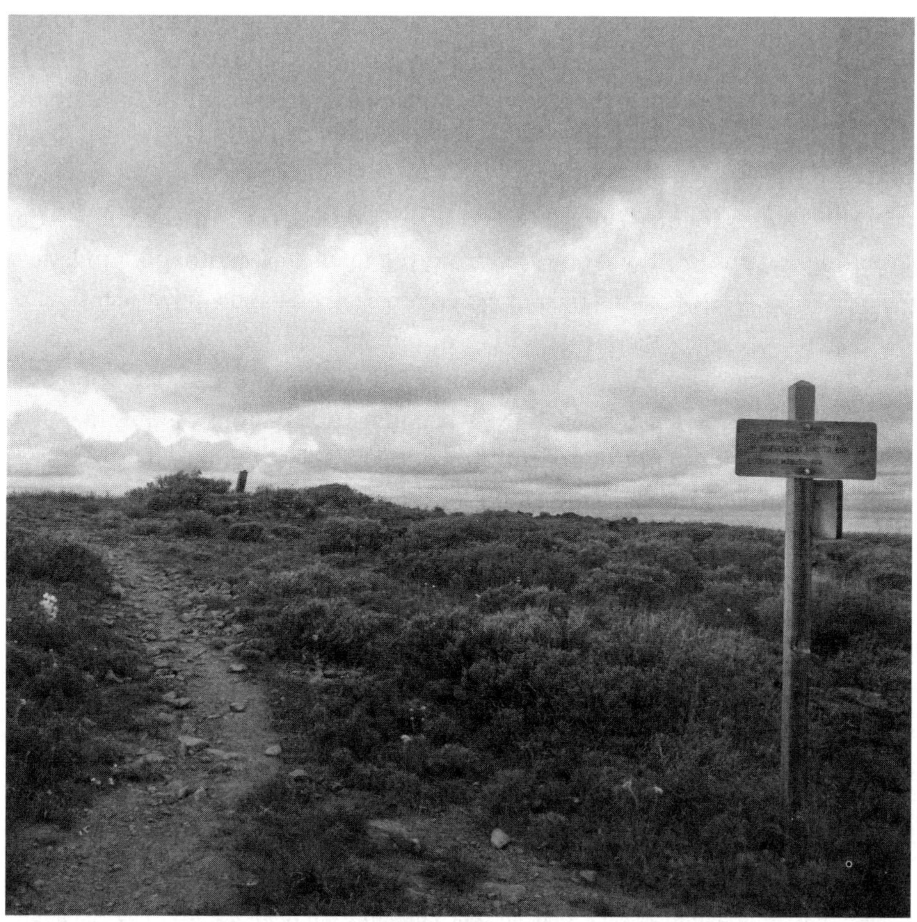

The trail bisects a stark High Desert landscape.

Brush Creek at 2.4 miles, continue along the rolling plateau to a marked junction with the Line Butte Tie Trail at 3.5 miles. Follow signs pointing to the summit and take in the views of the Cascades to your left as you steadily climb to the high point of the loop.

Shortly after the 4-mile marker, reach the summit and the former lookout site for which the mountain is named. Though the structure is no longer there, a crumbling lava rock wall lining the periphery of the location spurs the imagination of how the entire area once appeared. Views from here are expansive, and this is a perfect spot to catch your breath and reward yourself for the 1,000-foot climb.

If you have time and desire to extend the run a bit, continue from the summit junction straight on 808 along the rim of the plateau for even more views.

When you're ready to return, follow Lookout Mountain Trail 804 toward the snow shelter to continue along the intended loop. In a quick quarter-mile downhill, turn right to explore the rustic shelter—a popular rest stop and warming station for cross-country skiers and snowshoers during the winter season. After exploring the hut, continue downhill from the main trail another 0.4 mile to a Y-junction. Stay left for the Lookout Mountain Trail 804 and enjoy the fast, runnable trail as it snakes its way back into the pine forest at the base of the plateau.

Zigzag your way back downhill, crossing a few small creeks before turning a corner to find an abandoned three-story mine building on the hillside. Just beyond the log bridge in front of the structure is a collapsed mineshaft complete with ore cart rails. Though the impulse to explore may be high, it's best to resist the urge as the mining site was once used for processing mercury, a dangerous and highly toxic element.

From the mining site, continue along the trail for another quarter-mile to an unmarked junction at 6.9 miles. A short uphill brings you back to the trailhead and your car, completing the loop.

DIRECTIONS

From Prineville, take US 26 east toward the Ochoco Mountains and John Day. About 16 miles from town, turn right onto Ochoco Creek Road/Forest Road 23, following signs for Walton Lake and Lookout Mountain. Follow this road for 8 miles. Just beyond the Ochoco Ranger Station, turn right onto Canyon Creek Road/FR 42 and follow the paved road to the Round Mountain South Trailhead near the saddle. If you'd like to extend the run 2 miles and add more elevation, park here. Otherwise, continue up rough dirt Lookout Mountain Road/FR 4205 for another mile to the Independent Mine Trailhead.

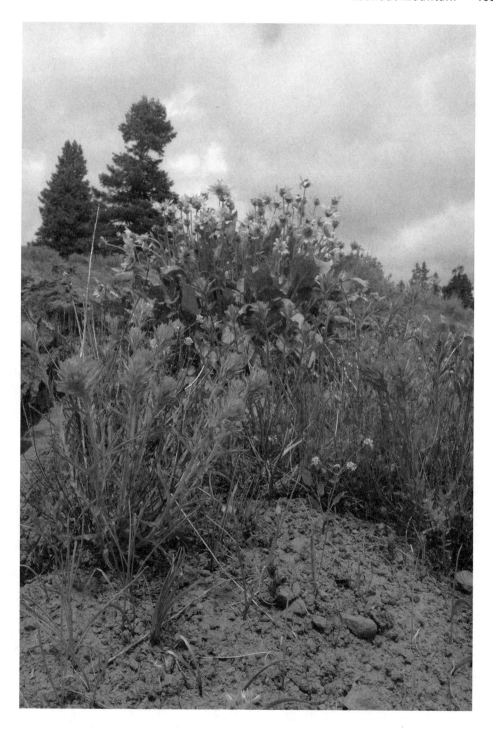

A riot of color: balsamroot and Indian paintbrush

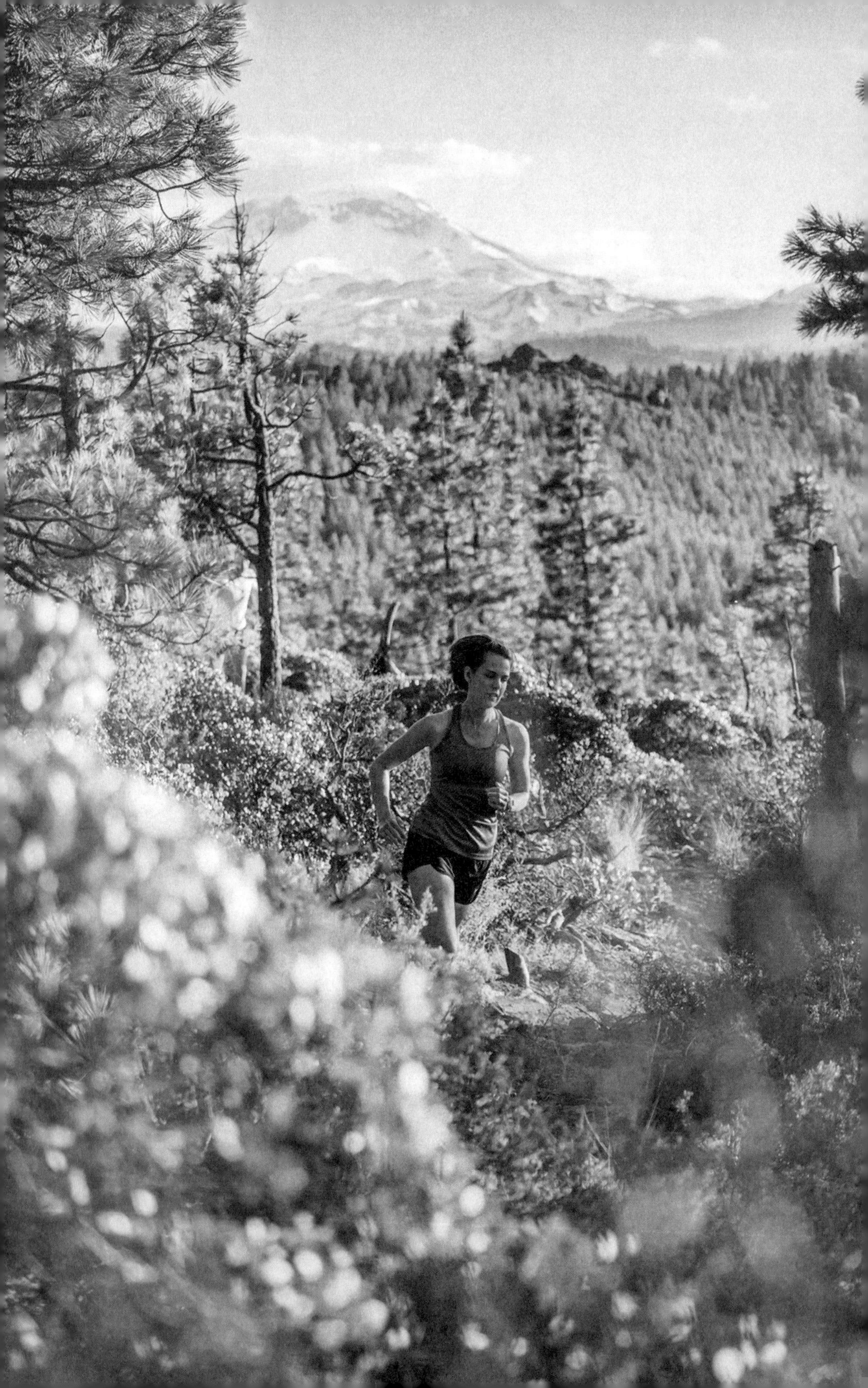

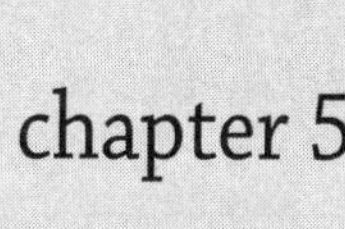

chapter 5

FALL RUNS

FALL TRAIL LIST

OPPOSITE: *Running along the ridgeline* PHOTO: NATE WYETH

43 Metolius River

TRAIL DETAILS AT A GLANCE

- **DISTANCE** 5.6-mile loop • **GPS TRAILHEAD COORDINATES** N44° 31.342' W121° 37.926'
- **DIFFICULTY** 2 • **SCENERY** 7 • **CROWDS** 6
- **SEASON** Year-round, sunrise–sunset • **ELEVATION** +/–96'
- **USERS** Hikers, runners
- **CONTACTS** Sisters Ranger District, Deschutes National Forest; 541-549-7700, **www.fs.usda.gov/deschutes;** Wizard Falls Fish Hatchery, 541-595-6611, **tinyurl.com/wizardfalls**
- **PERMITS/FEES** None
- **RECOMMENDED MAP** *Sisters & Redmond High Desert Trail Map* by Adventure Maps, Inc. ($12, **adventuremaps.net**) • **DOGS** Yes (leashed only)

THE METOLIUS RIVER IS THE MOST MAGICAL OF ALL RIVERS in the state of Oregon. Originating from two clusters of substantial underground springs at the base of Black Butte, the river appears to rise fully formed from underground. Though the headwaters are impressive, the rest of the river is even more spectacular. The waters of the Metolius are clean and clear, and the river and idyllic woods on each side create a stunning backdrop. A National Wild and Scenic River, the Metolius is best described as a scene from the Brad Pitt film *A River Runs Through It.*

On the upper stretches of the river, accessible and well-maintained trails on both sides make the river an ideal spot for hiking, fly fishing, and running throughout the year. Though the run can be started in many locations, an ideal spot is at the Wizard Falls Fish Hatchery, which makes for a fun and interesting destination on its own. Wizard Falls is run by the Oregon Department of Fish and Wildlife and offers a parklike setting complete with viewing ponds, interpretive signage, and pleasant spots for a picnic. The hatchery rears Atlantic salmon, brook trout, cutthroat trout, kokanee, and rainbow trout for fishing programs around the state and has an incubation program for spring Chinook salmon.

Begin the run on the west side of the river, near the fish hatchery. Ignore the upriver trail on the opposite side of the road and instead look for a RIVER TRAIL sign 20 yards past the bathrooms and a strand of Douglas-firs. Just beyond the hatchery, the trail begins to hug the banks of the river, flowing in and out with the

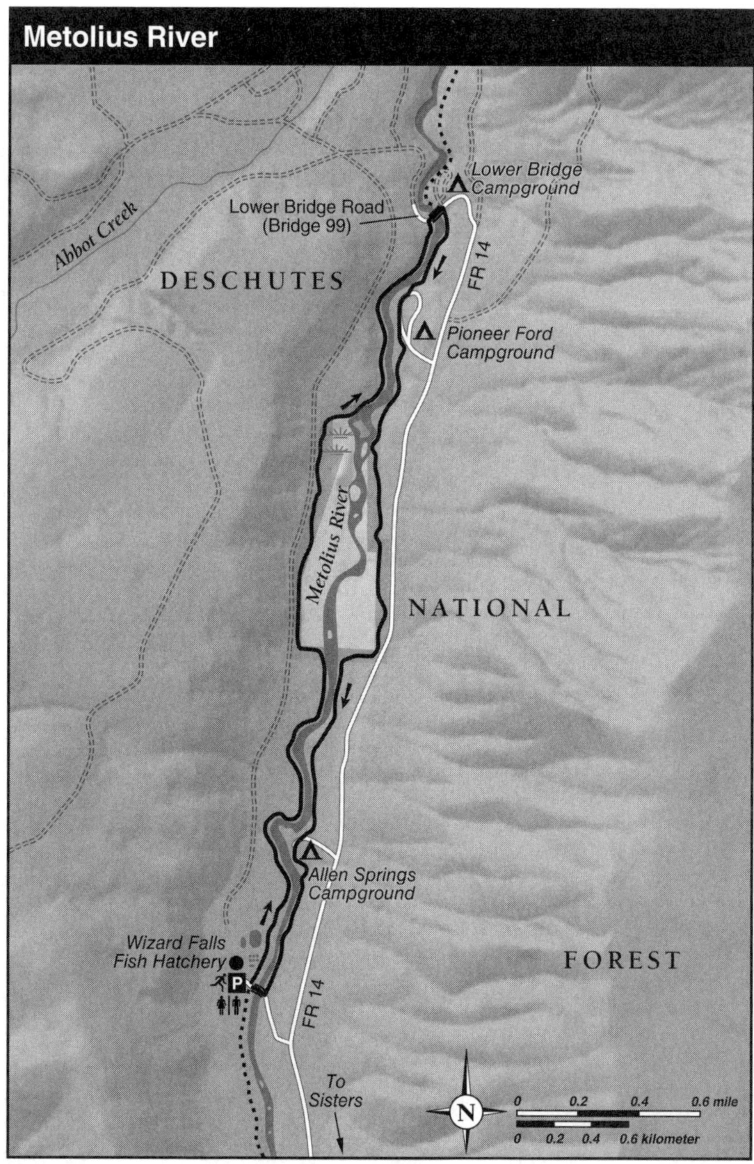

contours of the scenic river. Immediately you feel like you're transported to a film location or a photo shoot.

After 1.2 miles, the trail veers sharply left from the banks, avoiding a parcel of private property. A barely readable sign, along with a very noticeable fence, blocks the way along the bank. Instead, turn left and run slightly uphill for a short stint before continuing to parallel the river from afar. As you begin to round the

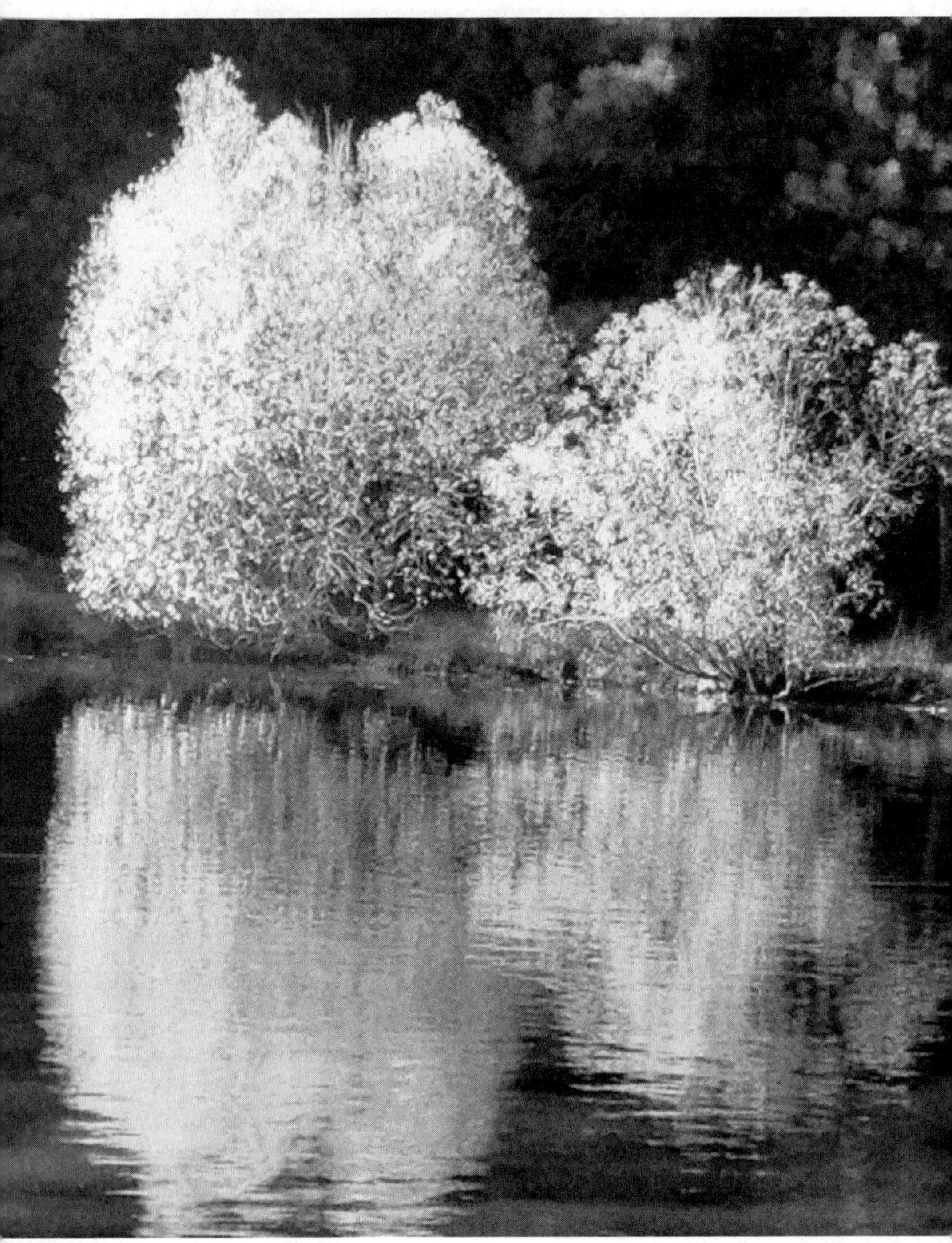

Fall color reflects off the Metolius.

corner looping around the property and back toward the river, keep your eyes out for a misty, murky swamp far below the trail to your right. During summer months, you'll hear the area long before you see it, with hundreds of croaking frogs calling it home.

Back along the riverbanks, continue downstream until mile 2.8, when you emerge from the trail onto Lower Bridge Road (Bridge 99). Cross the bridge here to the opposite side of the river and pick up the trail going back south toward the hatchery. Approximately a quarter-mile later, you hit your first of multiple campgrounds. Run on the paved loop road through Pioneer Campground and look for Campsite 19, which is also the host. Just past the site, the doubletrack trail starts on your right.

At 3.7 miles, the trail begins to veer away from the river, again skirting private property. After crossing multiple gravel driveways, run up the singletrack as it parallels a fence until 4.3 miles, when it ducks back toward the river on the right. Several signs help point the way at this confusing area.

Back along the river, the trail soon dumps you out into Allen Springs Campground near Campsite 4. Follow the paved loop road through the campground until Campsite 14, where you'll take a hard right toward the river, looking for the singletrack. From here, continue along the riverbank, taking in the scenery until you reach the hatchery bridge to complete the loop and your run.

DIRECTIONS

Drive northwest from Bend about 28 miles on US 20. Near Milepost 91, turn right on Forest Road 14 at the METOLIUS RIVER/CAMP SHERMAN sign. After 2.7 miles, bear right to stay on FR 14, heading east and then north. In another 1.7 miles, bear right again to stay on FR 14 and drive north about 6 miles, past the campgrounds, until the signs for Wizard Falls Fish Hatchery. Then turn left, crossing the river, and find the trailhead near the parking area for the hatchery.

44 Metolius Preserve

TRAIL DETAILS AT A GLANCE

- **DISTANCE** 3.7-mile loop
- **GPS TRAILHEAD COORDINATES** N44° 26.698' W121° 40.840'
- **DIFFICULTY** 3 • **SCENERY** 5 • **CROWDS** 4
- **SEASON** Year-round, sunrise–sunset • **ELEVATION** +/–94' • **USERS** Hikers, runners
- **CONTACT** Deschutes Land Trust, 541-330-0017, **deschuteslandtrust.org**
- **PERMITS/FEES** None
- **RECOMMENDED MAP** *Sisters & Redmond High Desert Trail Map* by Adventure Maps, Inc. ($12, **adventuremaps.net**) • **DOGS** Yes (leashed only)

A SIMPLE CONVERSATION between two fishermen started the land purchase that today forms the Metolius Preserve. That 2003 meeting between a board member from the Deschutes Basin Land Trust and the chairman of Willamette Industries initiated a plan to conserve habitat for the return of salmon to the Deschutes Basin. More than a decade later, not only are the Chinook salmon and various species of trout returning, but many hikers, mountain bikers, and trail runners are as well.

The Metolius Preserve encompasses over 1,240 acres of ponderosa pine–forested land, along with three different branches of Fish Creek—an important migratory route and habitat for spawning salmon. Today the preserve features more than 10 miles of newly developed trails open nearly year-round. The singletrack trails and former fire roads make for easy and tranquil trail running through an area that crosses the North, Middle, and South Forks of Lake Creek.

Note: The Metolius Preserve trails are still being established, and work remains to be done on more-permanent signs and guides. For now, be sure to have a map handy when running in the area, and keep your eyes peeled for temporary signage on trees and stakes.

Begin the run at the north end of the preserve off of Forest Road 1216 (Suttle–Sherman Road). From the trailhead parking lot, take the wide doubletrack path back west toward the way you drove in. A quick 100 yards later, turn left on the obvious but unmarked singletrack—there should be a temporary sign on the tree by the junction. Weave in and out of ponderosa pines on the newly formed path before crossing a nice, sturdy bridge over North Fork Fish Creek at 0.25 mile.

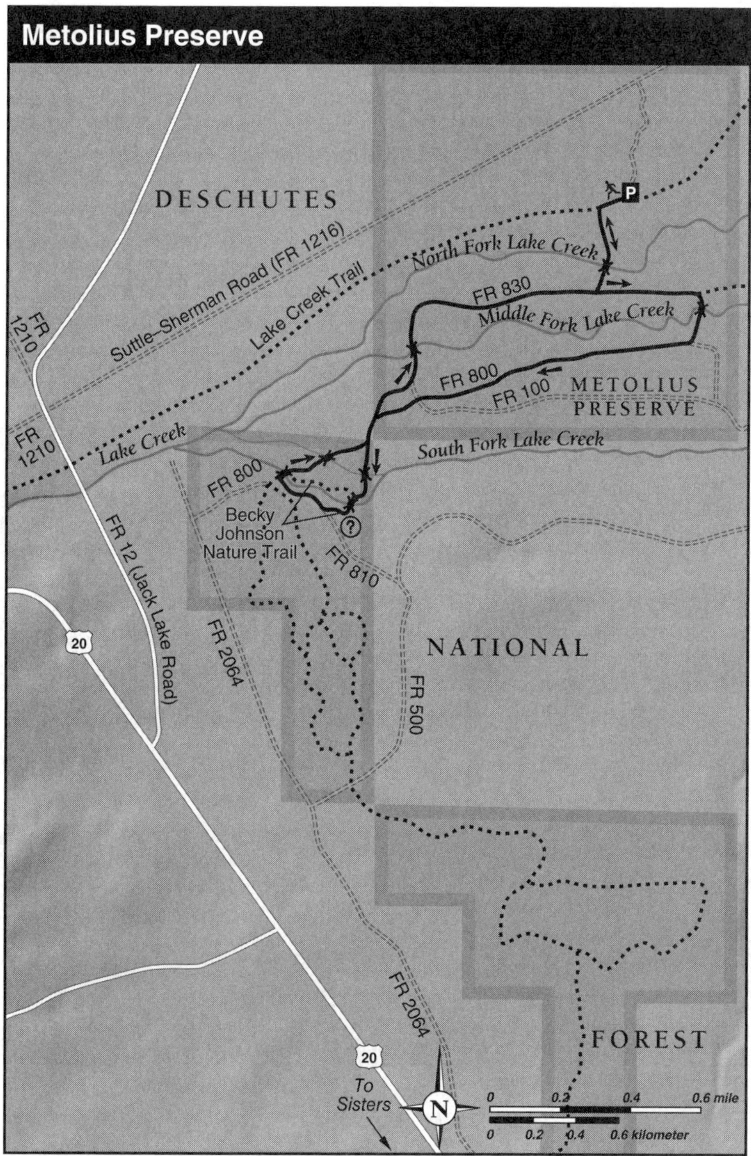

Shortly after, turn left at a junction with an old jeep road to begin the upper loop portion of the run.

Run down the rocky, sandy jeep road, keeping right at 0.5 mile at the fork. A short time later, at 0.6 mile, turn right at the obvious singletrack marked by a temporary sign. Cross another picturesque bridge 20 yards after the junction, taking you over the Middle Fork of Fish Creek. The trail then winds its way back

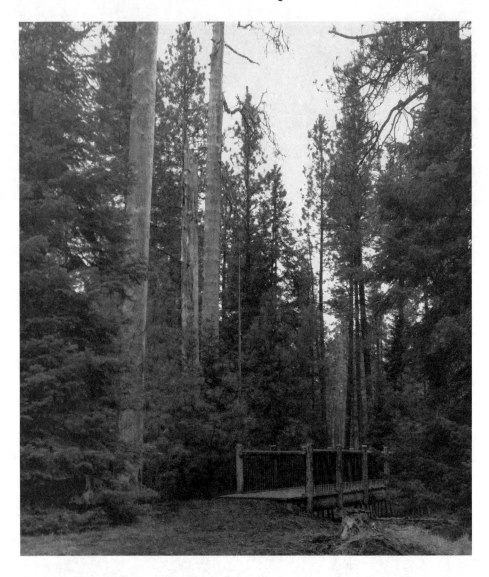

Footbridge over Middle Fork Lake Creek

on the loop through the viewless pine forests before spitting you out at a junction with multiple old roads.

Take a left here on the most obvious road (not Forest Road 100) and soon you'll pass Forest Road 801, which will be your return. For now, keep straight and veer left on the singletrack trail at 1.7 miles. The trail weaves in between the old-growth pines before looping back toward the South Fork Fish Creek. Cross a small footbridge and, a short time later, a pair of larger bridges over the main creek, and you'll soon see a large interpretive kiosk ahead.

From here, run along the Becky Johnson Nature Trail along the south side of Fish Creek and past several viewing platforms with signage describing the habitat and preserve. If you have time, it's worth it to check out the signage and read about the history of the creek and the area. At 2.1 miles, turn right and cross back over Fish Creek to begin making your way back. Ignore the creekside trail on the opposite back (the continuation of the 0.6-mile Becky Johnson Nature Trail loop) and instead continue straight. Soon you'll pass by the singletrack where you recently turned, completing the southern loop portion.

Keep left at the next several junctions and soon you'll hear the Middle Fork in the distance. After running over the creek via a culvert, the road turns sharply back east, and within a half-mile you'll reach the initial junction for the upper loop. From here, retrace your steps over the North Fork bridge and the short distance back to the trailhead.

DIRECTIONS

Drive 12 miles northwest of Sisters on US 20. Turn right just beyond Milepost 88, at the junction signed MT. JEFFERSON WILDERNESS TRAILHEADS, onto Jack Lake Road/ Forest Road 12. After 1 mile, turn right at the four-way intersection onto nicely graded gravel FR 1216/Suttle–Sherman Road and drive 1.8 miles until you see signs for Metolius Preserve on the right. The trailhead is 0.3 mile down this side road.

45 Black Butte

TRAIL DETAILS AT A GLANCE

- **DISTANCE** 4.7-mile loop
- **GPS TRAILHEAD COORDINATES** N44° 25.689' W121° 39.351'
- **DIFFICULTY** 5 • **SCENERY** 5 • **CROWDS** 3 • **SEASON** Year-round, sunrise–sunset
- **ELEVATION** +/–735' • **USERS** Hikers, runners
- **CONTACT** Sisters Ranger District, Deschutes National Forest; 541-549-7700, **www.fs.usda.gov/deschutes** • **PERMITS/FEES** None
- **RECOMMENDED MAP** *Mount Jefferson and Mount Washington Trails Illustrated Topographic Map* by National Geographic ($11.95, **natgeomaps.com**) • **DOGS** Yes (leashed only)

BLACK BUTTE'S 6,436-FOOT SUMMIT and nearly perfectly symmetrical shape make it one of Central Oregon's most recognized landmarks. Though much smaller in stature than the neighboring Cascades, the region's tallest butte is held in deep regard by locals, who have been hiking its flanks for over a century.

The popular Black Butte Trail was originally used to pack supplies up to the butte's first fire lookout in 1910. Local Camp Sherman residents began hiking the trail soon after in what historians say were post–dance hall night hikes timed to catch the morning sunrise from the summit. Over the years, sturdier fire lookouts were built, along with a still-existing cupola building in 1924 and a log cabin residence in 1979. Because the existing fire lookout tower is still in use by the US Forest Service, trail users are asked to respect the boundaries of the lookout and keep to the trail.

Though the Black Butte Trail is a long, steep up-and-down to the summit, trail runners can make good use of the USDA's Roads to Trails program and make a nice 5-mile loop from the Upper Butte and Lower Butte Trails. Those seeking extra views and a true quad-burner may continue along toward the summit for a total of 11.5 miles and a grinding 3,400-foot elevation gain.

Start the run from the lower trailhead for Black Butte Trail 4026. The first 0.75 mile is on a wide, shaded path through mature lodgepole and ponderosa pines with manzanita underbrush and a pine needle–covered forest floor. Several abandoned forest roads intersect the trail; however, signed posts urge you forward in the right direction. At 0.75 mile, turn left uphill on the hikers-only Black

Black Butte

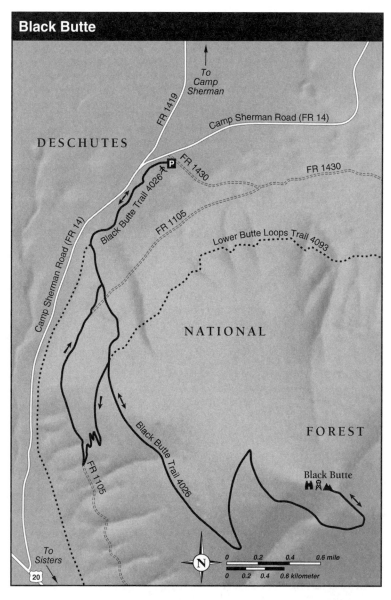

To Camp Sherman
FR 1419
Camp Sherman Road (FR 14)
DESCHUTES
FR 1430
FR 1430
Black Butte Trail 4026
FR 1105
Camp Sherman Road (FR 14)
Lower Butte Loops Trail 4093
NATIONAL
FOREST
Black Butte Trail 4026
FR 1105
Black Butte
To Sisters
20
N
0 0.2 0.4 0.6 mile
0 0.2 0.4 0.6 kilometer

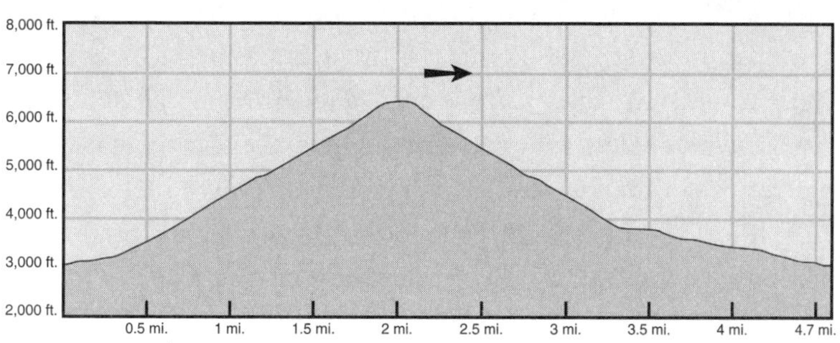

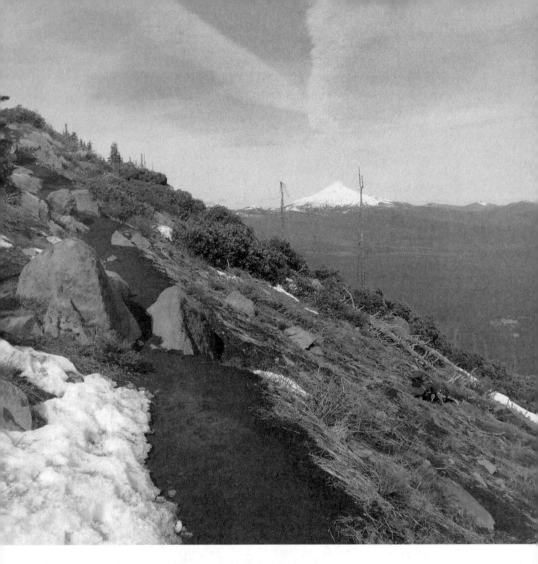

Mount Jefferson rises behind Black Butte.

Butte Trail. A quick quarter-mile later, cross Lower Butte Loops Trail 4093 and continue climbing along the singletrack.

Another half-mile of climbing brings you to a decision point. If you're looking for a longer, more strenuous run, continue along the Black Butte Trail, following signs toward the summit. The trail is a relentless uphill but rewards your efforts tenfold with endless views of Central Oregon and snowcapped mountains beyond. If you're out for a leisurely loop instead, turn right here on Upper Butte Loops Trail 4093.1. Though slightly more overgrown than its lower counterpart, the Upper Butte Loops Trail is still very obvious and discernible.

Run 0.5 mile on mostly viewless trail and look for signs around 2 miles pointing toward descending singletrack on your right. Follow this winding, needle-cushioned path as it switchbacks down to the Lower Butte Loops Trail 0.5 mile later. (*Note:* The junction with the Lower Butte Loops Trail is the only junction not signed on this route.) Turn right and run 1.2 miles to complete the Butte Loops Trail loop. Along the way, keep your eyes peeled for peeks of Three Fingered Jack and Mount Jefferson through the trees.

At 3.65 miles, turn left back onto the trail on which you came, Black Butte Trail 4026, descending back on singletrack until the junction with the first stretch of road converted to trail. At this point, simply turn right and retrace your steps to complete your run.

DIRECTIONS

Drive northwest from Bend about 28 miles on US 20. Near Milepost 91, turn right on Forest Road 14 at the METOLIUS RIVER/CAMP SHERMAN sign. About 2.7 miles later on FR 14/Camp Sherman Road, veer right at the Y-intersection toward the campgrounds. Take your first right 0.2 mile later. The Lower Black Butte Trailhead will be another 50 yards ahead, on your right.

Helpful signs point the way along the trail.

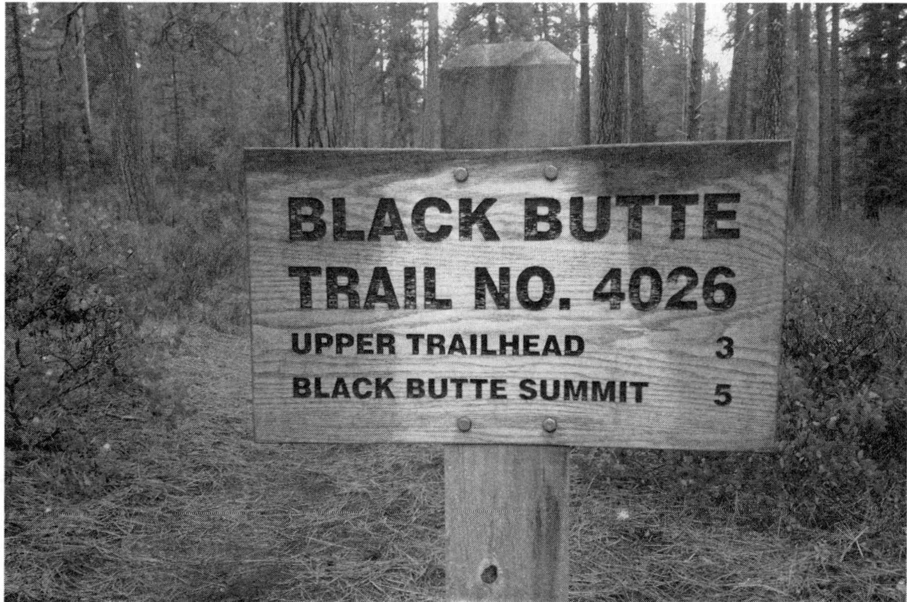
BLACK BUTTE
TRAIL NO. 4026
UPPER TRAILHEAD 3
BLACK BUTTE SUMMIT 5

46 Upper Peterson Ridge Trail

TRAIL DETAILS AT A GLANCE

- **DISTANCE** 7.1-mile loop
- **GPS TRAILHEAD COORDINATES** N44° 13.353' W121° 34.535'
- **DIFFICULTY** 3 • **SCENERY** 7 • **CROWDS** 5
- **SEASON** Year-round, sunrise–sunset • **ELEVATION** +/–440'
- **USERS** Hikers, runners, mountain bikers
- **CONTACT** Sisters Trail Alliance, 541-719-8822, **sisterstrails.com** • **PERMITS/FEES** None
- **RECOMMENDED MAP** *Sisters & Redmond High Desert Trail Map* by Adventure Maps, Inc. ($12, **adventuremaps.net**) • **DOGS** Yes (leashed only)

THE PETERSON RIDGE TRAIL (PRT) SYSTEM is a well-marked, meticulously maintained network of trails west of Sisters. Cared for by the Sisters Trail Alliance, the singletrack is fast, fun, and open nearly year-round with the exception of an occasional winter snowstorm. The trails on the upper portion are best in spring and fall when the dust has settled from summer and the moisture has dried up from winter.

Whereas the lower trails in the PRT network are mostly viewless, much of the western half of the upper trails parallels the ridge shelf—allowing expansive views of the Cascades on the horizon and the numerous rounded buttes closer at hand. Many of the trails are smooth singletrack through sparse forests of ponderosa and lodgepole pine with sagebrush dotting the forest floor. Though the loop can be run in either direction, the recommended route is counterclockwise for better views of the western horizon on the return.

To begin, find the upper trailhead opposite the parking area at mile 5.3 on Three Creeks Lake Road. Soon after the trailhead sign (maps are available here), keep right at the first marked junction—number 34—to continue along PRT East. The smooth singletrack weaves its way through heavy manzanita amidst a lightly burned pine forest before hitting Marker 28 within the first three-quarters of a mile. Keep right here on PRT East, avoiding the horse trail straight ahead. After dropping slightly, the trail levels out, and at 1.6 miles you begin to reel in the Eagle Rock 2 viewpoint on your right. It's worth venturing slightly off-trail here to climb the small rock formation for even better views beyond the ridge.

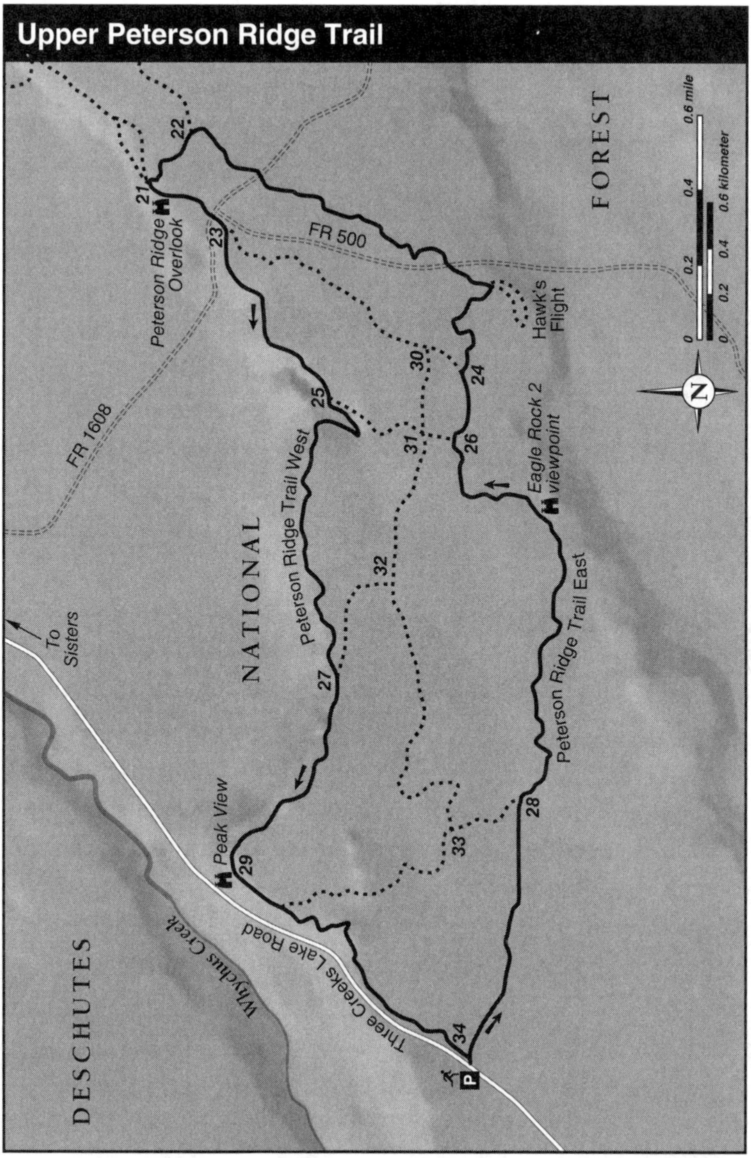

Upper Peterson Ridge Trail

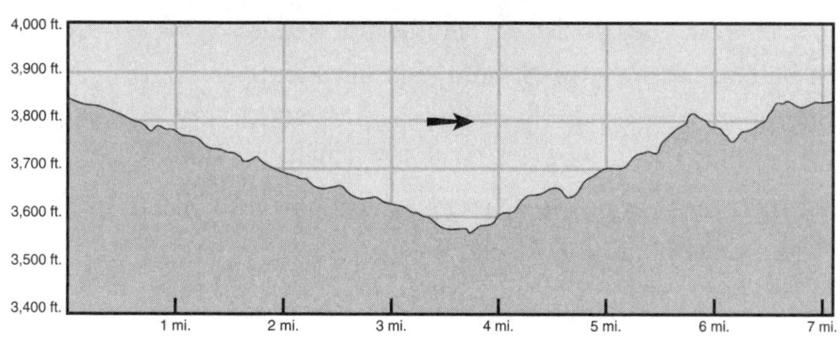

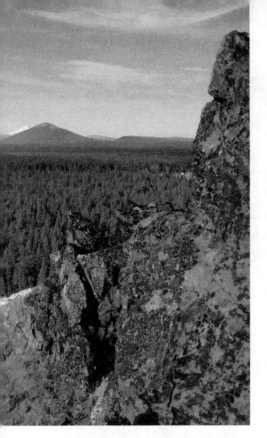

Mount Jefferson peeks around Black Butte.

Once back on the trail, continue along PRT East and pass Markers 26 and 24. At 2.5 miles, the trail skirts a rocky ridge with great views to the southeast. Ignore the unmarked trail (Hawk's Nest) and follow PRT East back through the trees before crossing a red-hued, crushed volcanic rock forest road. Less than a mile later, turn left at Marker 22 on the Turkey Hollow connector trail toward the Peterson Ridge Overlook. A quick 0.25 mile later, at Marker 21, turn right for 20 yards to take in the expansive views at the Peterson Ridge Overlook.

The overlook is a great spot to catch your breath while taking in the views of the Cascades. On clear, sunny days, runners can see Black Butte; Mount Washington; Three Fingered Jack; and North, Middle, and South Sisters. Though you most likely will not be alone at this viewpoint, it's an inspiring spot and one that makes you quickly realize the beauty of Central Oregon.

Back on the trail, retrace your steps to Marker 21 and continue along PRT West. Cross a forest road at 3.6 miles and turn right at Marker 23. Just over 0.5 mile later, pass Signpost 25 and drop into a small, scenic canyon for a quick dipsy-doo before resurfacing along the ridge with views of Black Butte pulling you forward along the trail.

For the next 2 miles, the trail closely parallels the ridgeline and views continue to present themselves on your right. As you make your way west along the trail, keep your eyes peeled for shy Mount Jefferson, which begins to poke out from behind Black Butte. Several rock outcroppings offer further opportunities for scenery, and the aptly named Peak View (Marker 29) even provides a soundtrack with the murmurs of Whychus Creek below the ridge. One final view worth noting is that of the Three Sisters, which appear to be within touching distance on clear days, at around 6 miles.

The remaining 0.75 mile is less exciting, though by now runners should have had their fill of scenery. The last stretch of trail parallels Three Creeks Lake Road before returning to the trailhead and your vehicle.

DIRECTIONS

From Bend, drive 21.8 miles northwest on US 20 toward Sisters. In downtown Sisters, turn left (south) on Elm Street, which turns into Three Creeks Lake Road. After 5.3 miles, just after you crest the hill, look for the signed trailhead on the left-hand side of the road. Limited parking is available opposite the trailhead on the other side of the road.

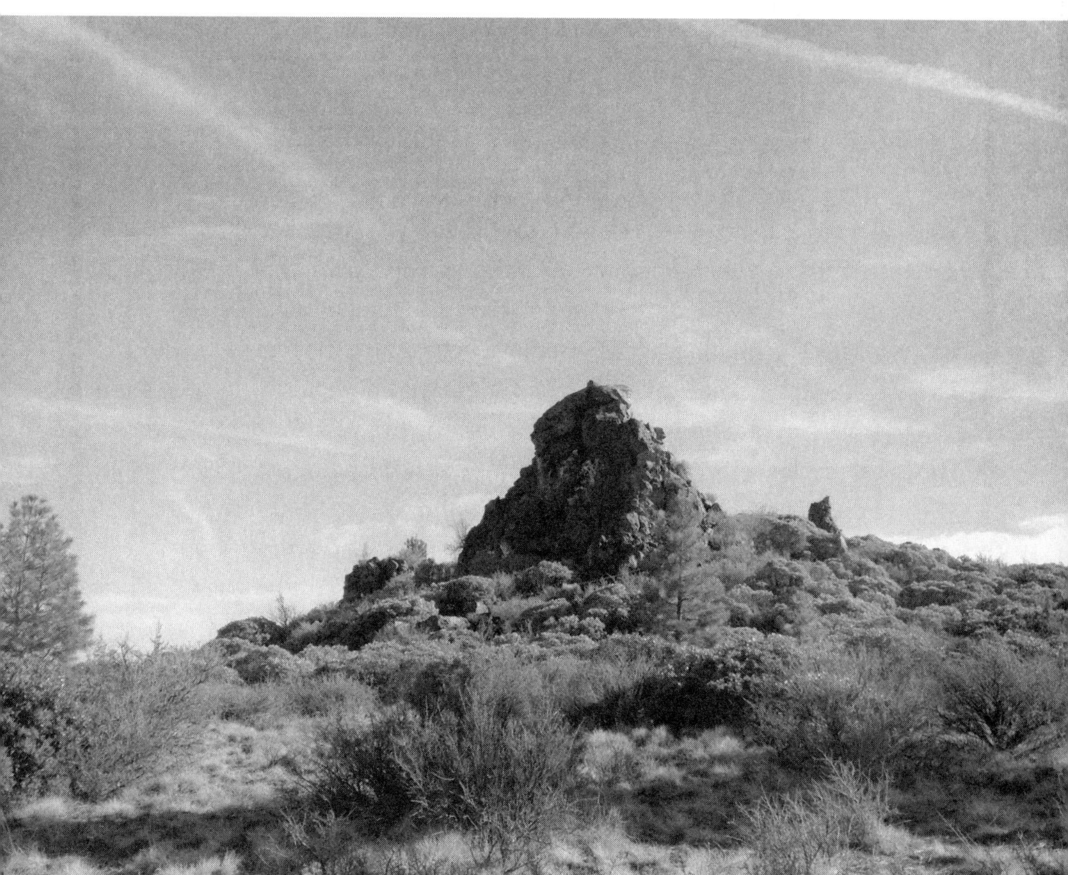

Eagle Rock 2

47 LaPine State Park:
NORTH LOOP

TRAIL DETAILS AT A GLANCE

- **DISTANCE** 7.8-mile loop
- **GPS TRAILHEAD COORDINATES** N43° 46.576' W121° 31.842'
- **DIFFICULTY** 3 • **SCENERY** 8 • **CROWDS** 6 • **SEASON** Year-round, sunrise–sunset
- **ELEVATION** +/–69' • **USERS** Hikers, runners, mountain bikers
- **CONTACT** LaPine State Park, 541-536-2071, **tinyurl.com/lapinestatepark**
- **PERMITS/FEES** None (day use is free)
- **RECOMMENDED MAP** PDF map at **tinyurl.com/lapinenorthmap** • **DOGS** Yes (leashed only)

LaPine State Park is an angler's haven, encompassing two of the best trout-fishing rivers in Central Oregon in the Upper Deschutes and Fall Rivers. On the North Loop run, you'll get to see both up close as you meander along the curves of each river for nearly half the loop. And though the park may be crowded during the summer months with campers and floaters splashing along the river, the trails also offer solitude and serenity as you move deeper into the forests.

The North Loop starts at McGregor Memorial Viewpoint, which is reached by the second right-hand turn after you cross the bridge into the park. The view here is spectacular, with the bending Deschutes River leading your eyes to Paulina Peak and the Newberry National Volcanic Monument in the distance.

Begin by running east (left) at the viewpoint, and within a quarter-mile you'll reach the first junction. Stay left, following the Fall River and McGregor Trail markers. Soon after, you'll reach another marker indicating the wraparound of the 1.5-mile McGregor Trail Loop. Stay straight and continue through the sub-alpine pine forest. After a forest road crossing, connect to doubletrack taking you past a ramshackle old cabin where you'll catch a glimpse of the Deschutes as it pops back into view through the trees to your right.

Around 1.6 miles, a short side trail leading down toward the river will take you toward the confluence of the Fall River and Deschutes, where you can spot great blue herons and egrets in the shallows. The lower trail joins back up within a

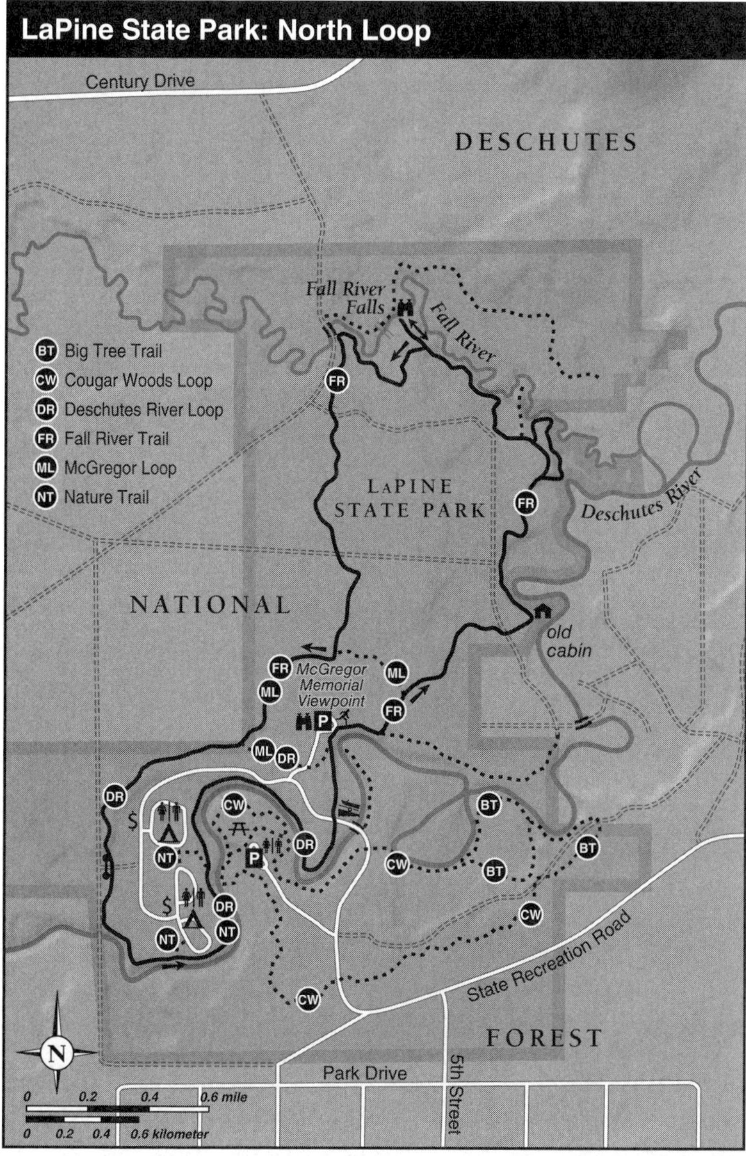

half-mile to the doubletrack and is worth checking out. Farther on, be sure to take the short side trail to the marked Fall River Falls viewpoint, which fans out into some of the most prized trout-fishing spots in Central Oregon.

Now following the Fall River, you'll soon come upon a parking area used by anglers and river admirers. Take a sharp left at the marked trailhead sign

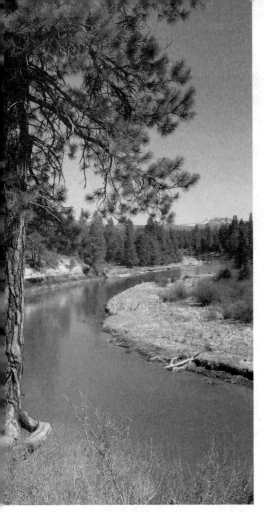

The Deschutes River with Paulina Peak on the horizon

and begin heading south and away from the Fall River, back through the trees toward the heart of the park. Eventually, you'll connect to the McGregor Loop junction, which merges again with the Fall River Loop.

After 3.2 miles, take a right at the marker toward Deschutes River Loop and away from the McGregor Loop/Fall River Loop return route. Passing a gate, you'll run along doubletrack until a sign points you back onto singletrack into the trees. As you get closer to the Deschutes River, the forest opens up, and you'll soon begin to smell campfires and hear the chatter of campers through the trees. Keep your eyes peeled for children and others on the trail at this point, as campers heavily populate it during the summer months. Continue along the river trail back toward your starting point to complete a loop of close to 8 miles.

DIRECTIONS

LaPine State Park is 22.4 miles southwest of Bend, about 5 miles west of US 97 on State Recreation Road. Look for signs on US 97 for the turnoff. The North Loop starts at McGregor Memorial Viewpoint, on the north side of the Deschutes River, which is reached by the second right-hand (north) turn after you cross the bridge into the park.

48 LaPine State Park: SOUTH LOOP

TRAIL DETAILS AT A GLANCE

- **DISTANCE** 3.9-mile loop
- **GPS TRAILHEAD COORDINATES** N43° 46.292' W121° 32.166'
- **DIFFICULTY** 3 • **SCENERY** 6 • **CROWDS** 6 • **SEASON** Year-round, sunrise–sunset
- **ELEVATION** +/–65' • **USERS** Hikers, runners, mountain bikers
- **CONTACT** LaPine State Park, 541-536-2071, **tinyurl.com/lapinestatepark**
- **PERMITS/FEES** None (day use is free)
- **RECOMMENDED MAP** PDF map at **tinyurl.com/lapinesouthmap** • **DOGS** Yes (leashed only)

THE STATE OF OREGON IS KNOWN FOR ITS TOWERING TIMBER, and LaPine State Park is home to one such ancient wooden giant. The approximately 500-year-old Oregon Heritage Tree, appropriately nicknamed the Big Tree, is the largest ponderosa pine in Oregon, with a whopping circumference of 28 feet 11 inches. It used to be the tallest as well, at 191 feet, until a storm took its crown (literally) down to its current 162-foot height. On the South Loop, you'll run by for a close-up of the famous pine, along with several great overlooks of the Deschutes River along the way.

Though the north side of the river houses the longer loops and campgrounds, the south side draws fewer crowds. Of course, both sides of the river can also be combined in whole or in parts to lengthen the run to your preference. Begin your loop at the day-use and picnic area. Follow the gravel walkway down to the river and look for the Cougar Woods Loop trailhead marker, just to the east of the restrooms.

From the picnic area, follow the singletrack along the scenic Deschutes River as it snakes its way around gentle curves toward the bridge. The trail hugs the slope in several areas and offers great views downstream. Continue the gradual uphill, where you'll reach a junction with the main park road and a fenced parking area on the other side. Stay right in the lot, toward the sign and the unmarked doubletrack trail. Note that on the opposite end of the parking lot (closer to the bridge), another trail continues along the river for a short distance before petering out.

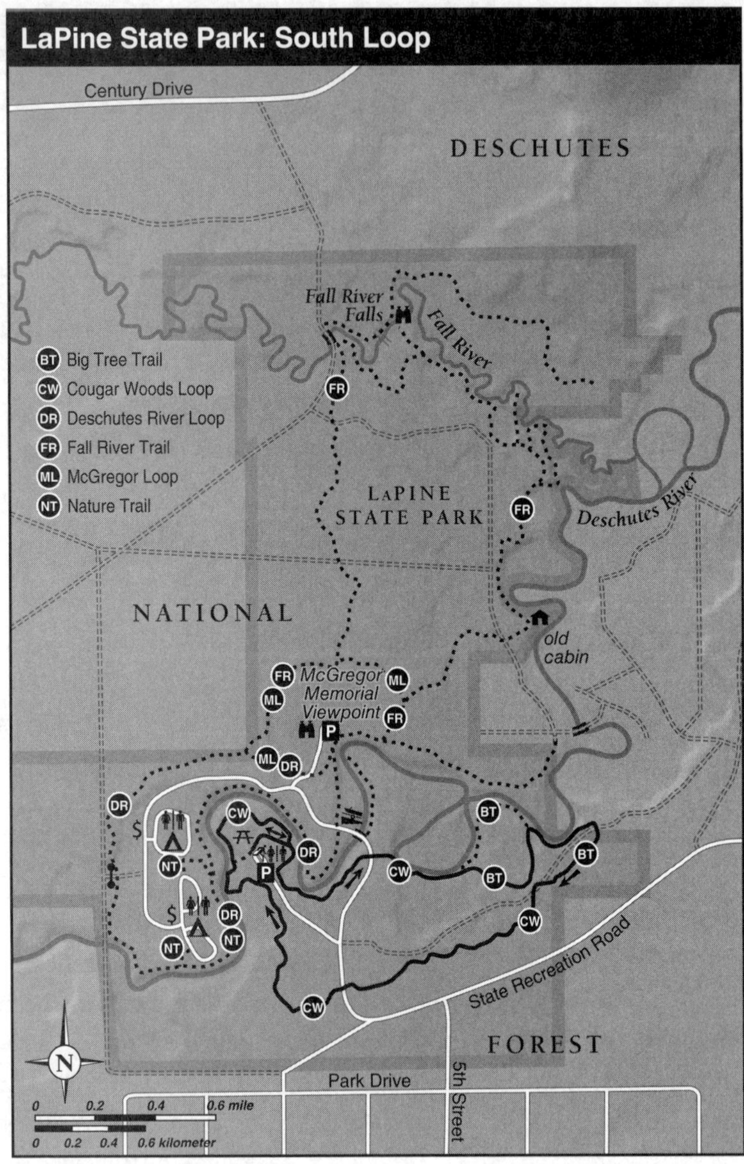

The smooth doubletrack takes you past a few more great views overlooking the Deschutes, and you'll stay right at an unmarked junction to veer toward the giant ponderosa pine known as the Big Tree. When you reach the parking lot, take a quick glance around to estimate the crowds. If the lot is busy, walking down the paved path toward the attraction is recommended. Once you've taken

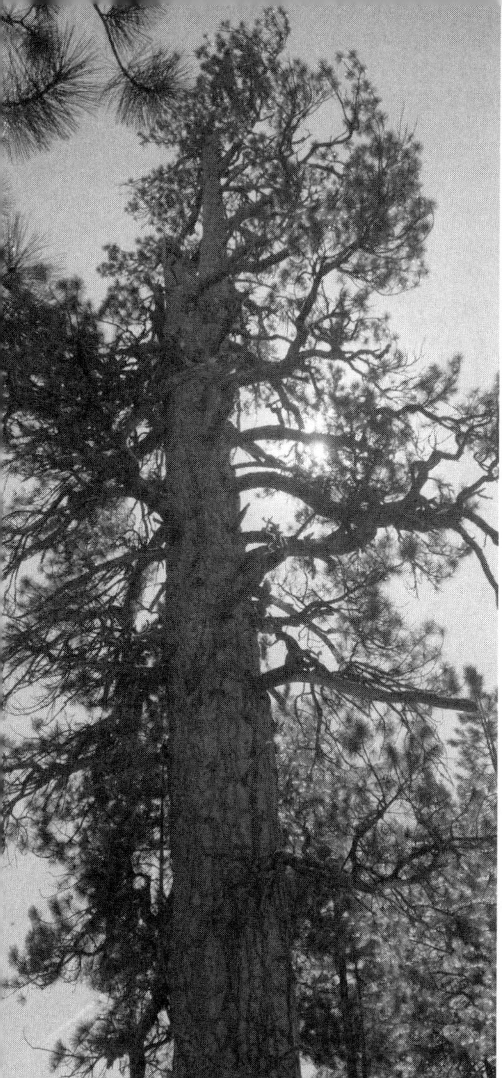

The Big Tree

in the sights, look for the Big Tree Trail marker pointing you to the right, along the river and uphill. This is a good place to pick up the run again.

The Big Tree Trail is relatively short, getting you back to the parking lot in about 0.75 mile. As you reenter the lot, look to your left to reconnect with the Cougar Woods Loop, which quickly takes you back into the trees and away from the crowds. Follow this trail back down to the park road, which you'll cross one more time before descending to the Deschutes River and back upstream to your starting point.

DIRECTIONS

LaPine State Park is 22.4 miles southwest of Bend, about 5 miles west of US 97 on State Recreation Road. Look for signs on US 97 for the turnoff. The South Loop starts at the day-use and picnic area, accessed by taking the first left about 0.25 mile after you enter the park.

49 Paulina Creek

TRAIL DETAILS AT A GLANCE

- **DISTANCE** 11.1-mile loop
- **GPS TRAILHEAD COORDINATES** N43° 42.996' W121° 22.638'
- **DIFFICULTY** 8 • **SCENERY** 7 • **CROWDS** 4
- **SEASON** June–October, sunrise–sunset
- **ELEVATION** +/–1,596'
- **USERS** Hikers, runners, mountain bikers
- **CONTACT** Newberry National Volcanic Monument, 541-383-5700, **tinyurl.com/newberrynvm**
- **PERMITS/FEES** None
- **RECOMMENDED MAP** *Bend, Oregon, Trail Map* by Adventure Maps, Inc. ($12, **adventuremaps.net**)
- **DOGS** Yes (leashed only)

PAULINA FALLS IS A SPECTACULAR SET OF TWO 80-FOOT WATERFALLS that cascade over a vertical drop of basalt rock into a set of boulders below. The falls, and the creek itself, are named after a Northern Paiute Indian chief who was known for his fierceness in battle and ability to evade enemy capture. Located a short quarter-mile from the outlet of Paulina Lake, and also close to the visitor center, Paulina Falls tends to be a popular spot among tourists and recreationalists throughout the summer. The good news, however, is that this is really the only crowded spot on the stream that, as a whole, is exceptionally scenic.

Over the course of this run, you'll follow the shores of Paulina Creek, gaining more than 1,500 feet in elevation in under 6 miles. Along the way, you'll see some exceptional river scenery, many more waterfalls beyond just Paulina Falls, and some great views of the Cascade range from Mount Thielsen all the way to Mount Hood.

The run begins at McKay Crossing Campground, a lovely campground that straddles Paulina Creek and the lesser-known Lower Paulina Falls. After checking out the first set of falls (near Campsite 9), cross the bridge into the day-use area and look for Peter Skene Ogden Trail 56 just to the right of the road.

The first mile of trail is fairly flat as it winds its way up through forests of ponderosa pine along the shores of the creek. In just under a mile, you emerge from the trees into an old burn area and a great example of new, second-growth forest. Smaller trees allow for great views of the creek, including a few small

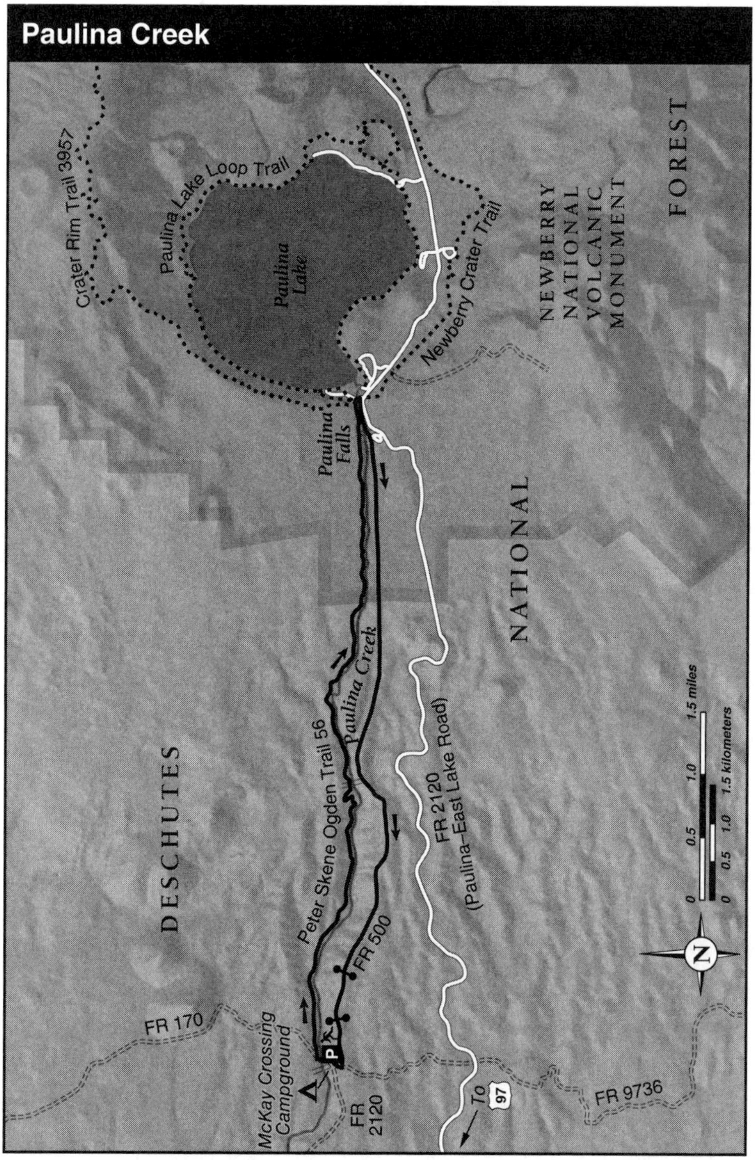

Paulina Creek
Crater Rim Trail 3957
Paulina Lake Loop Trail
Paulina Lake
Newberry Crater Trail
NEWBERRY
NATIONAL
VOLCANIC
MONUMENT
FOREST
Paulina Falls
NATIONAL
DESCHUTES
Paulina Creek
Peter Skene Ogden Trail 56
FR 2120
(Paulina–East Lake Road)
FR 500
FR 170
McKay Crossing Campground
P
FR 2120
To 97
FR 9736
0 0.5 1.0 1.5 miles
0 0.5 1.0 1.5 kilometers
N

7,000 ft.
6,500 ft.
6,000 ft.
5,500 ft.
5,000 ft.
4,500 ft.
4,000 ft.
2 mi.
4 mi.
6 mi.
8 mi.
10 mi.

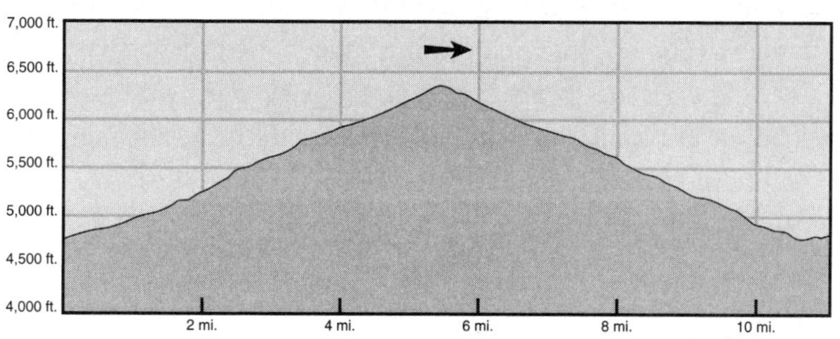

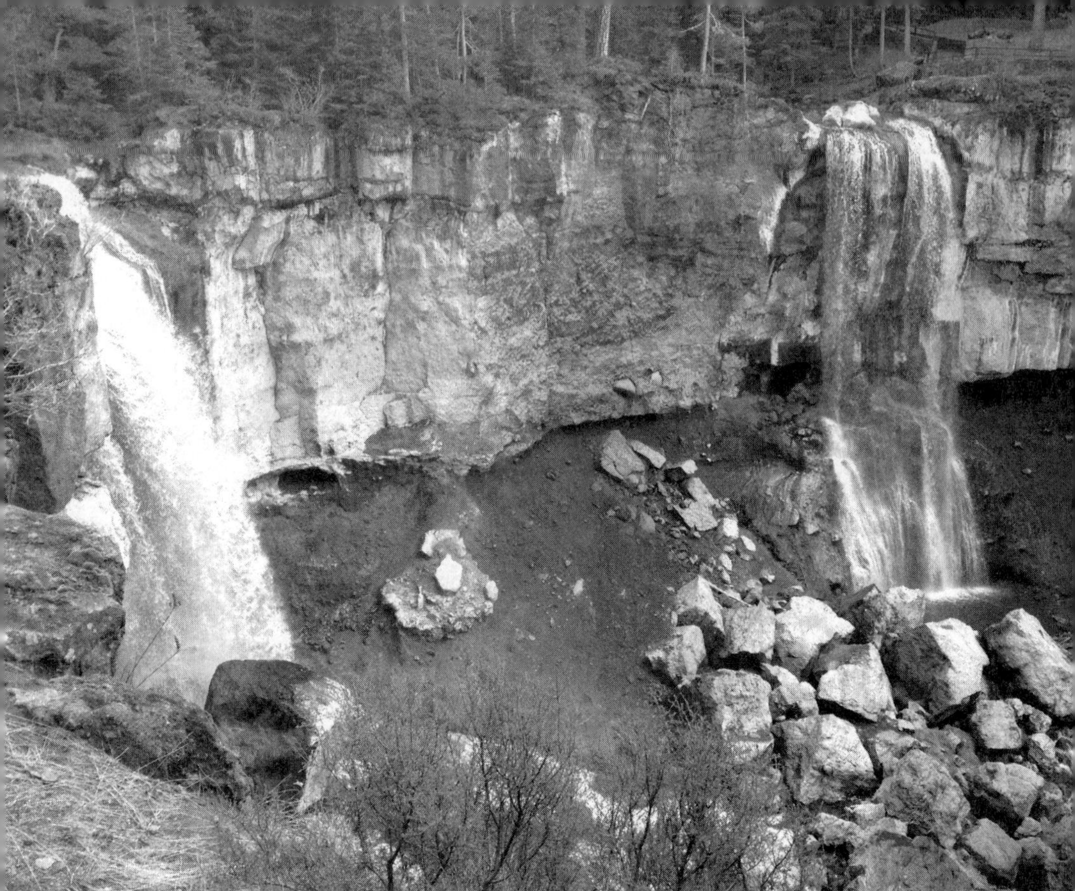

Paulina Falls

waterfalls and rapids. Keen eyes will also spot some gentle natural waterslides in the creek starting around 1.5 miles that are popular among local swimmers during the hot summer months.

Soon enough, the gentle grade begins to steepen and the river cuts a deeper channel into the landscape. A series of switchbacks helps lessen the grade, and several more waterfalls provide great excuses for a quick stop—including a set of spectacular double falls around the 2-mile marker. This pattern continues until 3.2 miles, when the singletrack empties onto an old jeep road. Before continuing, be sure to take a moment to check out the large fanned waterfall at the bend in the creek here. The best views are from a nice rogue campsite beside the water.

Back on the jeep trail, keep right and look for the unmarked singletrack as it ducks back into the forest 30 yards up. As you continue your ascent, Paulina Peak begins to emerge off in the distance on your right around 4 miles. Soon after, the forest begins to lose the underbrush and, at 5.5 miles, an unmarked but obvious side trail through the lodgepole pines directs you to the northern viewpoint of Paulina Falls.

A short distance later, Paulina Lake presents itself as the trail empties out at the junction with Crater Rim Trail 3957 and the Paulina Lake Loop Trail at 5.75 miles. Watching for cars and pedestrians, cross the bridge and look for signs denoting the continuation of the path on the other side of the creek. Begin your descent by taking a right and following the trail a quick quarter-mile to the much more crowded Paulina Falls viewpoint on the south side. An upper viewpoint and lower viewpoint provide a few different options for viewing the impressive falls.

Just beyond the sign for the lower falls but before the parking lot, take a slight right onto Forest Road 500—the wide, bumpy jeep road with the telephone poles. This will be your return route nearly all the way back to McKay Crossing. Though not nearly as scenic, the road is infrequently used in summertime and is mostly used during the winter as a snowmobile route. During the warmer months, the lack of rocks and obstacles makes for a fast, fun descent for runners.

Just beyond the junction with FR 550 at 8.1 miles, pass through a gate following the bike signs and continue along FR 500. A half-mile later, you'll pass by two side trails, the second of which points to the footbridge crossing Paulina Creek and connecting to the Peter Skene Ogden Trail on the other side—a great option for a much shorter loop beginning from 10 Mile Sno-Park.

Continue straight along FR 500, following the orange-diamond bike markers in the trees along the way. At 9.4 miles, reenter the burn area and be treated to spectacular views of the Cascades, in particular Mount Bachelor and South Sister. North and Middle Sister, along with Mount Jefferson and Mount Hood, are also visible in the distance. In another mile, reenter the trees and pass through a second gate at 10.8 miles before intersecting a logging road at 11.0 miles. Turn right here, following the road 0.1 mile down to McKay Crossing and your starting point.

DIRECTIONS

Travel south from Bend on US 97. After about 24 miles, look for signs for Newberry National Volcanic Monument and Paulina Lake. Turn left (east) on paved Paulina–East Lake Road (County Road 21/Forest Road 2120) and, after about 3 miles, look for signs for McKay Crossing Campground. Follow the gravel road 2.25 miles to the campground. The day-use area is just past the bridge over Paulina Creek.

50 Otter Bench Trail

TRAIL DETAILS AT A GLANCE

- **DISTANCE** 6.5-mile double loop
- **GPS TRAILHEAD COORDINATES** N44° 27.758' W121° 17.002'
- **DIFFICULTY** 4 • **SCENERY** 7 • **CROWDS** 2
- **SEASON** Year-round, sunrise–sunset • **ELEVATION** +/–574'
- **USERS** Hikers, runners, mountain bikers, horses
- **CONTACT** BLM Prineville District, 541-416-6700, **blm.gov/or/districts/prineville**
- **PERMITS/FEES** None
- **RECOMMENDED MAP** *Sisters & Redmond High Desert Trail Map* by Adventure Maps, Inc. ($12, **adventuremaps.net**) • **DOGS** Yes (leashed only)

THE OTTER BENCH TRAIL SYSTEM lies on a relatively flat shelf high above the Crooked River just north of where it drains into the Deschutes. This section of the Crooked River is on the list of National Wild and Scenic Rivers—and for good reason. The 400-foot-deep canyon offers some dramatic views, and classic High Desert sagebrush and juniper combine for a fitting backdrop to the trails that run along the rim of the gorge.

Open nearly year-round, the trail system is also an ideal choice for those seeking solitude. Most of the network was built in the last five years, and chances are very high that you will not run past another soul during your time here. The run is made up of two loops connected by singletrack in between, with multiple options for extending the total distance (and adding some steep elevation). In summary, if you're looking for bang for your buck and some alone time in the desert, this run is for you.

Find the trailhead at the far end of the parking lot and take a left onto the Otter Bench Trail. The right fork, the Horny Hollow Trail, will be the return loop. (*Note:* The Horny Hollow Trail is closed seasonally from February 1 through August 31 due to raptor nesting.) The trail gently climbs through wheatgrass and sagebrush as it rolls its way along the shelf. Views soon begin to emerge of the canyon and, in short glimpses, the Crooked River far below. During wintertime, this area tends to be colder since it lies in the shade of the rimrock wall to the west.

At 1.7 miles, a four-way junction appears and marks the second leg of the run. Continuing along for the double loop, keep left to connect to the Opal Canyon Trail

Otter Bench Trail

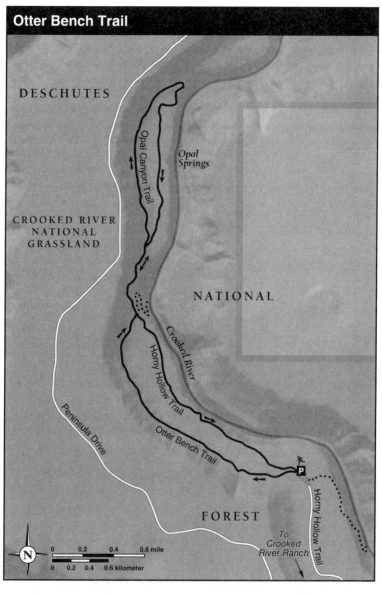

DESCHUTES
CROOKED RIVER NATIONAL GRASSLAND
NATIONAL
FOREST
Opal Canyon Trail
Opal Springs
Crooked River
Horny Hollow Trail
Otter Bench Trail
Peninsula Drive
To Crooked River Ranch
Horny Hollow Trail
N
0 0.2 0.4 0.6 mile
0 0.2 0.4 0.6 kilometer

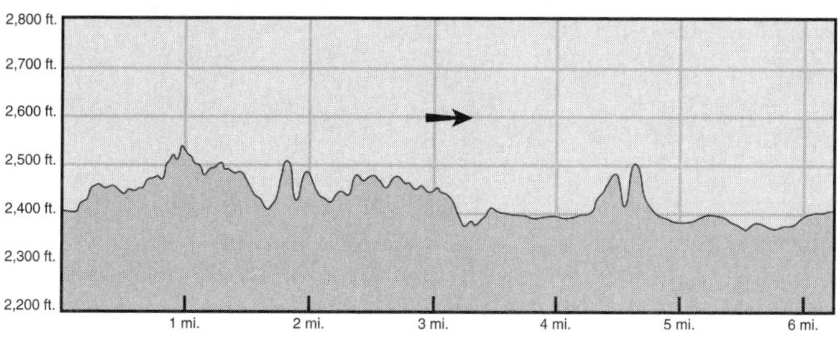

loop. After a brief climb, the trail emerges along the precipitous edge of the canyon, providing outstanding scenery and views far into the canyon below. Circling hawks and raptors overhead seem to add to the dramatic feel, while a multitude of animal tracks identify the presence of the numerous creatures that call the area home.

In 0.5 mile, keep left at an unmarked intersection, which will be your return on the second loop. The trail continues along the western edge of the shelf and eventually begins to make the turn back north around mile 3.3. The views get even better during the next quarter-mile as the trail hugs the rim, making its way north. Along with views into the canyon, you'll also notice at this point a few industrial buildings on the opposite side of the river, marring the tranquil High Desert scenery.

The trail soon cuts back up and away from the rim to make its way back to the singletrack and complete the second loop at 4.5 miles. From here, retrace your steps along the narrow trail high along the canyon rim for the half-mile to the four-way junction and the top of the first loop. Take the Horny Hollow Trail, a decommissioned Bureau of Land Management road, to complete your run.

DIRECTIONS

From Bend, drive north on US 97 about 20 miles. Just north of the town of Terrebonne, turn left on Lower Bridge Market Road, following the signs for Crooked River Ranch. In 2.2 miles, turn right on NW 43rd Street. After 1.8 miles, turn left on NW Chinook Drive. Follow this road for 5 miles to SW Horny Hollow Trail, keeping straight where Hill Road switchbacks left and then bearing left where Ranch House Road forks right. Follow Horny Hollow Trail 1.8 miles to the paved road's end, where the trailhead parking lot is located.

OPPOSITE: *Marked singletrack carves its way through tall wheatgrass.*

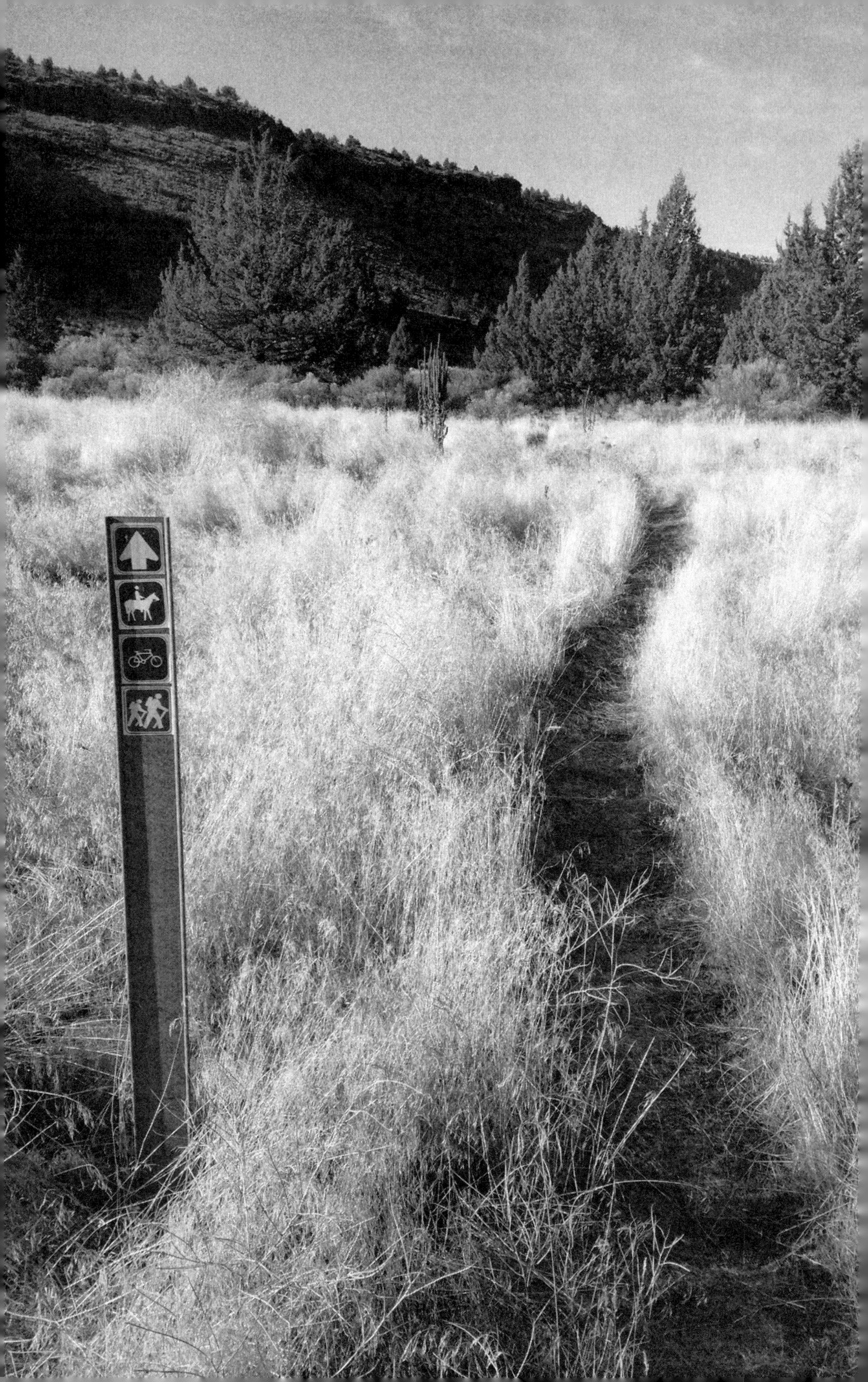

APPENDIX A

MANAGING AGENCIES

- **BEND PARK AND RECREATION DISTRICT**
  799 SW Columbia St.
  Bend, OR 97702
  541-389-7275, **bendparksandrec.org**
  TRAILS COVERED Archie Briggs Canyon, Entrada River Loop, Old Mill Loop, Shevlin Park Loop Trail

- **BUREAU OF LAND MANAGEMENT, PRINEVILLE DISTRICT**
  3050 NE 3rd St.
  Prineville, OR 97754
  541-416-6700, **blm.gov/or/districts/prineville**
  TRAILS COVERED Badlands Rock, Horse Ridge, Larry Chitwood Trail, Maston, Otter Bench Trail, Tumalo Canal Historic Area, Tumulus Trail

- **DESCHUTES LAND TRUST**
  210 NW Irving Ave., Ste. 102
  Bend, OR 97703
  541-330-0017, **deschuteslandtrust.org**
  TRAILS COVERED Metolius Preserve, Whychus Canyon Preserve

- **DESCHUTES NATIONAL FOREST** **www.fs.usda.gov/deschutes**

  Bend–Fort Rock Ranger District
  63095 Deschutes Market Rd.
  Bend, OR 97701, 541-383-4000
  TRAILS COVERED Ben's Trail, Broken Top, Green Lakes, Horse Butte, Horse Lake, Lemish Lake, Moraine Lake, Phil's Trail, Sisters Mirror Lake, Swampy Lakes, Three Shelters Loop, Tumalo Falls

Newberry National Volcanic Monument

County Road 21/Forest Road 21, near La Pine, Oregon

541-383-5700, **tinyurl.com/newberrynvm**

TRAILS COVERED Paulina Creek, Paulina Lake

Sisters Ranger District

Pine Street and US 20

Sisters, OR 97759

541-549-7700

TRAILS COVERED Black Butte, Matthieu Lakes, Metolius River, Obsidian Trail, Suttle Lake

- **OCHOCO NATIONAL FOREST**

www.fs.usda.gov/ochoco

Crooked River National Grassland

274 SW 4th St.

Madras, OR 97741

541-416-6640

TRAILS COVERED Gray Butte

Lookout Mountain Ranger District

3160 NE 3rd St.

Prineville, OR 97754

541-416-6500

TRAILS COVERED Lookout Mountain

- **OREGON STATE PARKS**

725 Summer St. NE, Ste. C

Salem, OR 97301, 800-551-6949, **oregonstateparks.org**

TRAILS COVERED The Cove Palisades State Park, LaPine State Park (North and South Loops), Pilot Butte State Park, Smith Rock State Park

- **REDMOND AREA PARK AND RECREATION DISTRICT**

465 SW Rimrock Dr.

Redmond, OR 97756

541-548-7275, **raprd.org**

TRAILS COVERED Radlands

MANAGING AGENCIES *(continued)*

- **SISTERS TRAIL ALLIANCE**

  PO Box 1871
  Sisters, OR 97759
  541-719-8822, **sisterstrails.com**
  TRAILS COVERED Lower Peterson Ridge Trail, Upper Peterson Ridge Trail

- **WILLAMETTE NATIONAL FOREST**

  www.fs.usda.gov/willamette

  Detroit Ranger District

  44125 N. Santiam Highway SE
  Detroit, OR 97342
  503-854-3366
  TRAILS COVERED Canyon Creek Meadows, Duffy Lake, Eight Lakes Basin

  McKenzie River Ranger District

  57600 McKenzie Highway (OR 126)
  McKenzie Bridge, OR 97701
  541-822-3381
  TRAILS COVERED Clear Lake, McKenzie River, Patjens Lakes, Scott Lake

  Sweet Home Ranger District

  4431 US 20
  Sweet Home, OR 97386
  541-367-5168
  TRAILS COVERED Iron Mountain

APPENDIX B

RUNNING CLUBS AND GROUPS

- **CENTRAL OREGON RUNNING KLUB**
  PO Box 415
  Bend, OR 97709, 541-317-1882
  centraloregonrunningklub.org, centraloregonrunningklub@gmail.com
- **MADRAS RUNNERS**
  sites.google.com/site/madrasrunners, madrasrunners@hotmail.com
- **REDMOND OREGON RUNNING KLUB**
  CONTACT: Dan Edwards
  541-419-0889, **facebook.com/redmondoregonrunningklub,**
  rundanorun1985@gmail.com

APPENDIX C

RUNNING STORES

- **FLEET FEET BEND**
  1320 NW Galveston Ave., #1
  Bend, OR 97701
  541-389-1601, **fleetfeetbend.com**

- **FOOTZONE**
  845 NW Wall St.
  Bend, OR 97701
  541-317-3568, **footzonebend.com**

APPENDIX D

CENTRAL OREGON RACE CALENDAR

- **JANUARY**

Madass Run, Madras

541-325-1064 or 541-325-6090

sites.google.com/site/madass2010, monstan@hotmail.com

- **MARCH**

Mastondon 10-ish Miler

CONTACT: "SuperDave" Thomason, SuperFit Productions

541-317-3568, **tinyurl.com/mastondon, superdave@footzonebend.com**

- **APRIL**

Horse Butte 10-Miler

CONTACT: "SuperDave" Thomason, SuperFit Productions

541-317-3568, **superfitproductions.com/races/horse-butte-10-miler, superdave@footzonebend.com**

Hot Springs Trail Runs

CONTACT: Pink Buffalo Racing, PO Box 5404, Eugene, OR 97405

541-731-3507, **tinyurl.com/hotspringstrailruns, pinkbuffaloracing.com/ContactUs.html**

Peterson Ridge Rumble

petersonridgerumble.com (click "Contact" to send e-mail)

(Continued on next page)

CENTRAL OREGON RACE CALENDAR

- **MAY**

Smith Rock Ascent

CONTACT: Go Beyond Racing, 6107 SW Murray Blvd., #283, Beaverton, OR 97008
gobeyondracing.com/races/smith-rock-ascent, gobeyondracing.com/contact

- **JUNE**

Dirty Half Marathon

CONTACT: "SuperDave" Thomason, SuperFit Productions, 541-317-3568
footzonebend.com/happenings/dirty-half, superdave@footzonebend.com

- **AUGUST**

Haulin' Aspen

CONTACT: Lay It Out Events, 704 NW Georgia St., Bend, OR 97701
541-323-0964, **haulinaspen.com** (click "Contact Us" to send e-mail)

Monkey Face Half Marathon

CONTACT: Pink Buffalo Racing, PO Box 5404, Eugene, OR 97405, 541-731-3507
tinyurl.com/monkeyfacehalf, pinkbuffaloracing.com/ContactUs.html

- **SEPTEMBER**

Bigfoot and Dirtyfoot 10K

CONTACT: Central Oregon Running Klub, c/o Footzone, 845 NW Wall St., Bend OR 97701, **tinyurl.com/bigfootraces, karisstrang@gmail.com**

Flagline 50K and High Alpine Half

CONTACT: "SuperDave" Thomason, SuperFit Productions, 541-317-3568
superfitproductions.com/races/flagline-50k, superdave@footzonebend.com

- **OCTOBER**

SuperDave's Down and Dirty Half

CONTACT: "SuperDave" Thomason, SuperFit Productions, 541-317-3568
tinyurl.com/superdavesdowndirty, superdave@footzonebend.com

- **DECEMBER**

Canyon Rumble Frozen Half

541-325-1064 or 541-325-6090
tinyurl.com/canyonrumble, monstan@hotmail.com

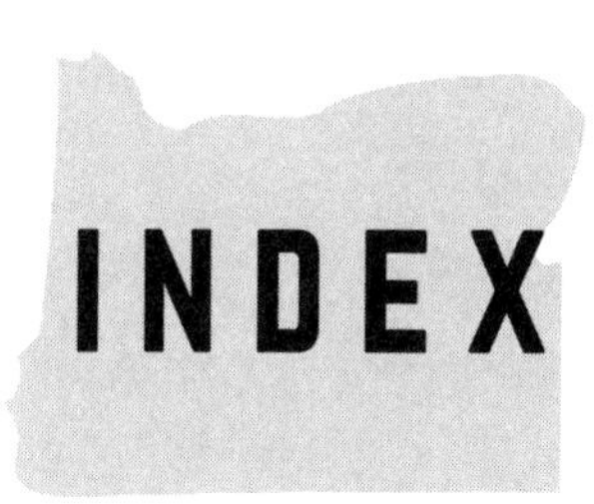

INDEX

ABOUT THE AUTHOR

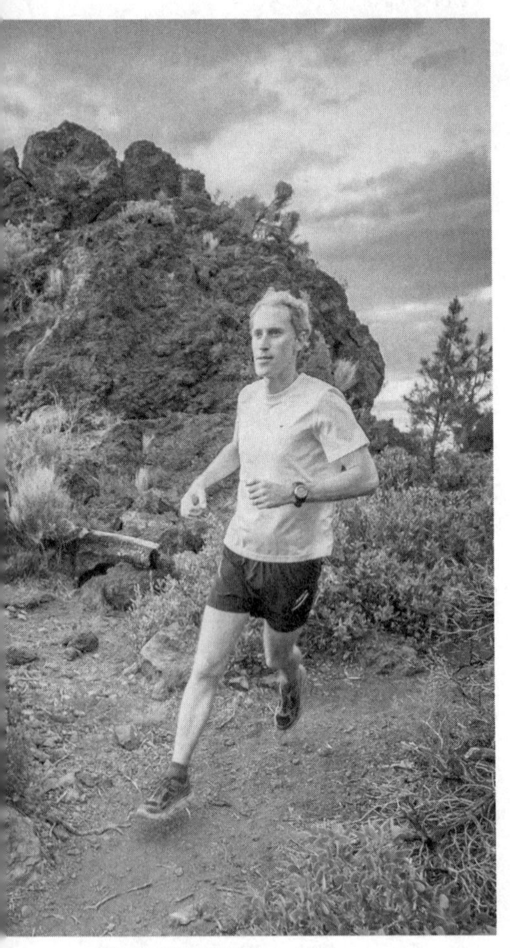

PHOTO: NATE WYETH

LUCAS ALBERG is a native Kansan who ventured west after college in pursuit of outdoor adventure in the mountains. A distance runner since his youth, Lucas took to trail running when he moved to Portland in 2001. After exhausting the trails in the northwest part of the state, he moved to the sunnier side of the Cascade Mountains and Bend in 2011. Since then, he has been eagerly exploring Central Oregon's diverse geography and gobbling up miles on the area's vast network of trails.

Outside of running, Lucas enjoys mountain biking, hiking, backpacking, cross-country skiing, and camping with his lovely wife, Rae, and son, Loren. A longtime musician, Lucas has written and recorded two albums with his band, The Beautiful Train Wrecks, and has found time to play hundreds of shows across the Pacific Northwest. Lucas currently serves as PR manager for a Bend-based outdoor company.